Effects of Mycotoxins on the Intestine

Effects of Mycotoxins on the Intestine

Special Issue Editors

Isabelle P. Oswald
Philippe Pinton
Imourana Alassane-Kpembi

MDPI • Basel • Beijing • Wuhan • Barcelona • Belgrade

MDPI

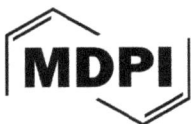

Special Issue Editors
Isabelle P. Oswald
INRA
France

Philippe Pinton
INRA
France

Imourana Alassane-Kpembi
INRA
France

Editorial Office
MDPI
St. Alban-Anlage 66
4052 Basel, Switzerland

This is a reprint of articles from the Special Issue published online in the open access journal *Toxins* (ISSN 2072-6651) from 2017 to 2019 (available at: https://www.mdpi.com/journal/toxins/special_issues/mycotoxins_intestine)

For citation purposes, cite each article independently as indicated on the article page online and as indicated below:

LastName, A.A.; LastName, B.B.; LastName, C.C. Article Title. *Journal Name* **Year**, *Article Number*, Page Range.

ISBN 978-3-03897-782-7 (Pbk)
ISBN 978-3-03897-783-4 (PDF)

Cover image courtesy of Isabelle P. Oswald, Philippe Pinton and Imourana Alassane-Kpembi.

Contents

About the Special Issue Editors

Isabelle P. Oswald is a research director at the French National Institute for Agricultural Research (INRA). She is the head of the head of the INRA Research Center in Food Toxicology, Toxalim in Toulouse, France. This laboratory develops an expertise in Food and Feed toxicology applied to agro-resources—especially pesticides, food contact materials, and mycotoxins. It characterizes the molecular, cellular, and physiological impacts of these contaminants. Within this research center, Isabelle Oswald is heading a group of 20 persons (7 scientists, 2 post-doctoral fellows, 7 PhD students, and 4 technicians) working on the biosynthesis and toxicity of mycotoxins. Isabelle Oswald is an author and co-author of more than 200 international publications, and in 2018 she was among the top 1% highly cited researchers in the Web of Science. She is an expert for EFSA, (the European Food Safety Authority) and ANSES (the French Agency for Food, Environmental and Occupational Health & Safety). In 2010 she was awarded the title of Knight of the Agricultural merit, and last December she received the "Laurier de l'INRA", a Lifetime Achievement Award, from her work on mycotoxins.

Philippe Pinton is an Engineer in the Toxalim Research Center in Food Toxicology (INRA, Toulouse, France). He spent eight years in the Atomic Energy Commission (CEA) in research teams working on radiochemistry and radiobiology. He then joined the French National Institute for Agricultural Research (INRA) and was initially involved in pig genome mapping, based on chromosomal in situ hybridization. Concerned by the effects of food contaminants on health, he joined Toxalim. He has been working on the toxicology of mycotoxins since 2000. His work mainly focuses on the effects of mycotoxins, when present alone or in combination, on the intestinal barrier. He has developed innovative tools to study mycotoxin toxicity (intestinal explants, laser microdissection, etc.). He defended his PhD in 2012 at Toulouse University. Philippe Pinton is authors or co-author of 70 international publications. He supervises PhD students in different projects and is an expert at ILSI (International Life Sciences Institute). Recently, he obtained grants from the French National Research Agency (ANR). The "ExpoMycoPig" project aims at identifying biomarkers of pig exposure to the most common mycotoxins, while the "EmergingMyco" project will improve our knowledge on the occurrence and toxicity of emerging mycotoxins.

Imourana Alassane-Kpembi is an adjunct professor of veterinary toxicology at Université d'Abomey-Calavi (BENIN), and a research fellow in the French National Institute for Agricultural Research INRA in Toulouse. His work focuses on the effects of natural exposure to mycotoxins (chronic, low doses, and multi-exposures) on the intestinal health of farm animals. Dr. Imourana Alassane-Kpembi received his PhD in 2013 from Université de Toulouse, and his doctorate in veterinary medicine in 2004 from Université Cheikh Anta Diop de Dakar.

Preface to "Effects of Mycotoxins on the Intestine"

Mycotoxins are secondary metabolites produced by several fungal species. They can contaminate human food and animal feed, and have been a threat for thousands of years. The gastrointestinal tract is the first target when ingesting mycotoxin-contaminated food or feed. As unlikely as it sounds, the investigations concerning the effects of mycotoxins on the intestine are still in their early stages. This book gathers the most recent advances related to the characterization of the intestinal toxicity of mycotoxins. The substantial data assembled on the damage caused to a number of histological structures and functions of the intestine remove any remaining doubt about this organ being a primary target for the toxicity of mycotoxins. An interesting overview of the detrimental effects of mycotoxins on the gut-hosted microbiota—now regarded as a fully-fledged organ associated with the gut—is also given.

The emergence of the intestine as a critical target for mycotoxin toxicity concurrently raises the question of the suitability of current regulations to protect against alterations of this organ. Finally, the unavoidable presence of mycotoxins in animal feed, despite continuing efforts to keep the risk under control, calls for the implementation of new detoxification strategies whose efficacy still needs to be assessed, especially considering intestinal toxicity as a relevant endpoint. All those questions are addressed by outstanding contributions in this book.

We hope that this book which correlates papers from the Special Issue "Effect of Mycotoxins on the Intestine" in the open access journal Toxins from MDPI will further stimulate research interest in this field and increase our understanding of the toxicity of these fascinating fungal metabolites.

Isabelle P. Oswald, Philippe Pinton, Imourana Alassane-Kpembi
Special Issue Editors

toxins

Editorial

Effects of Mycotoxins on the Intestine

Imourana Alassane-Kpembi [1,2], Philippe Pinton [1] and Isabelle P. Oswald [1,*]

[1] Toxalim (Research Centre in Food Toxicology), Université de Toulouse, INRA, ENVT, INP-Purpan, UPS, 31027 Toulouse, France; imourana.alassane-kpembi@inra.fr (I.A.-K.); philippe.pinton@inra.fr (P.P.)
[2] Ecole Polytechnique d'Abomey-Calavi, Université d'Abomey-Calavi, 01BP2009 Abomey-Calavi, Bénin
[*] Correspondence: Isabelle.oswald@inra.fr

Received: 22 February 2019; Accepted: 10 March 2019; Published: 13 March 2019

The gastrointestinal tract is the first physiological barrier against food contaminants, as well as the first target for these toxicants. As prominent food and feed contaminants, mycotoxins frequently come into contact with the intestinal mucosa, and awareness of their potentially deleterious effects is increasing [1,2]. Even though the mucosa is a major functional element of intestinal integrity, increasing evidence suggests that other constituents, such as mucus and microbiota, are also involved [3]. This special issue reports on recent progress in the characterization of the intestinal toxicity of mycotoxins.

Substantial data have been assembled on the damage caused by mycotoxins to a number of histological structures and functions of the intestinal tissue. Mycotoxins, with chemical structures as diverse as aflatoxins, ochratoxin, and deoxynivalenol (DON), have been shown to impair intestinal permeability in species as different as humans, fish, and pigs, removing any remaining doubt about global mycotoxin-driven alteration of the intestinal barrier function [4–6]. The mucus and its goblet cell producers are underestimated players that have long escaped the attention of the mycotoxicology community when assessing the barrier function [3,7]. A light and electron microscopy study by Przybylska-Gornowicz et al. [8] investigated the fate of goblet cells and their mucus production in a pig colon exposed to the *Fusarium* toxins, DON and zearalenone (ZEN), at supposedly non-toxic levels.

Enteric neurons involved in many regulatory processes, connected with all aspects of intestinal physiology, have also been underestimated, and the question of whether mycotoxins could target the enteric nervous system (ENS) deserves attention. Makowska et al. [9] demonstrated that following the exposure of pigs to low doses of the T-2 toxin, even the ENS undergoes adaptive and reparative processes, possibly resulting in changes in the chemical coding of the neurons and nerve fibers in the porcine stomach and duodenum.

An overview of the detrimental effects of mycotoxins on the intestine could not ignore the gut-hosted microbiota that are now regarded as a fully fledged organ associated with the gut [10]. Yang et al. [11] reported dramatic changes in mouse-digestive microbiota, following long-term feeding with aflatoxin B_1. Reddy et al. [12] analyzed the colon content of pigs fed with DON or ZEN and reported that both mycotoxins favored the abundance of the *Lactobacillus* genus, suggesting that members of this genus could play a key role in the detoxification of dietary DON and ZEN in pigs. Also in pigs, dietary fumonisin B_1 (FB_1) was shown to hinder the age-related dynamic of fecal microbiota, starting from 15 days of exposure [13].

The emergence of the intestine as a critical target for mycotoxin toxicity concurrently raises the question of the suitability of current regulations to protect against alterations of this organ. Maruo et al. [14] concluded that ergot alkaloids that contaminate feed, but at rates under the current EU regulatory limits, still damage the intestine. Likewise, Cieplinska et al. [15] reported that the cecal water obtained from pigs fed ZEN at no-observed-adverse-effect-level (NOAEL) and below, still had a significant genotoxic effect, highlighting the need for further investigation into the specific sensitivity of the intestine to mycotoxins.

Finally, the unavoidable presence of mycotoxins in animal feed, despite continuing efforts to keep the risk under control, calls for the implementation of new detoxification strategies, whose efficacy still needs to be assessed [16]. To that end, the intestinal toxicity of mycotoxins offers several possibilities. Alassane-Kpembi et al. [17] performed a whole-transcriptome analysis to decipher the early response of the small intestine to the deleterious effects of DON after administration of the *Saccharomyces cerevisiae* boulardii strain CNCM I-1079. These authors reported that applying the yeast significantly reduced the overall impact of DON on the transcriptome, and specifically reversed a number of signaling pathways triggering inflammation, oxidative stress, and lipid metabolism. Likewise, the oxidative stress and mitochondrial apoptosis induced by ZEN in pig intestinal epithelial cells were reported to be alleviated by application of N-Acetylcysteine [18]. Dietary supplementation with the *Clostridium* sp. WJ06 strain as a DON detoxification strategy in pigs also appears to be of potential interest, as Li et al. [19] showed that this bacterial strain significantly attenuated the toxicity of DON, while simultaneously modulating the intestinal micro-ecosystem of growing pigs. Hypothesizing that the toxicity of mycotoxins can be counteracted through specific adjustments of the composition of intestinal microflora, Zheng et al. [20] explored the effects of administering hydrogen-rich water and lactulose, two hydrogen-producing prebiotics, on the microbiota imbalance induced by *Fusarium* mycotoxins in piglets. These authors showed that providing functional hydrogen to the pig gut could protect the animal against the imbalance of intestinal communities of microbiota, and protect it from a reduction in the production of short-chain fatty acids and a higher rate of diarrhea induced by a mix of *Fusarium* mycotoxins. Conversely, despite their broadly acknowledged gut health promoting action, chito-oligosaccharides had no remediating effect against the intestinal toxicity of DON [21].

This special issue contains original contributions that advance our knowledge of the intestinal toxicity of mycotoxins. Most of the studies focus on fusariotoxins, but the toxicity of aflatoxins and ergot alkaloids is also addressed. Mycotoxin toxicity is investigated on different cellular targets (epithelial cells, goblet cells, and neurons), markers (oxidative stress, permeability), and the intestinal bacterial flora. The use of the pig model was recurrent in in vivo studies, making it possible to envisage dual valorization of the present findings in biomedical and agricultural research. An original contribution on salmon provides useful information for this breeding species, which remains poorly investigated in the field of mycotoxicology. The outcomes of this special issue improve the characterization of the deleterious effects of mycotoxins on the intestine and identify potential solutions to mitigate these effects. The different detoxification strategies described here will certainly attract the attention of the scientific community.

Acknowledgments: The editors are grateful to all the authors who contributed to this special issue. They are also mindful that without the rigorous and selfless evaluation of the submitted manuscripts by expert peer reviewers, this special issue would not be possible. The valuable contributions, organization, and editorial support of the MDPI management team and staff are greatly appreciated.

Conflicts of Interest: The authors declare no conflict of interest.

References

1. Pinton, P.; Oswald, I.P. Effect of deoxynivalenol and other type b trichothecenes on the intestine: A review. *Toxins* **2014**, *6*, 1615–1643. [CrossRef]
2. Akbari, P.; Braber, S.; Varasteh, S.; Alizadeh, A.; Garssen, J.; Fink-Gremmels, J. The intestinal barrier as an emerging target in the toxicological assessment of mycotoxins. *Arch. Toxicol.* **2017**, *91*, 1007–1029. [CrossRef] [PubMed]
3. Robert, H.; Payros, D.; Pinton, P.; Theodorou, V.; Mercier-Bonin, M.; Oswald, I.P. Impact of mycotoxins on the intestine: Are mucus and microbiota new targets? *J. Toxicol. Environ. Health B Crit. Rev.* **2017**, *20*, 249–275. [CrossRef] [PubMed]
4. Gao, Y.; Li, S.; Wang, J.; Luo, C.; Zhao, S.; Zheng, N. Modulation of intestinal epithelial permeability in differentiated caco-2 cells exposed to aflatoxin M_1 and ochratoxin a individually or collectively. *Toxins* **2017**, *10*, 13. [CrossRef]

5.   Moldal, T.; Bernhoft, A.; Rosenlund, G.; Kaldhusdal, M.; Koppang, E.O. Dietary deoxynivalenol (DON) may impair the epithelial barrier and modulate the cytokine signaling in the intestine of atlantic salmon (*Salmo salar*). *Toxins* **2018**, *10*, 376. [CrossRef] [PubMed]

6.   Pasternak, J.A.; Aiyer, V.I.A.; Hamonic, G.; Beaulieu, A.D.; Columbus, D.A.; Wilson, H.L. Molecular and physiological effects on the small intestine of weaner pigs following feeding with deoxynivalenol-contaminated feed. *Toxins* **2018**, *10*, 40. [CrossRef]

7.   Pinton, P.; Graziani, F.; Pujol, A.; Nicoletti, C.; Paris, O.; Ernouf, P.; Di Pasquale, E.; Perrier, J.; Oswald, I.P.; Maresca, M. Deoxynivalenol inhibits the expression by goblet cells of intestinal mucins through a pkr and map kinase dependent repression of the resistin-like molecule beta. *Mol. Nutr. Food Res.* **2015**, *59*, 1076–1087. [CrossRef] [PubMed]

8.   Przybylska-Gornowicz, B.; Lewczuk, B.; Prusik, M.; Hanuszewska, M.; Petrusewicz-Kosinska, M.; Gajecka, M.; Zielonka, L.; Gajecki, M. The effects of deoxynivalenol and zearalenone on the pig large intestine. A light and electron microscopy study. *Toxins* **2018**, *10*, 148.

9.   Makowska, K.; Obremski, K.; Gonkowski, S. The impact of T-2 toxin on vasoactive intestinal polypeptide-like immunoreactive (VIP-LI) nerve structures in the wall of the porcine stomach and duodenum. *Toxins* **2018**, *10*, 138. [CrossRef]

10. O'Hara, A.M.; Shanahan, F. The gut flora as a forgotten organ. *Embo. Rep.* **2006**, *7*, 688–693. [CrossRef]

11. Yang, X.A.; Liu, L.L.; Chen, J.; Xiao, A.P. Response of intestinal bacterial flora to the long-term feeding of aflatoxin B$_1$ (AFB$_1$) in mice. *Toxins* **2017**, *9*, 317. [CrossRef]

12. Reddy, K.E.; Jeong, J.Y.; Song, J.; Lee, Y.; Lee, H.J.; Kim, D.W.; Jung, H.J.; Kim, K.H.; Kim, M.; Oh, Y.K.; et al. Colon microbiome of pigs fed diet contaminated with commercial purified deoxynivalenol and zearalenone. *Toxins* **2018**, *10*, 347. [CrossRef] [PubMed]

13. Mateos, I.; Combes, S.; Pascal, G.; Cauquil, L.; Barilly, C.; Cossalter, A.M.; Laffitte, J.; Botti, S.; Pinton, P.; Oswald, I.P. Fumonisin-exposure impairs age-related ecological succession of bacterial species in weaned pig gut microbiota. *Toxins* **2018**, *10*, 230. [CrossRef]

14. Maruo, V.M.; Bracarense, A.P.; Metayer, J.P.; Vilarino, M.; Oswald, I.P.; Pinton, P. Ergot alkaloids at doses close to EU regulatory limits induce alterations of the liver and intestine. *Toxins* **2018**, *10*, 183. [CrossRef] [PubMed]

15. Cieplinska, K.; Gajecka, M.; Nowak, A.; Dabrowski, M.; Zielonka, L.; Gajecki, M.T. The genotoxicity of caecal water in gilts exposed to low doses of zearalenone. *Toxins* **2018**, *10*, 350. [CrossRef] [PubMed]

16. Hassan, Y.I.; Zhou, T. Promising detoxification strategies to mitigate mycotoxins in food and feed. *Toxins* **2018**, *10*, 116. [CrossRef]

17. Alassane-Kpembi, I.; Pinton, P.; Hupe, J.F.; Neves, M.; Lippi, Y.; Combes, S.; Castex, M.; Oswald, I.P. *Saccharomyces cerevisiae* boulardii reduces the deoxynivalenol-induced alteration of the intestinal transcriptome. *Toxins* **2018**, *10*, 199. [CrossRef] [PubMed]

18. Wang, J.; Li, M.; Zhang, W.; Gu, A.; Dong, J.; Li, J.; Shan, A. Protective effect of n-acetylcysteine against oxidative stress induced by zearalenone via mitochondrial apoptosis pathway in SIEC02 cells. *Toxins* **2018**, *10*, 407. [CrossRef]

19. Li, F.; Wang, J.; Huang, L.; Chen, H.; Wang, C. Effects of adding *Clostridium* sp. WJ06 on intestinal morphology and microbial diversity of growing pigs fed with natural deoxynivalenol contaminated wheat. *Toxins* **2017**, *9*, 383.

20. Zheng, W.; Ji, X.; Zhang, Q.; Yao, W. Intestinal microbiota ecological response to oral administrations of hydrogen-rich water and lactulose in female piglets fed a fusarium toxin-contaminated diet. *Toxins* **2018**, *10*, 246. [CrossRef] [PubMed]

21. Gerez, J.; Buck, L.; Marutani, V.H.; Calliari, C.M.; Bracarense, A.P. Low levels of chito-oligosaccharides are not effective in reducing deoxynivalenol toxicity in swine jejunal explants. *Toxins* **2018**, *10*, 276. [CrossRef] [PubMed]

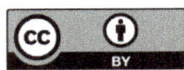

toxins

MDPI

Article

Modulation of Intestinal Epithelial Permeability in Differentiated Caco-2 Cells Exposed to Aflatoxin M1 and Ochratoxin A Individually or Collectively

Yanan Gao [1,2,3,†], Songli Li [1,2,3,†], Jiaqi Wang [1,2,3], Chaochao Luo [1,2,3], Shengguo Zhao [1,2,3] and Nan Zheng [1,2,3,*]

1   Ministry of Agriculture Laboratory of Quality & Safety Control for Risk Assessment for Dairy Products (Beijing), Institute of Animal Science, Chinese Academy of Agricultural Sciences, Beijing 100193, China; gyn758521@126.com (Y.G.); Lisongli@caas.cn (S.L.); wang-jia-qi@263.net (J.W.); luochaochao839505@163.com (C.L.); zhaoshengguo1984@163.com (S.Z.)
2   Ministry of Agriculture-Milk and Dairy Product Inspection Center, Beijing 100193, China
3   State Key Laboratory of Animal Nutrition, Institute of Animal Science, Chinese Academy of Agricultural Sciences, Beijing 100193, China
*   Correspondence: zhengnan_1908@126.com; Tel.: +86-010-6281-6069
†   These authors contributed equally to the work.

Received: 10 November 2017; Accepted: 25 December 2017; Published: 27 December 2017

Abstract: Aflatoxin M1 (AFM1) and ochratoxin A (OTA) are mycotoxins commonly found in milk; however, their effects on intestinal epithelial cells have not been reported. In the present study, we show that AFM1 (0.12 and 12 µM) and OTA (0.2 and 20 µM) individually or collectively increased the paracellular flux of lucifer yellow and fluorescein isothiocyanate (FITC)-dextrans (4 and 40 kDa) and decreased transepithelial electrical resistance values in differentiated Caco-2 cells after 48 h of exposure, indicating increased epithelial permeability. Immunoblotting and immunofluorescent analysis revealed that AFM1, OTA, and their combination decreased the expression levels of tight junction (TJ) proteins and disrupted their structures, namely, claudin-3, claudin-4, occludin, and zonula occludens-1 (ZO-1), and p44/42 mitogen-activated protein kinase (MAPK) partially involved in the mycotoxins-induced disruption of intestinal barrier. The effects of a combination of AFM1 and OTA on intestinal barrier function were more significant ($p < 0.05$) than those of AFM1 and OTA alone, yielding additive or synergistic effects. The additive or synergistic effects of AFM1 and OTA on intestinal barrier function might affect human health, especially in children, and toxin risks should be considered.

Keywords: aflatoxin M1; ochratoxin A; intestinal epithelial cells; tight junction; permeability

---

1. Introduction

Human exposure to mycotoxins not only can occur through direct dermal contact and inhalation of contaminated agricultural products, but also could occur through the consumption of foods of animal origin, such as milk and eggs, which were obtained from animals fed with mycotoxin-contaminated material [1]. Given that milk supplies the general public with a large quantity of essential nutrients, it is a part of the prevailing diet for all age groups. The largest consumers of milk are children because milk is vital for their growth and development. Thus, mycotoxin-contaminated milk can produce detrimental effects on their health [2]. Moreover, the presence of multiple mycotoxins in milk is likely. In raw milk from China, we identified several mycotoxins, including aflatoxin M1 (AFM1), ochratoxin A (OTA), zearalenone (ZEA), and α-zearalenol (α-ZOL) [3]. In raw bulk milk produced in northwest France in 2003, AFM1 was found in 3 out of 264 samples at levels of 26 ng/L or less, and OTA was detected in three samples at levels of 5 to 8 ng/L [4]. For infant milk formulas produced in Italy, AFM1

5. Moldal, T.; Bernhoft, A.; Rosenlund, G.; Kaldhusdal, M.; Koppang, E.O. Dietary deoxynivalenol (DON) may impair the epithelial barrier and modulate the cytokine signaling in the intestine of atlantic salmon (*Salmo salar*). *Toxins* **2018**, *10*, 376. [CrossRef] [PubMed]
6. Pasternak, J.A.; Aiyer, V.I.A.; Hamonic, G.; Beaulieu, A.D.; Columbus, D.A.; Wilson, H.L. Molecular and physiological effects on the small intestine of weaner pigs following feeding with deoxynivalenol-contaminated feed. *Toxins* **2018**, *10*, 40. [CrossRef]
7. Pinton, P.; Graziani, F.; Pujol, A.; Nicoletti, C.; Paris, O.; Ernouf, P.; Di Pasquale, E.; Perrier, J.; Oswald, I.P.; Maresca, M. Deoxynivalenol inhibits the expression by goblet cells of intestinal mucins through a pkr and map kinase dependent repression of the resistin-like molecule beta. *Mol. Nutr. Food Res.* **2015**, *59*, 1076–1087. [CrossRef] [PubMed]
8. Przybylska-Gornowicz, B.; Lewczuk, B.; Prusik, M.; Hanuszewska, M.; Petrusewicz-Kosinska, M.; Gajecka, M.; Zielonka, L.; Gajecki, M. The effects of deoxynivalenol and zearalenone on the pig large intestine. A light and electron microscopy study. *Toxins* **2018**, *10*, 148.
9. Makowska, K.; Obremski, K.; Gonkowski, S. The impact of T-2 toxin on vasoactive intestinal polypeptide-like immunoreactive (VIP-LI) nerve structures in the wall of the porcine stomach and duodenum. *Toxins* **2018**, *10*, 138. [CrossRef]
10. O'Hara, A.M.; Shanahan, F. The gut flora as a forgotten organ. *Embo. Rep.* **2006**, *7*, 688–693. [CrossRef]
11. Yang, X.A.; Liu, L.L.; Chen, J.; Xiao, A.P. Response of intestinal bacterial flora to the long-term feeding of aflatoxin B_1 (AFB$_1$) in mice. *Toxins* **2017**, *9*, 317. [CrossRef]
12. Reddy, K.E.; Jeong, J.Y.; Song, J.; Lee, Y.; Lee, H.J.; Kim, D.W.; Jung, H.J.; Kim, K.H.; Kim, M.; Oh, Y.K.; et al. Colon microbiome of pigs fed diet contaminated with commercial purified deoxynivalenol and zearalenone. *Toxins* **2018**, *10*, 347. [CrossRef] [PubMed]
13. Mateos, I.; Combes, S.; Pascal, G.; Cauquil, L.; Barilly, C.; Cossalter, A.M.; Laffitte, J.; Botti, S.; Pinton, P.; Oswald, I.P. Fumonisin-exposure impairs age-related ecological succession of bacterial species in weaned pig gut microbiota. *Toxins* **2018**, *10*, 230. [CrossRef]
14. Maruo, V.M.; Bracarense, A.P.; Metayer, J.P.; Vilarino, M.; Oswald, I.P.; Pinton, P. Ergot alkaloids at doses close to EU regulatory limits induce alterations of the liver and intestine. *Toxins* **2018**, *10*, 183. [CrossRef] [PubMed]
15. Cieplinska, K.; Gajecka, M.; Nowak, A.; Dabrowski, M.; Zielonka, L.; Gajecki, M.T. The genotoxicity of caecal water in gilts exposed to low doses of zearalenone. *Toxins* **2018**, *10*, 350. [CrossRef] [PubMed]
16. Hassan, Y.I.; Zhou, T. Promising detoxification strategies to mitigate mycotoxins in food and feed. *Toxins* **2018**, *10*, 116. [CrossRef]
17. Alassane-Kpembi, I.; Pinton, P.; Hupe, J.F.; Neves, M.; Lippi, Y.; Combes, S.; Castex, M.; Oswald, I.P. *Saccharomyces cerevisiae* boulardii reduces the deoxynivalenol-induced alteration of the intestinal transcriptome. *Toxins* **2018**, *10*, 199. [CrossRef] [PubMed]
18. Wang, J.; Li, M.; Zhang, W.; Gu, A.; Dong, J.; Li, J.; Shan, A. Protective effect of n-acetylcysteine against oxidative stress induced by zearalenone via mitochondrial apoptosis pathway in SIEC02 cells. *Toxins* **2018**, *10*, 407. [CrossRef]
19. Li, F.; Wang, J.; Huang, L.; Chen, H.; Wang, C. Effects of adding *Clostridium* sp. WJ06 on intestinal morphology and microbial diversity of growing pigs fed with natural deoxynivalenol contaminated wheat. *Toxins* **2017**, *9*, 383.
20. Zheng, W.; Ji, X.; Zhang, Q.; Yao, W. Intestinal microbiota ecological response to oral administrations of hydrogen-rich water and lactulose in female piglets fed a fusarium toxin-contaminated diet. *Toxins* **2018**, *10*, 246. [CrossRef] [PubMed]
21. Gerez, J.; Buck, L.; Marutani, V.H.; Calliari, C.M.; Bracarense, A.P. Low levels of chito-oligosaccharides are not effective in reducing deoxynivalenol toxicity in swine jejunal explants. *Toxins* **2018**, *10*, 276. [CrossRef] [PubMed]

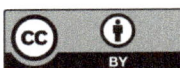

toxins

MDPI

Article

Modulation of Intestinal Epithelial Permeability in Differentiated Caco-2 Cells Exposed to Aflatoxin M1 and Ochratoxin A Individually or Collectively

Yanan Gao [1,2,3,†], Songli Li [1,2,3,†], Jiaqi Wang [1,2,3], Chaochao Luo [1,2,3], Shengguo Zhao [1,2,3] and Nan Zheng [1,2,3,*]

[1] Ministry of Agriculture Laboratory of Quality & Safety Control for Risk Assessment for Dairy Products (Beijing), Institute of Animal Science, Chinese Academy of Agricultural Sciences, Beijing 100193, China; gyn758521@126.com (Y.G.); Lisongli@caas.cn (S.L.); wang-jia-qi@263.net (J.W.); luochaochao839505@163.com (C.L.); zhaoshengguo1984@163.com (S.Z.)
[2] Ministry of Agriculture-Milk and Dairy Product Inspection Center, Beijing 100193, China
[3] State Key Laboratory of Animal Nutrition, Institute of Animal Science, Chinese Academy of Agricultural Sciences, Beijing 100193, China
* Correspondence: zhengnan_1908@126.com; Tel.: +86-010-6281-6069
† These authors contributed equally to the work.

Received: 10 November 2017; Accepted: 25 December 2017; Published: 27 December 2017

Abstract: Aflatoxin M1 (AFM1) and ochratoxin A (OTA) are mycotoxins commonly found in milk; however, their effects on intestinal epithelial cells have not been reported. In the present study, we show that AFM1 (0.12 and 12 µM) and OTA (0.2 and 20 µM) individually or collectively increased the paracellular flux of lucifer yellow and fluorescein isothiocyanate (FITC)-dextrans (4 and 40 kDa) and decreased transepithelial electrical resistance values in differentiated Caco-2 cells after 48 h of exposure, indicating increased epithelial permeability. Immunoblotting and immunofluorescent analysis revealed that AFM1, OTA, and their combination decreased the expression levels of tight junction (TJ) proteins and disrupted their structures, namely, claudin-3, claudin-4, occludin, and zonula occludens-1 (ZO-1), and p44/42 mitogen-activated protein kinase (MAPK) partially involved in the mycotoxins-induced disruption of intestinal barrier. The effects of a combination of AFM1 and OTA on intestinal barrier function were more significant ($p < 0.05$) than those of AFM1 and OTA alone, yielding additive or synergistic effects. The additive or synergistic effects of AFM1 and OTA on intestinal barrier function might affect human health, especially in children, and toxin risks should be considered.

Keywords: aflatoxin M1; ochratoxin A; intestinal epithelial cells; tight junction; permeability

1. Introduction

Human exposure to mycotoxins not only can occur through direct dermal contact and inhalation of contaminated agricultural products, but also could occur through the consumption of foods of animal origin, such as milk and eggs, which were obtained from animals fed with mycotoxin-contaminated material [1]. Given that milk supplies the general public with a large quantity of essential nutrients, it is a part of the prevailing diet for all age groups. The largest consumers of milk are children because milk is vital for their growth and development. Thus, mycotoxin-contaminated milk can produce detrimental effects on their health [2]. Moreover, the presence of multiple mycotoxins in milk is likely. In raw milk from China, we identified several mycotoxins, including aflatoxin M1 (AFM1), ochratoxin A (OTA), zearalenone (ZEA), and α-zearalenol (α-ZOL) [3]. In raw bulk milk produced in northwest France in 2003, AFM1 was found in 3 out of 264 samples at levels of 26 ng/L or less, and OTA was detected in three samples at levels of 5 to 8 ng/L [4]. For infant milk formulas produced in Italy, AFM1 was found in 2 out of 185 samples (concentration range, 11.8 ng/L to 15.3 ng/L), while OTA was detected in 133 (72%) samples (concentration range, 35.1 to 689.5 ng/L) [5]. In a recent analysis of baby food (flours and milk powder) in Portugal, AFM1 and OTA were detected in 2 out of 27 samples, AFM1 was detected in two samples, OTA was detected in seven samples, and aflatoxin B1 (AFB1) and OTA were detected in one sample. For these samples, the AFM1 concentration was 0.017–0.041 µg/kg, and the OTA concentration was 0.034–0.212 µg/kg [6]. Considering the well demonstrated cytotoxic, genotoxic, and carcinogenic effects of AFM1, the International Agency for Research of Cancer (IARC) changed its carcinogenicity classification from Group 2 to Group 1 [7]. Furthermore, AFM1 is the only mycotoxin with an established maximum residue limit (MRL) in milk worldwide. The established MRL of AFM1 is 0.05 µg/kg in the European Union (EU) and 0.5 µg/kg in China and the United States of America (USA). We previously showed that OTA exerts a toxicity similar to that of AFM1 on human intestinal cells [8]. Furthermore, the IARC has classified OTA as a Group 2B carcinogen, suggesting that it is a possible human carcinogen [7]. Although there is no MRL for OTA in milk, a provisional tolerable weekly intake (PTWI) of 100 ng kg^{-1} body weight was established [9]. Hence, it is important to determine the toxicological effects of AFM1 and OTA on human health.

The gastrointestinal tract (GIT) is the first tissue barrier to come into contact with food contaminants, such as mycotoxins [10,11], and intestinal epithelial cells are most affected [12,13]. The GIT barrier is constituted by intercellular tight junction (TJ) proteins that localize to the apical domain of epithelial cells, where they selectively limit the passage of large molecules, ions, solutes, and water [14,15]. TJs are comprised of several multiprotein complexes that include transmembrane proteins (e.g., claudin, occludin, and junctional adhesion molecule (JAM) and cytoplasmic scaffolding proteins (e.g., zonula occludens (ZO)-1, ZO-2, and ZO-3) [16–19]. Therefore, it is likely that the defects in intestinal epithelial barrier function caused by mycotoxins are associated with the disruption of TJ integrity. Among the cell lines used as models of TJ function, the Food and Drug Administration (FDA) has recognized the Caco-2 cell line, originally isolated from human colon adenocarcinoma, as a reference model to assess the effects of drugs and toxins on intestinal barrier function [20]. A previous study showed that results obtained from this cell line are reproducible and applicable to in vivo data [21]. After culturing Caco-2 cells for 16–22 days, differentiated monolayers are established, mimicking the small intestine epithelial layer in that they form a polarized monolayer with functional TJs [22].

Presently, there is a growing awareness of the adverse effects of various mycotoxins on the intestine and the disruption of intestinal integrity in differentiated Caco-2 cells [23]. Romero et al. [24] reported that OTA decreased transepithelial electrical resistance (TEER) values and claudin-3, claudin-4, and occludin mRNA expression levels, and other studies demonstrated that treatment with OTA reduced intestinal barrier function in humans [25–27]. In addition, low concentrations of AFM1, added to either the apical or basal compartment of transwell chambers, significantly decreased TEER values [28]. The effects of mycotoxins on cells can be characterized as synergistic, additive, or antagonistic, and these effects might adversely affect human health. In addition, the contamination of aflatoxin B1 (AFB1) and OTA has been frequently observed in cereals and beans, and their concentrations in such foods are generally higher than that in milk. Wangikar et al. [29] demonstrated that AFB1 and OTA have antagonistic interaction in New Zealand White rabbits regarding their teratogenic effect. Huang et al. [30] reported that the mixture of AFB1, OTA, and ZEA exerted the greatest adverse effects on dairy goats, indicating the serious negative effects of the combinations of mycotoxins. We previously demonstrated synergistic and additive cytotoxic effects for OTA, ZEA, and/or α-ZOL with AFM1, except that AFM1 and ZEA produced an antagonistic effect on the proliferation of Caco-2 cells by isobologram analysis [8]. In recent decades, isobologram analysis has become the most commonly used approach to evaluate the interactive effects between chemical substances. Practical limitations exist in the combination analysis based on *Loewe Additivity* [31]. Estimation of dose–effect curves for the drugs being combined requires a certain amount of data and can rapidly become expensive as well as experimentally and computationally demanding, and makes the analysis of drug combination prohibitive [32]. *Loewe Additivity* model becomes unusable when a dose–effect curve is not available or difficult to model [33].

Previous studies have reported an association of epithelial barrier function with mitogen-activated protein kinases (MAPK) [34,35], which are responsible for intracellular signaling pathway. More importantly, MAPK are considered to play a vital role in inflammatory responses of epithelial cells and includes there subfamilies-p44/42 extracellular signal regulated kinase (ERK), p38 and c-Jun *N*-terminal Kinase (JNK). A mechanistic study demonstrated that the undermined epithelial barrier induced by deoxynivalenol (DON), which was reflected by the drop TEER values and reduced expression level of claudin-4 protein, was associated with the activation of ERK signaling pathway [36]. Though numerous studies have been reported that DON-induced intestinal barrier dysfunction was seen with the activation of MAPK signaling pathway, the underlying mechanisms of compromised intestinal barrier caused by AFM1 and OTA yet to be illustrated. With regard to intestinal barrier integrity, one study focused on the mycotoxin special DON, while another study examined the effects of DON and FB1 on the intestine of piglets [37,38]. Hence, it is crucial to understand the individual and combined effects of AFM1 and OTA on the structure and function of the gut. The purpose of this study was to investigate the individual and combined effects of AFM1 and OTA on intestinal permeability and to define the underlying mechanism(s). We hypothesized that (i) a combination of AFM1 and OTA, which frequently occur simultaneously in milk, might significantly affect intestinal permeability and TJ function and produce a variety of interactive effects, (ii) the decreased expression of TJ proteins leads to an increased epithelial permeability, and (iii) the decreased TJ proteins expression level mediated through modulation of MAPK. To address these hypotheses, we carried out TEER measurements, paracellular tracer flux assays, and related protein expression experiments in differentiated Caco-2 cells exposed to different concentrations of AFM1 and OTA individually and collectively.

2. Results

2.1. Effects of AFM1 and OTA Individually or Collectively on the TEER Values of Caco-2 Cell Monolayers

The baseline TEER values of Caco-2 cell monolayers (on day 21 post-seeding) varied from 1411 to 1645 $\Omega \cdot cm^2$. The culture of these monolayers in Dulbecco's modified Eagle Medium (DMEM) containing 1% (v/v) methanol (control) did not significantly alter the initial TEER values over a period of 48 h. After 48 h of exposure to mycotoxins, the TEER values of Caco-2 cells exposed to non-cytotoxic concentrations of AFM1 (0.12 µM) and OTA (0.2 µM) individually or collectively were not significantly different ($p > 0.05$) from those of control cells. However, the TEER values of cells exposed to cytotoxic concentrations of AFM1 (12 µM) or the combination of AFM1 (12 µM) and OTA (20 µM) collectively were significantly lower ($p < 0.05$) than those of control cells. Furthermore, the TEER values of cells exposed to cytotoxic concentrations of AFM1 and OTA collectively were lower than those of cells exposed to AFM1 and OTA individually, although the difference between them were not significant ($p > 0.05$) (Figure 1).

2.2. Effects of AFM1 and OTA Individually or Collectively on the Permeability of Caco-2 Cell Monolayers

The effects of non-cytotoxic and cytotoxic concentrations of AFM1 and OTA individually or collectively on intestinal permeability were investigated by measuring the paracellular flux of fluorescent tracers with different molecular weights (lucifer yellow (LY) and FITC-dextran) across Caco-2 cell monolayers. Except for the non-cytotoxic concentration of AFM1, which did not significantly affect ($p > 0.05$) the paracellular flux of LY (Figure 2a), mycotoxins significantly increased ($p < 0.05$) the paracellular flux of LY and FITC-dextran (4 and 40 kDa) across cell monolayers (Figure 2). For individual mycotoxins, the paracellular flux of LY and FITC-dextran (4 and 40 kDa) across cell monolayers was significantly higher ($p < 0.05$) after treatment with non-cytotoxic and cytotoxic concentrations of OTA than after similar concentrations of AFM1 (Figure 2). With regard to the combined use of AFM1 and OTA, both mycotoxins exerted a more significant effect ($p < 0.05$) on intestinal permeability than the individual mycotoxins (Figure 2).

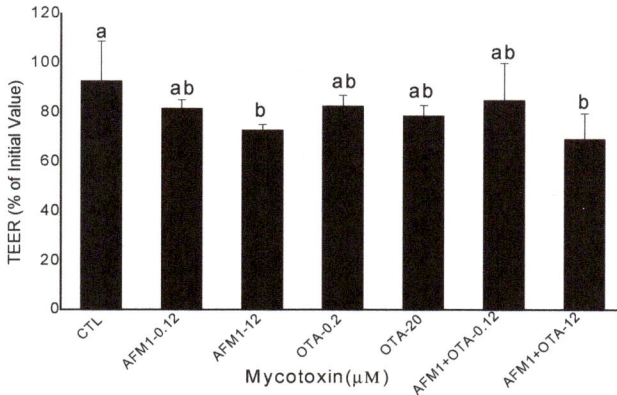

Figure 1. Changes in transepithelial electrical resistance (TEER) values in differentiated Caco-2 cells after treatment with different concentrations of aflatoxin M1 (AFM1) and ochratoxin A (OTA) individually or collectively (AFM1+OTA) for 48 h compared with the initial value. Results are expressed as the mean ± SEM of three independent experiments. TEER was measured before and after mycotoxin treatment for each condition. Different letters (a,b) indicate significant differences in TEER ($p < 0.05$). TEER, transepithelial electrical resistance. AFM1-0.12 represents AFM1 at 0.12 μM, AFM1-12 represents AFM1 at 12 μM, OTA-0.2 represents OTA at 0.2 μM, OTA-20 represents OTA at 20 μM, AFM1+OTA-0.12 represents the combination of AFM1 (0.12 μM) and OTA (0.2 μM), AFM1+OTA-12 represents the combination of AFM1 (12 μM) and OTA (20 μM).

2.3. Effects of ATM1 and OTA Individually or Collectively on TJ Protein Levels in Caco-2 Cell Monolayers

To investigate the mechanism by which mycotoxins increase the permeability of Caco-2 cell monolayers, the levels of TJ proteins were quantified by Western blot analysis. Occludin and ZO-1 levels in Caco-2 cells exposed to non-cytotoxic and cytotoxic concentrations of AFM1 and OTA individually or collectively were significantly lower ($p < 0.05$) than those in control cells. By contrast, claudin-3 and claudin-4 levels in cells exposed to OTA, but not ATM1, or both mycotoxins were significantly lower ($p < 0.05$) than those in control cells (Figure 3). The negative effects of OTA on the levels of claudin, occludin, and ZO-1 were significantly greater ($p < 0.05$) than those of AFM1. Furthermore, the negative effects of AFM1 and OTA collectively were greater than those of AFM1 and OTA individually. The decrease in claudins, occludin, and ZO-1 expression in cells exposed to non-cytotoxic concentrations of AFM1 and OTA was not significantly different ($p > 0.05$) from that in cells exposed to cytotoxic concentrations.

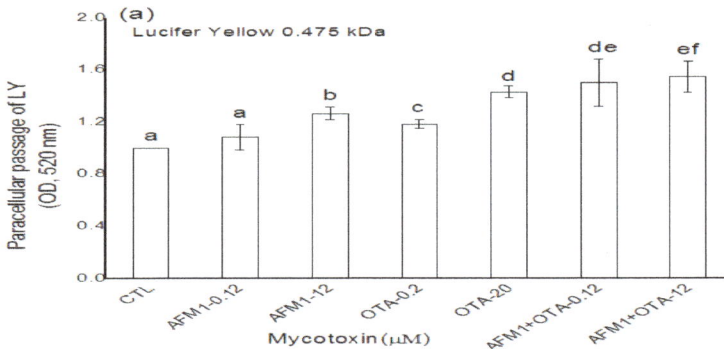

Figure 2. *Cont.*

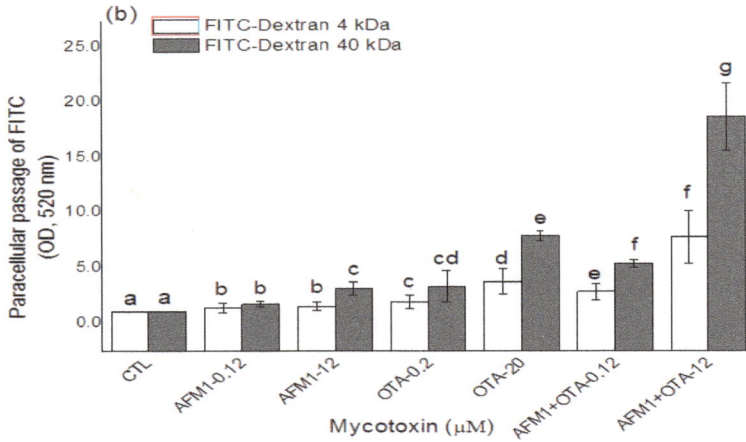

Figure 2. Mycotoxin increased the permeability of the Caco-2 cell monolayer. Caco-2 cells were cultured on transwell chambers and stimulated for 48 h with different concentrations of AFM1, OTA, and AFM1+OTA added to apical and basal compartments. Subsequently, the paracellular flux of lucifer yellow (LY) (0.457 kDa; (**a**)) and fluorescein isothiocyanate (FITC)-dextran (4 and 40 kDa; (**b**)) from the apical to the basal compartment was assessed. Results are expressed as the mean ± SEM of three independent experiments with three replicates. Different letters (a–g) indicate significant differences in FITC ($p < 0.05$). AFM1-0.12 represents AFM1 at 0.12 μM, AFM1-12 represents AFM1 at 12 μM, OTA-0.2 represents OTA at 0.2 μM, OTA-20 represents OTA at 20 μM, AFM1+OTA-0.12 represents the combination of AFM1 (0.12 μM) and OTA (0.2 μM), AFM1+OTA-12 represents the combination of AFM1 (12 μM) and OTA (20 μM).

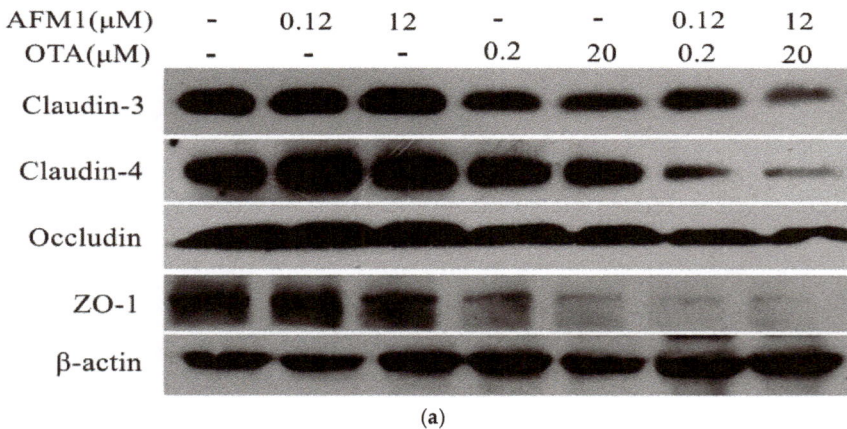

(**a**)

Figure 3. *Cont.*

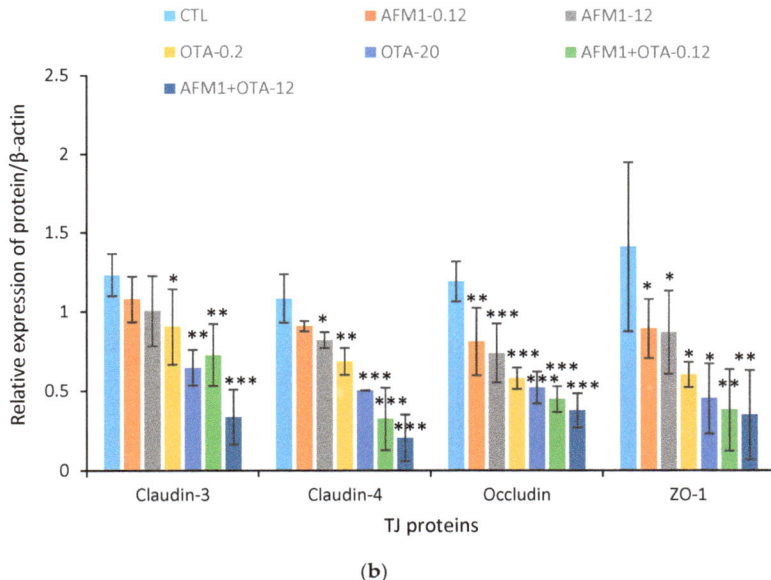

(b)

Figure 3. Effects of different concentrations of AFM1, OTA, and AFM1+OTA on TJ protein levels in Caco-2 cells after 48 h of exposure. (**a**) Cell proteins (20 µg) were separated by sodium dodecyl sulfate polyacrylamide gel electrophoresis (SDS-PAGE) and immunoblotted first for tight junction (TJ) proteins, and second for human β-actin; (**b**) the intensities of the TJ proteins were quantified with ImageJ software (Version 2.1.0, National Institutes of Health, Bethesda, MD, USA, 2006). Values were normalized to the loading control (human β-actin) and expressed relative to the negative control (untreated cells). Results are expressed as the mean ± Standard Error of Mean (SEM), $n = 3$–5. M-0.12 represents AFM1 at 0.12 µM, M-12 represents AFM1 at 12 µM, O-0.2 represents OTA at 0.2 µM, O-20 represents OTA at 20 µM, M+O-0.12 represents the combination of AFM1 (0.12 µM) and OTA (0.2 µM), M+O-12 represents the combination of AFM1 (12 µM) and OTA (20 µM). * $p < 0.05$; ** $p < 0.001$; *** $p < 0.000$.

2.4. Effects of AFM1 and OTA Individually or Collectively on TJ Protein Localization in Caco-2 Cell Monolayers

The localization of TJ proteins was assessed by immunofluorescent staining. In confluent Caco-2 cells not exposed to mycotoxins, claudin-3, claudin-4, occludin, and ZO-1 localized at the plasma membrane and resembled a cobblestone pattern. There was no significant difference in the localization of claudin-3 and ZO-1 in cells exposed to non-cytotoxic concentrations of mycotoxins individually or collectively. Furthermore, claudin-3 and ZO-1 were hardly detected in cells exposed to cytotoxic concentrations of AFM1 and OTA individually or collectively, suggesting that claudin-3 and ZO-1 protein synthesis was affected. Mycotoxins also affected claudin-4, as evidenced by a faint immunofluorescent signal and a discontinuous cobblestone pattern unlike in control cells. Although there was no difference in the localization of occludin in cells exposed to a non- or cytotoxic concentration of AFM1 and a non-cytotoxic concentration of OTA, a cytotoxic concentration of OTA and non- or cytotoxic concentrations of AFM1 and OTA disrupted the continuous cobblestone pattern. Indeed, the individual use of mycotoxins did not significantly affect the localization of occludin in differentiated Caco-2 cells, while the combined use of mycotoxins, especially at cytotoxic concentrations, undermined the integrity of the cobblestone pattern of occludin (Figure 4).

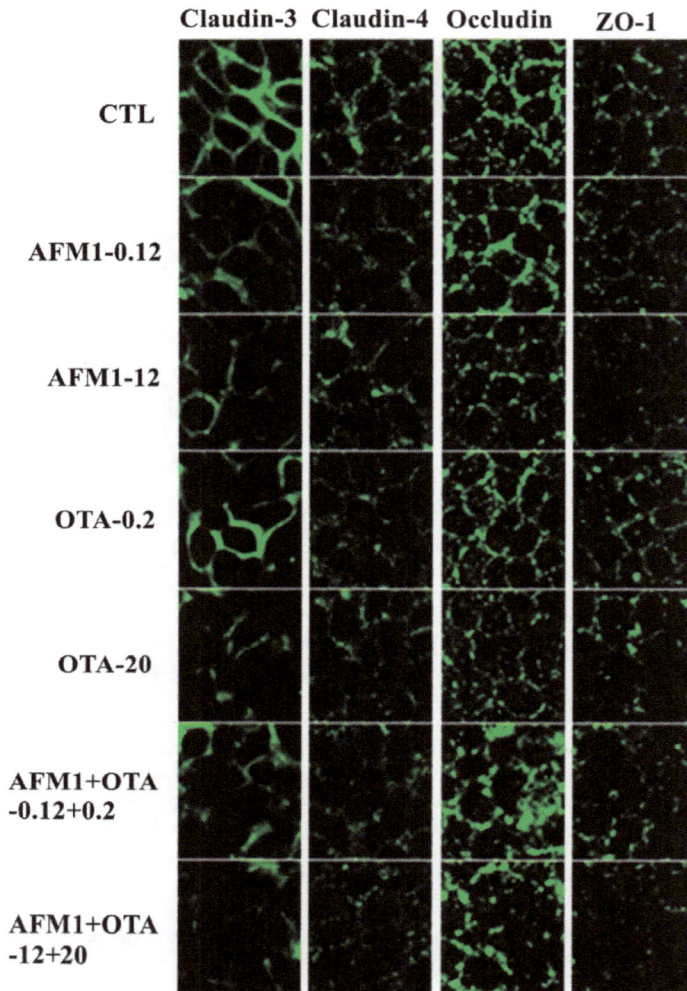

Figure 4. Effects of AFM1 and OTA on the localization of TJ proteins. Differentiated Caco-2 cells were cultured on transwell chambers for 21 days. The cells were then treated for 48 h with different concentrations of AFM1 and OTA added to apical and basal compartments, followed by fixation and staining with an anti-claudin-3, anti-claudin-4, anti-occludin, or anti-zonula occludens-1 (ZO-1) antibody, as described in Section 2.

2.5. The Interactive Effects of the Combination of AFM1 and OTA

After assessing the interactive effects of AFM1 and OTA at different concentrations on TEER, according to the analysis for interactions described in Section 4.10, we found an antagonistic effect between non-cytotoxic concentrations of AFM1 and OTA, and the measured value was 20.8% ($p < 0.05$) higher than the expected value. However, an additive effect was found at cytotoxic concentrations of the mycotoxins, with a non-significant difference ($p > 0.05$) between the measured and expected values (Figure 5a).

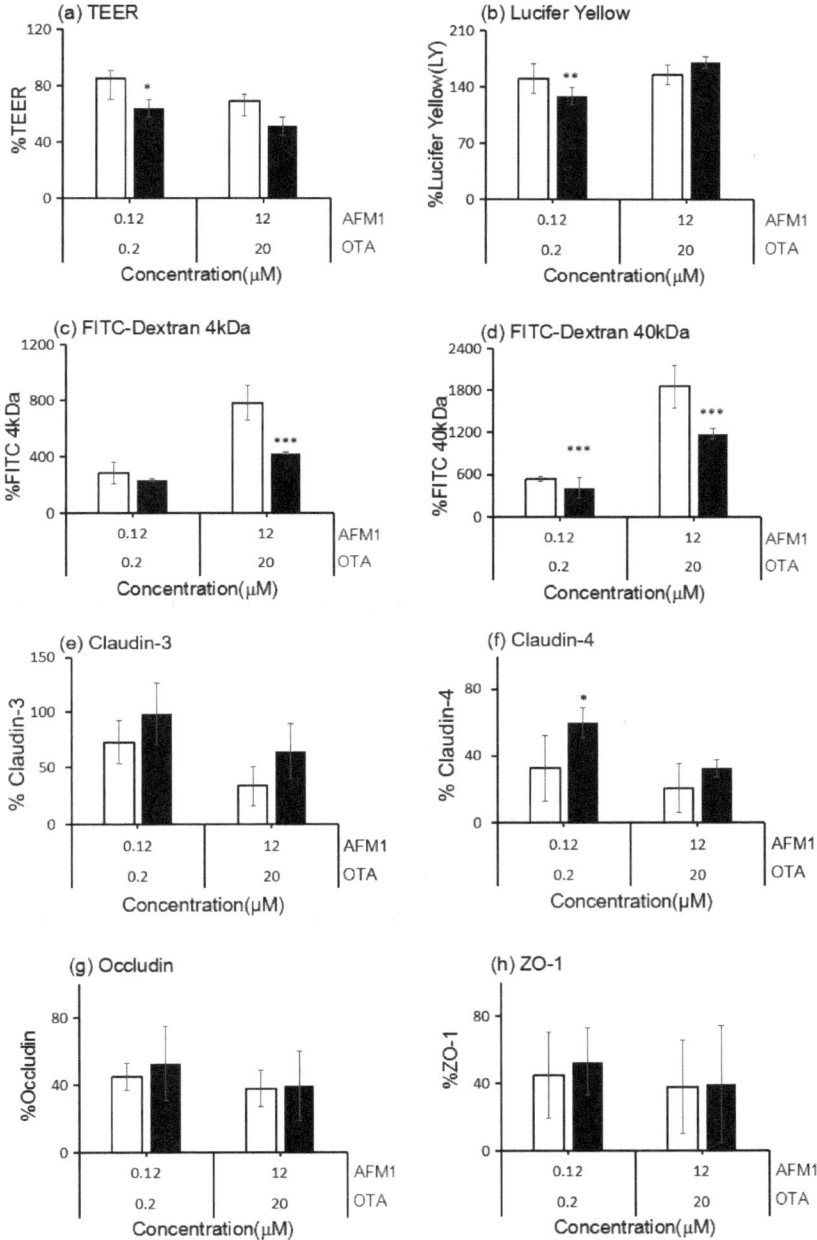

Figure 5. Interactive cytotoxic effects of binary combinations of AFM1 and OTA in differentiated Caco-2 cells after exposure for 48 h (**a–h**). After the exposure to mycotoxins, TEER, FITC-dextran (4 and 40 kDa) paracellular flux, and TJ protein expression were measured. There were no significant interactive effects for claudin-3, occludin, and ZO-1 expression. Data are expressed as a percentage of the untreated control for each parameter. White bars represent the measured values, and dark bars represent the expected values. * $p < 0.05$; ** $p < 0.001$; *** $p < 0.000$ represent both significant synergistic and antagonist effects.

Synergistic effects were observed for the paracellular flux of LY after treatment with non-cytotoxic concentrations of AFM1 and OTA collectively (with a 21.5% difference over the expected values, $p < 0.05$), the paracellular flux of FITC-dextran (4 kDa) after treatment with cytotoxic concentrations of both mycotoxins (with a 357.0% difference over the expected values, $p < 0.05$), and the paracellular flux of FITC-dextran (40 kDa) after treatment with non-cytotoxic and cytotoxic concentrations of both mycotoxins (with a 129.8% and 679.0% difference over the expected values, respectively, $p < 0.05$) (Figure 5b–d, respectively). Additive effects were observed for the paracellular flux of LY after treatment with cytotoxic concentrations of both mycotoxins ($p > 0.05$) and the paracellular flux of FITC-dextran (4 kDa) after treatment with non-cytotoxic concentrations of both mycotoxins ($p > 0.05$) (Figure 5b,c, respectively).

The additive effects of AFM1 and OTA were evident on claudin-3, occludin, and ZO-1 expression, with no significant difference between the measured and expected values (Figure 5e,g,h). Synergistic effects were observed for claudin-4 expression after treatment of Caco-2 cells with a non-cytotoxic concentration of both mycotoxins, with a 27.4% ($p < 0.05$) decrease compared with the expected values, and additive effects were shown at cytotoxic concentrations of both mycotoxins (Figure 5f).

2.6. Correlations between TJ Junction and Intestinal Permeability

To understand the significance of the changes in TJ protein levels and intestinal permeability following exposure to mycotoxins, the correlations among TEER values, the permeability of fluorescent tracers (LY, FITC-dextran (4 kDa), and FITC-dextran (40 kDa)), and the levels of TJ proteins (claudin-3, claudin-4, occludin, and ZO-1) were evaluated. Significantly negative ($p < 0.000$) correlations were found between the TEER values and the three fluorescent tracers, and a significantly positive ($p < 0.05$) correlation was found between LY and FITC-dextran (40 kDa). In addition, there were significantly positive ($p < 0.000$) correlations between the TEER values and the four TJ proteins. There were also significantly negative ($p < 0.05$) correlations between FITC-dextran (40 kDa) and the four TJ proteins, although there were no significant ($p > 0.05$) correlations between LY or FITC-dextran (4 kDa) and claudin-3, claudin-4, occludin, or ZO-1. The significant correlations between the TEER values or FITC-dextran (40 kDa) and the TJ proteins suggest that an increased epithelial permeability associates with the disruption of TJ integrity (Figure 6).

To further investigate the role of TJs in intestinal epithelial permeability, we silenced occludin, a representative TJ protein, in Caco-2 cells. Occludin knockdown in transfected cells was confirmed by immunoblotting (Figure S1a). More specially, the expression level of occludin of siRNA group were significantly lower than that in control and NC group, indicating that the effects of occludin knockdown was creditable. In addition, the TEER values in occludin-silenced cells were significantly lower ($p < 0.05$) than those in control and NC-silenced cells (Figure S1b), indicating that occludin plays an important role in TJ integrity. These results also indicate that TJs contribute to the maintenance of epithelial permeability.

2.7. AFM1 and OTA Induce Barrier Dysfunction via MAPK-Dependent Mechanism

In order to identity intracellular signaling pathways related to AFM1 and OTA-induced downregulation of TJ proteins, the MAPK pathway was measured in differentiated Caco-2 cells treated with these mycotoxins individually or collectively. Cells were pretreated specific pharmacological inhibitors for the related molecules (p44/42 (U-0126), JNK (SP600125), p38 (SB203580)) for 1 h, followed by a 30 min exposure of AFM1 and OTA. The immunoblotting results showed that the combined mycotoxins led to a more significant activation of p44/42 MAPK than these individually and the pretreatment of inhibitor U-0126 prevented individual and combined AFM1 and OTA-induced p44/42 MAPK phosphorylation (Figure 7), while the mycotoxin-induced phosphorylation of p38 and JNK MAPK was not affected by the corresponding inhibitors (data not shown).

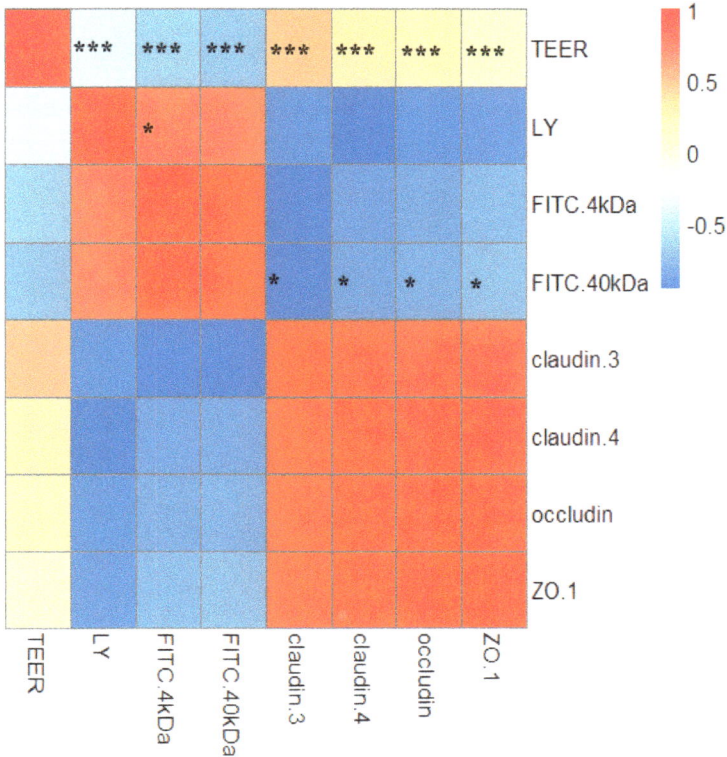

Figure 6. Heat map showing correlations among TEER, FITC-dextran (4 and 40 kDa), and TJ proteins (claudin-3, claudin-4, occludin, and ZO-1) for differentiated Caco-2 cells taking into account data from all of the experiments performed in this study. The heat map is a visual representation of correlated values between each pair of parameters denoted by the corresponding row and the column of the matrix. Red represents a positive correlation, yellow represents a low correlation, and blue represents a negative correlation, as shown in the color key. Statistical significance was analyzed by Spearman's correlations. The number scale to the right represents the correlation coefficients. The higher the number, the higher the correlation. * $p < 0.05$ and *** $p < 0.000$. (For an interpretation of the references to the color in this figure, the reader is referred to the web version of the article.).

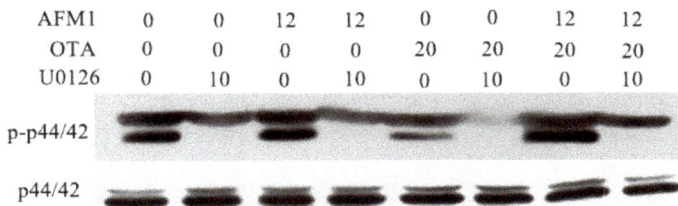

Figure 7. U-0126 monoethanolate (U-0126) (10 μM) counteracted AFM1 (12 μM) and OTA (20 μM)-induced p44/42 mitogen-activated protein kinase (MAPK) (extracellular regulated protein kinases 1/2, [ERK] 1/2). Differentiated Caco-2 cells were either pretreated with U-0126 or complete cultivation medium for 1 h before addition of individual and combined AFM1 and OTA for 30 min. Phosphorylation of p44/42 MAPK was determined by immunoblotting.

3. Discussion

It is common to find co-contamination of mycotoxins in milk, which has been reported worldwide, instead of the occurrence of individual mycotoxins [3]. However, most studies mainly focused on the toxic effects of individual mycotoxins. Given that the intestine functions as the initial barrier against mycotoxins, and that it could be exposed to high doses of these toxins, little is known about the interaction of mycotoxins with the human intestinal epithelium [39]. Thus, it is essential to determine the combined effects of mycotoxins on the intestinal barrier. In this study, we investigated the effects of AFM1 and OTA, which are common mycotoxins found in milk, on differentiated Caco-2 cells that resemble epithelial cells of the small intestine to determine the underlying mechanisms of the dysfunction of the intestinal barrier caused by mycotoxins and to discover whether they have additive, synergistic or antagonistic effects.

TEER values and the paracellular flux of tracers (LY, FITC-dextran) are vital parameters in the study of epithelial barrier integrity. In this study, a dose-dependent decrease in TEER of the differentiated Caco-2 monolayer was observed after 48 h of AFM1 and/or OTA treatment. This is in agreement with previous studies [28,40–42] that reported individual mycotoxins, such as AFM1, AFB1, OTA, patulin (PAT), and FB1, to decrease TEER values in Caco-2 cells and to disrupt barrier function. A previous study has illustrated that a reduction in TEER can however be caused by different events including: (i) increase in paracellular permeability to ions; (ii) changes in transcellular ion flux through altered plasma membrane channels or pumps; or (iii) uncontrolled cell death within the monolayer [43]. From this angle, the reduced cell viability induced by AFM1 and OTA at higher concentration may play a role in the change of TEER values and cell monolayer permeability. Indeed, after 48 h of exposure, AFM1 and OTA individually or collectively induced a significant increase in the translocation of LY and FITC-dextran from the apical to the basal compartment. These findings are consistent with the data of Akbari et al. [44] and Pinton et al. [45], demonstrating that DON increased the paracellular permeability to FITC-dextran in Caco-2 cells and intestinal epithelial cell lines from porcine (IPEC-1) cells.

TJs are comprised of multiple protein complexes located at the apical domain of lateral membranes of intestinal epithelial cells. The integral components of TJ complexes are the four transmembrane proteins, namely, occludin, claudins, JAMs, and tricellulin, as well as ZO-1, which anchors the transmembrane proteins to the perijunctional actomyosin ring [15]. To our best knowledge, there are few studies that report the effects of AFM1 or OTA on the integrity of the intestinal barrier. Romero et al. [24] showed that, after 24 h of exposure to OTA, claudin-3, claudin-4, and occludin mRNA expression decreased in differentiated Caco-2 cells. McLaughlin et al. [42] reported that OTA reduced claudin-3 and claudin-4 protein levels after 24 h of exposure. Although there was a moderate decrease in TEER values in the presence of low concentrations of AFM1 added to either the apical or basal compartment of transwell chambers, occludin and ZO-1 localization was relatively unchanged in Caco-2 cells [28]. By Western blotting and immunofluorescent microscopy, we demonstrate for the first time the loss of TJ proteins (claudin-3, claudin-4, occludin, and ZO-1) from cells. Furthermore, the emphasis for Western blotting and immunofluorescent staining of tight junction proteins are different. The focus of Western blotting analysis is to measure the change of proteins expression level induced by mycotoxins, while the aim of immunofluorescent staining is to determine the effect of mycotoxins on the cellular localization of cell adhesion molecules. Thereby, the different objective of these two experiments could explain that the trend between Figures 3 and 4 is not closely coincident. The marked loss of ZO-1 could be explained by the fact that ZO-1 links TJ proteins to the actin cytoskeleton, which is critical for the maintenance of the structure and function of the TJ barrier. Defective barrier integrity may contribute to various intestinal and systemic inflammatory diseases. Clinical studies showed that, in patients with Crohn's disease (CD), the expression of claudin-3 and occludin was decreased [46]. Thus, further studies are needed to understand the mechanisms behind this AFM1/OTA-induced decrease in TJ permeability.

There is considerable evidence showing that disrupted intestinal permeability is related to the decreased expression and translocation of TJ proteins. Watari et al. [47] demonstrated that homoharringtonine (HHT) increased the paracellular flux of FITC-dextrans (4 and 40 kDa) and reduced the protein levels of claudin-3, claudin-5, and claudin-7 in Caco-2 cells. Akbari et al. [41] reported that DON increased the paracellular flux of LY and FITC-dextran (4 kDa) and decreased the levels of claudin-1, claudin-3, and claudin-4. Romero et al. [24] reported decreased TEER values with decreased claudin-3 and occludin mRNA expression levels in Caco-2 cells exposed to AFB1, FB1, T2, and OTA at concentrations up to 100 µM for seven days. In the present study, the increased intestinal permeability caused by AFM1 and OTA was concomitant with the reduced expression of claudin-3, claudin-4, occludin, and ZO-1. Indeed, significant correlations were observed between TEER values/FITC-dextran (40 kDa) and the four TJ proteins, which were assessed by Spearman's correlations. Therefore, we concluded that the mechanism by which these mycotoxins reduce the barrier properties of Caco-2 cells appears to be via altering the expression levels and/or distribution of specific TJ proteins, namely, claudin-3, claudin-4, occludin, and ZO-1.

Emerging evidence have demonstrated involvement of MAPK signaling in the compromised barrier function caused by TJ proteins. For example, the reduced expression of occludin and ZO-1 in human gastric epithelial cells may underlie clopidogrel-induced gastric mucosal injury, which involves the activation of the p38 MAPK pathway [48]. DON-induced MAPK activation decreased the expression of claudin in the disrupted intestinal barrier [36]. Recently, one study reported that arsenic downregulated TJ protein claudin through p38 MAPK in HT29 intestinal epithelial cell line [49]. Thus, it is reasonable to conclude that mycotoxin-induced MAPK pathway activation decreases the expression of TJ proteins, which in turn reduces the barrier function of the intestine as evaluated by TEER and paracellular permeability. In the present study, we examined the extent to which the activation of MAPK regulate barrier disruption of AFM1 and OTA. The results showed that only p44/42 MAPK play an important role in mediating the expression level of TJs, especially for their combination, and this finding is in accordance with literature reporting the regulation of TJs structure and function is often regulated by this MAPK [50]. To further investigate whether p44/42 activation mediates intestinal barrier effects of AFM1 and OTA individually or collectively, differentiated Caco-2 cells exposed to these mycotoxins in the absence and presence of U-0126. According to our study, pretreatment with U-0126 in differentiated Caco-2 cells and then subsequent with mycotoxins in the presence of the inhibitor significantly reduced the adverse effects induced by AFM1 and OTA individually or collectively, indicating that the activation of p44/42 MAPK is partially involved in these mycotoxins-induced barrier disruption.

One of the aims of the present study was to assess the combined effects of AFM1 and OTA. In this study, non-cytotoxic concentrations of AFM1 and OTA exerted antagonistic effects on the TEER, while these mycotoxins at the same concentrations exerted synergistic effects on the paracellular flux of LY and FITC-dextran (40 kDa) and the expression of claudin-4. All other interactions of AFM1 and OTA at different concentrations with regard to epithelial permeability were additive. It is commonly assumed that mycotoxins with the same mode of action and/or the same cellular target exert a synergistic or additive effect when present together [51]. Studies demonstrated that exposure to AFM1 and OTA resulted in oxidative DNA damage, which represents the predominant mechanism for cytotoxicity [52–54]. This might explain the synergistic and additive interaction effects that we observed in this study. The antagonistic effect of AFM1 and OTA may be explained by the competition for glutathione (GSH) in cells. Since electrophiles generated from the metabolism of OTA with hydroquinone–quinone reduce GSH to produce GSH conjugates, the hydroxyl group of AFM1 can also be conjugated with GSH [55–57]. Indeed, the interactive effects were different depending on the concentrations and exposure time used, the endpoint assessed, or the species applied. Furthermore, the deeper mechanisms underlying the mycotoxin-induced dysfunction of intestinal barrier need to be explored.

In summary, we herewith present a detailed in vitro investigation of AFM1 and OTA individually or collectively on intestinal barrier integrity. Furthermore, the present study for the first time shows that AFM1 and OTA impaired the intestinal barrier as evaluated by increased TEER values and permeability tracer flux, which was associated with the perturbation of TJ complexes, including claudins, occludin and ZO-1, and p44/42 MAPK at least partially involved in the detrimental effects of integrity of TJs caused by AFM1 and OTA. Indeed, AFM1 and OTA exerted different interactive effects, depending on the endpoints of intestinal permeability assessed. These findings may explain some of the observed adverse effects on the GIT in vivo caused by these mycotoxins. The special molecular mechanisms that p44/42 MAPK influence the mycotoxin-mediated TJ disruption need to be clarified and further studies would be required to confirm these finding in vivo cases.

4. Materials and Methods

4.1. Chemicals and Reagents

AFM1 (structural formula, $C_{17}H_{12}O_7$; molecular weight, 328) and OTA (structural formula, $C_{20}H_{18}ClNO_6$; molecular weight, 403) were purchased from Fermentek, Ltd. (Jerusalem, Israel). Mycotoxins were dissolved in methanol as previously described [58,59]. AFM1 and OTA were dissolved in methanol to final concentrations of 400 µg/mL and 5000 µg/mL, respectively. Both stock solutions were stored at $-20\,^\circ$C. Dulbecco's modified Eagle medium (DMEM), fetal bovine serum (FBS), antibiotics (100 units/mL penicillin and 100 µg/mL streptomycin), nonessential amino acids (NEAA) were purchased from Life Technologies (Carlsbad, CA, USA). An Enhanced Cell Counting Kit-8, radio immunoprecipitation assay (RIPA) lysis buffer, immunofluorescent staining blocking buffer, primary and secondary antibody dilution buffer were purchased from Beyotime Biotechnology (Shanghai, China). Protease inhibitors, lucifer yellow (LY) and fluorescein isothiocyanate (FITC)-dextran were purchased from Sigma-Aldrich (St. Louis, MO, USA). Rabbit anti-claudin-3 and rabbit anti-claudin-4 were purchased from Abcam (Cambridge, MA, USA). Rabbit anti-ZO-1 and rabbit anti-occludin were purchased from Thermo Scientific (Waltham, MA, USA). Rabbit anti-β-actin was purchased from Cell Signaling Technology (Trask Lane Danvers MA, USA). Goat anti-rabbit IgG conjugated to horseradish peroxidase and Alexa Fluor 488 mouse anti-rabbit IgG were purchased from Bioss Antibodies (Beijing, China). Three MAPK-specific inhibitors (SB-203580, U-0126 and SP-600125) were purchased from Sigma-Aldrich, and their stock solutions were prepared with dimethyl sulfoxide (DMSO).

4.2. Cell Culture and Differentiation

The human colon adenocarcinoma Caco-2 cell line (passage number, 18) was obtained from American Type Culture Collection (ATCC) (Manassas, VA, USA). The cells were cultured in DMEM containing 4.5 g/L glucose, 10% FBS, antibiotics (100 units/mL penicillin and 100 µg/mL streptomycin), and 1% NEAA at 37 °C in a humidified atmosphere of 5% CO_2 in air.

In the present study, Caco-2 cells plated at a passage number (passage number, 23–35) similar to that reported by Watari et al. [47] were cultured in 6- or 12-well transwell chambers (Corning, NY, USA) at a density of 4×10^4 cells/cm^2, and the medium was replaced every other day until 21 days. The mean TEER value was $1528 \pm 117\ \Omega\cdot$cm^2 (Figure S2), which exceeded the TEER cut-off value of $300\ \Omega\cdot$cm^2, as measured by a Millicell-ERS volt-ohm meter (Millipore, Temecula, CA, USA). The differentiated Caco-2 cells were then used for TEER measurement, permeability tracer flux assay, Western blot analysis, and immunofluorescent staining.

4.3. Cytotoxicity Assay

The effects of mycotoxins on the proliferation of intestinal cells were determined using the Enhanced Cell Counting Kit (CCK)-8 according to the manufacturer's instructions. Caco-2 cells were seeded at 6×10^4 cells/well in 100 µL of complete proliferation medium in 96-well plates. After 24 h of culture, AFM1 (0.012, 0.12, 1.2, 6, and 12 µM) and OTA (0.02, 0.2, 2, 10, and 20 µM), which were prepared by adding DMEM, were added. After 48 h, 100 μL of CCK-8 Reagent was added per well, and the cells were incubated for 2 h. The absorbance was measured at 450 nm using an automated ELISA reader (Thermo Scientific, Waltham, MA, USA). Results were expressed as the percentage of cell survival (%) with respect to the control. Based on the cell viability results (Figure S3), 0.12 μM was selected as the non-cytotoxic AFM1 concentration and 12 μM as the cytotoxic concentration, and the corresponding concentrations of OTA (0.2 and 20 μM) were chosen. In all subsequent experiments, AFM1 at 0.12 and 12 μM, and OTA at 0.2 and 20 μM, were used.

4.4. TEER Measurement

The measurement of TEER across epithelial cell monolayers is one of the best ways to evaluate the integrity of the TJ barrier in Caco-2 models [20]. Caco-2 cells were cultured on transwell chambers as described in Section 4.2. Cells were challenged for 48 h with increasing concentrations of AFM1 (0.12 and 12 μM) or OTA (0.2 and 20 μM), which were added to apical and basal compartments of transwell chambers. Binary combinations (AFM1/OTA) were also tested using identical concentrations and exposure time. Results were expressed relative to the initial TEER value for each insert and presented as the mean ± standard error of the mean (SEM) of five independent experiments.

4.5. Permeability Tracer Flux Assay

In addition to TEER measurement, the paracellular flux of tracers across the cell monolayer also reflects the permeability of intestinal barrier. The most common paracellular tracers used in in vitro models are fluorescent compounds (e.g., LY) or fluorescently labeled compounds (e.g., FITC-dextran and FITC-inulin). To determine whether mycotoxins individually and collectively affect the size selectivity of the permeability barrier, different molecular size tracers were used. Caco-2 cell monolayers were cultured on transwell chambers to confluency and treated with AFM1 and OTA individually or collectively for 48 h as described in Section 4.4. The membrane-impermeable tracers LY and FITC conjugated-dextran with a molecular mass of 4 or 40 kDa were dissolved in phosphate-buffered saline (PBS) to a final concentration of 100 μg/mL. In this study, these tracers were added to the apical compartment for 4 h. The fluorescent intensity in the basal compartment was measured with an automated ELISA reader. The excitation and emission wavelengths were 410 and 520 nm, respectively, for LY, and 490 and 520 nm for FITC-dextran.

4.6. Western Blot Analysis

Immunoblot assays were conducted to examine the expression of TJ proteins claudin-3, claudin-4, occludin and ZO-1 as well as the phosphorylation status of MAPK proteins ERK, p38 and JNK. For TJ proteins analysis, Caco-2 cell monolayers were cultured on transwell chambers and incubated for 48 h with increasing concentrations of AFM1 and OTA, which were added to apical and basal compartments. Caco-2 cells were lysed with RIPA lysis buffer containing protease inhibitors. Equal amounts of protein were combined with a nonreducing buffer, heat-denatured, electrophoresed on sodium dodecyl sulfate (SDS)-polyacrylamide gels, and electroblotted onto polyvinylidene difluoride membranes. The membranes were blocked with 5% skim milk in PBS for 1.5 h at room temperature. Subsequently, rabbit anti-claudin-3, rabbit anti-claudin-4, rabbit anti-ZO-1, rabbit anti-occludin, and rabbit anti-β-actin antibodies were diluted according to the manufacturers' instructions and incubated with membranes for 3 h at room temperature. Goat anti-rabbit IgG conjugated to horseradish peroxidase was applied for 1 h at room temperature. Peroxidase activity was visualized on a radiographic film using enhanced chemiluminescence reagents. Signal intensities were determined by densitometry using ImageJ 2× software (Version 2.1.0, National Institutes of Health, Bethesda, MD, USA, 2006), and values were normalized to the loading control (human β-actin). In the kinase phosphorylation assay, after 21 days for culturing differentiated Caco-2 cells, the cells were treated with serum-free medium for 12 h. After 12 h, cells were washed and treated first with or without 10 μM three inhibitors for 1 h and then with 12 μM AFM1 or/and 20 μM OTA for 30 min. Whole cell lysates were collected, normalized for total proteins, and analyzed for the levels of phosphorylated ERK, p38 and JNK proteins.

4.7. Immunofluorescent Staining

The localization of TJ proteins was assessed by confocal microscopy. Confluent Caco-2 cells were incubated for 48 h with AFM1 and OTA individually or collectively by adding to apical and basal compartments. The cells were fixed with 4% paraformaldehyde for 10 min at 4 °C and then permeabilized with 0.1% Triton X-100 in PBS for 5 min. The cells were incubated in blocking buffer for 1.5 h, followed by incubation with an anti-claudin-3, anti-claudin-4, anti-occludin, or anti-ZO-1 antibody diluted in primary antibody dilution buffer for 1.5 h. The cells were then incubated with Alexa Fluor 488 mouse anti-rabbit IgG diluted in secondary antibody dilution buffer for 45 min at 37 °C in the dark. The cells were observed under a LSM780 immunofluorescent microscope (Carl Zeiss, Inc., Thornwood, NY, USA).

4.8. Downregulation of Occludin by siRNA

Occludin small interfering RNA (occludin siRNA; GenePharma) and negative control (NC) siRNA were transiently transfected into differentiated Caco-2 cells using OptiMEM siRNA transfection medium and Lipofectin 2000 siRNA transfection reagent according to the manufacturer's instructions. The primer sequences were GCGUUGGUGAUCUUUGUUATT (sense) and UAACAAAGAUCACCAACGCTT (antisense). The transfection medium containing the siRNA and siRNA transfection reagent was mixed with serum-free culture medium and incubated with the differentiated Caco-2 cells. The medium was replaced after 6 h, and cells were incubated for an additional 24 h, and then TEER values were determined. Cells were then collected and lysed, and occludin expression was examined.

4.9. Comparison between Expected and Measured Endpoints

To compare the expected values (expressed as %) with the measured values (expressed as %), the expected value was calculated by the addition of the mean after exposure to one (or two) substance(s) with the mean value obtained after exposure to the second or third substance [60]:

$$\text{mean (expected for AFM1+OTA)} = \text{mean (AFM1)} + \text{mean (OTA)} - 100\%, \tag{1}$$

$$\% \text{ difference} = |\text{mean (expected for AFM1+OTA)} - \text{mean (measured for AFM1+OTA)}|, \tag{2}$$

Taking the TEER value from the combined use of AFM1 and OTA at non-cytotoxic concentrations as an example, the mean measured TEER value was 84.9%, and, according to the calculation, the mean expected TEER value was 64.1%. Hence, the % difference was 20.8%:

$$\text{SEM (expected for AFM1+OTA)} = [(\text{SEM for AFM1})^2 + (\text{SEM for OTA})^2]^{1/2}, \tag{3}$$

4.10. Analysis for Interactions and Correlations

We previously used isobologram analysis, which is a quantitative method to measure the interaction of the combined use of mycotoxins [8]. However, the weakness of this approach is that it requires specialized software to calculate the combination index (CI) value. To analyze the interactive effects without this technical tool, expected and measured endpoints were compared.

The impaired intestinal barrier led to the situation that TEER values, as well as the expression of claudin-3, claudin-4, occludin, and ZO-1, decreased, while LY, FITC-4 kDa, and FITC-40 kDa increased. Synergistic effects were defined as those produced by various chemicals that were greater than the sum of their individual effects. Antagonistic effects were defined as those produced by various chemicals that were lower than the sum of each role.

The significance of difference in expected and measured values was calculated using an unpaired *t*-test, with $p < 0.05$ being considered statistically significant. The results were interpreted as follows:

Additive effects were defined as measured values for endpoints that were not significantly above or below the expected values ($p > 0.05$).

Synergistic effects were defined as measured values that were significantly lower than the expected values for endpoints TEER, claudin-3, claudin-4, occludin, and ZO-1 and significantly higher than for endpoints LY, FITC-4 kDa, and FITC-40 kDa.

Antagonistic effects were defined as measured values that were significantly higher than the expected values for endpoints TEER, claudin-3, claudin-4, occludin, and ZO-1 and significantly lower than the endpoints LY, FITC-4 kDa, and FITC-40 kDa.

Correlations among TEER values, the paracellular flux of LY, FITC-dextran (4 kDa), or FITC-dextran (40 kDa), and the levels of claudin-3, claudin-4, occludin, or ZO-1 in differentiated Caco-2 cells treated with AFM1 and OTA individually or collectively were assessed by Spearman's correlations (nonparametric).

4.11. Statistical Analysis

Statistical analysis was performed using SAS 9.2 software (Cary, NC, USA). Data were expressed as the mean $\pm$ SEM of three independent experiments. Differences between groups were analyzed by one-way analysis of variance (ANOVA), followed by the Tukey Honestly Significant Difference (HSD) test for multiple comparisons. Statistically significant cytotoxic effects are represented by * $p < 0.05$; ** $p < 0.001$; and *** $p < 0.0001$.

Supplementary Materials: The following are available online at www.mdpi.com/2072-6651/10/1/12/s1, Figure S1: Mycotoxins disrupt intestinal epithelial permeability by affecting occludin expression, Figure S2: Transepithelial electrical resistance values ($\Omega \times cm^2$) in differentiated Caco-2 cells were measured at different time points until 21 days, Figure S3: Concentration–response bar charts for AFM1 and OTA in Caco-2 cells after 48 h of exposure. Results are expressed as the mean $\pm$ SEM of three independent experiments with five replicates.

Acknowledgments: This study was supported by the National Natural Science Foundation of China (31501399), the Special Fund for Agro-Scientific Research in the Public Interest (201403071), the Project of Risk Assessment on Raw Milk (GJFP2016008), the Foundation of Institute of Animal Science (2017ywf-zd-1), the State Key Laboratory of Animal Nutrition (2004DA125184G1611), and the National Key R&D Program of China (2017YFD0500500).

Author Contributions: The experiments were conceived and designed by Yanan Gao, Songli Li, Jiaqi Wang, and Nan Zheng. The experiments and data analysis were performed by Yanan Gao, Chaochao Luo, and Shengguo Zhao. The paper was written by Yanan Gao and Nan Zheng.

Conflicts of Interest: The authors declare that there are no conflicts of interest.

References

1. Capriotti, A.L.; Caruso, G.; Cavaliere, C.; Foglia, P.; Samperi, R.; Laganà, A. Multiclass mycotoxin analysis in food, environmental and biological matrices with chromatography/mass spectrometry. *Mass Spectrom. Rev.* **2012**, *31*, 466–503. [CrossRef] [PubMed]

2. Flores-Flores, M.E.; Lizarraga, E.; López de Cerain, A.; González-Peñas, E. Presence of mycotoxins in animal milk: A review. *Food Control* **2015**, *53*, 163–176. [CrossRef]

3. Huang, L.C.; Zheng, N.; Zheng, B.Q.; Wen, F.; Cheng, J.B.; Han, R.W.; Xu, X.M.; Li, S.L.; Wang, J.Q. Simultaneous determination of aflatoxin M1, ochratoxin A, zearalenone and alpha-zearalenol in milk by UHPLC-MS/MS. *Food Chem.* **2014**, *146*, 242–249. [CrossRef] [PubMed]

4. Boudra, H.; Barnouin, J.; Dragacci, S.; Morgavi, D.P. Aflatoxin M1 and ochratoxin a in raw bulk milk from French dairy herds. *J. Dairy Sci.* **2007**, *90*, 3197–3201. [CrossRef] [PubMed]

5. Meucci, V.; Razzuoli, E.; Soldani, G.; Massart, F. Mycotoxin detection in infant formula milks in Italy. *Food Addit. Contam.* **2010**, *27*, 64–71. [CrossRef] [PubMed]

6. Alvito, P.C.; Sizoo, E.A.; Almeida, C.M.M.; van Egmond, H.P. Occurrence of Aflatoxins and Ochratoxin A in Baby Foods in Portugal. *Food Anal. Methods* **2008**, *3*, 22–30. [CrossRef]

7. Botta, A.; Martinez, V.; Mitjans, M.; Balboa, E.; Conde, E.; Vinardell, M.P. Erythrocytes and cell line-based assays to evaluate the cytoprotective activity of antioxidant components obtained from natural sources. *Toxicol. In Vitro* **2014**, *28*, 120–124. [CrossRef] [PubMed]

8. Gao, Y.N.; Wang, J.Q.; Li, S.L.; Zhang, Y.D.; Zheng, N. Aflatoxin M1 cytotoxicity against human intestinal Caco-2 cells is enhanced in the presence of other mycotoxins. *Food Chem. Toxicol.* **2016**, *96*, 79–89. [CrossRef] [PubMed]

9. Bondy, G.S.; Pestka, J.J. Immunomodulation by fungal toxins. *J. Toxicol. Environ. Health B* **2000**, *3*, 109–143.

10. Galarza-Seeber, R.; Latorre, J.D.; Bielke, L.R.; Kuttappan, V.A.; Wolfenden, A.D.; Hernandez-Velasco, X.; Merino-Guzman, R.; Vicente, J.L.; Donoghue, A.; Cross, D.; et al. Leaky Gut and Mycotoxins: Aflatoxin B1 Does Not Increase Gut Permeability in Broiler Chickens. *Front. Vet. Sci.* **2016**, *3*, 10. [CrossRef] [PubMed]

11. Gambacorta, L.; Pinton, P.; Avantaggiato, G.; Oswald, I.P.; Solfrizzo, M. Grape Pomace, an Agricultural Byproduct Reducing Mycotoxin Absorption: In Vivo Assessment in Pig Using Urinary Biomarkers. *J. Agric. Food Chem.* **2016**, *64*, 6762–6771. [CrossRef] [PubMed]

12. Grenier, B.; Applegate, T.J. Modulation of intestinal functions following mycotoxin ingestion: Meta-analysis of published experiments in animals. *Toxins* **2013**, *5*, 396–430. [CrossRef] [PubMed]

13. Maresca, M.; Mahfoud, R.; Garmy, N.; Fantini, J. The mycotoxin deoxynivalenol affects nutrient absorption in human intestinal epithelial cells. *J. Nutr.* **2002**, *132*, 2723–2731. [PubMed]

14. Qasim, M.; Rahman, H.; Ahmed, R.; Oellerich, M.; Asif, A.R. Mycophenolic acid mediated disruption of the intestinal epithelial tight junctions. *Exp. Cell Res.* **2014**, *322*, 277–289. [CrossRef] [PubMed]

15. Suzuki, T. Regulation of intestinal epithelial permeability by tight junctions. *Cell. Mol. Life Sci.* **2013**, *70*, 631–659. [CrossRef] [PubMed]

16. Gonzalez-Mariscal, L.; Betanzos, A.; Avila-Flores, A. MAGUK proteins: structure and role in the tight junction. *Semin. Cell Dev. Biol.* **2000**, *11*, 315–324. [CrossRef] [PubMed]

17. Furuse, M.; Hirase, T.; Itoh, M.; Nagafuchi, A.; Yonemura, S.; Tsukita, S. Occludin: A Novel Integral Membrane Protein Localizing at Tight Junctions. *J. Cell Biol.* **1993**, *123*, 1777–1788. [CrossRef] [PubMed]

18. Martin-Padura, I.; Lostaglio, S.; Schneemann, M.; Williams, L.; Romano, M.; Fruscella, P.; Panzeri, C.; Stoppacciaro, A.; Ruco, L.; Villa, A.; et al. Junctional Adhesion Molecule, a Novel Member of the Immunoglobulin Superfamily That Distributes at Intercellular Junctions and Modulates Monocyte Transmigration. *J. Cell Biol.* **1998**, *142*, 117–127. [CrossRef] [PubMed]

19. Mitic, L.L.; Anderson, J.M. Molecular architecture of tight junctions. *Annu. Rev. Physiol.* **1998**, *60*, 121–142. [CrossRef] [PubMed]

20. Akbari, P.; Braber, S.; Varasteh, S.; Alizadeh, A.; Garssen, J.; Fink-Gremmels, J. The intestinal barrier as an emerging target in the toxicological assessment of mycotoxins. *Arch. Toxicol.* **2017**, *91*, 1007–1029. [CrossRef] [PubMed]

21. Artursson, P.; Karlsson, J. Correlation between oral drug absorption in humans and apparent drug permeability coefficients in human intestinal epithelial (Caco-2) cells. *Biochem. Biophys. Res. Commun.* **1991**, *175*, 880–885. [CrossRef]

22. Artursson, P.; Palm, K.; Luthman, K. Caco-2 monolayers in experimental and theoretical predictions of drug transport. *Adv. Drug Deliv. Rev.* **2012**, *64*, 280–289. [CrossRef]

23. Assuncao, R.; Ferreira, M.; Martins, C.; Diaz, I.; Padilla, B.; Dupont, D.; Braganca, M.; Alvito, P. Applicability of in vitro methods to study patulin bioaccessibility and its effects on intestinal membrane integrity. *J. Toxicol. Environ. Health A* **2014**, *77*, 983–992. [CrossRef] [PubMed]

24. Romero, A.; Ares, I.; Ramos, E.; Castellano, V.; Martinez, M.; Martinez-Larranaga, M.R.; Anadon, A.; Martinez, M.A. Mycotoxins modify the barrier function of Caco-2 cells through differential gene expression of specific claudin isoforms: Protective effect of illite mineral clay. *Toxicology* **2016**, *353–354*, 21–33. [CrossRef] [PubMed]

25. Lambert, D.; Padfield, P.J.; McLaughlin, J.; Cannell, S.; O'Neill, C.A. Ochratoxin A displaces claudins from detergent resistant membrane microdomains. *Biochem. Biophys. Res. Commun.* **2007**, *358*, 632–636. [CrossRef] [PubMed]

26. Maresca, M.; Yahi, N.; Younes-Sakr, L.; Boyron, M.; Caporiccio, B.; Fantini, J. Both direct and indirect effects account for the pro-inflammatory activity of enteropathogenic mycotoxins on the human intestinal epithelium: Stimulation of interleukin-8 secretion, potentiation of interleukin-1beta effect and increase in the transepithelial passage of commensal bacteria. *Toxicol. Appl. Pharmacol.* **2008**, *228*, 84–92. [PubMed]

27. Ranaldi, G.; Mancini, E.; Ferruzza, S.; Sambuy, Y.; Perozzi, G. Effects of red wine on ochratoxin A toxicity in intestinal Caco-2/TC7 cells. *Toxicol. In Vitro* **2007**, *21*, 204–210. [CrossRef] [PubMed]
28. Caloni, F.; Cortinovis, C.; Pizzo, F.; De Angelis, I. Transport of Aflatoxin M(1) in Human Intestinal Caco-2/TC7 Cells. *Front. Pharmacol.* **2012**, *3*, 111. [CrossRef] [PubMed]
29. Wangikar, P.B.; Dwivedi, P.; Neeraji, S.; Sharma, A.K.; Telang, A.G. Teratogenic effects in rabbits of simultaneous exposure to ochratoxin A and aflatoxin B1 with special reference to microscopic effects. *Toxcology* **2005**, *215*, 37–47. [CrossRef] [PubMed]
30. Huang, S.; Zheng, N.; Fan, C.; Cheng, M.; Wang, S.; Jabar, A.; Wang, J.; Cheng, J. Effects of Aflatoxin B1 combined with Ochratoxin A and/or Zearalenone on Metabolism, Immune Function, and Antioxidant Status in Lactating Dairy Goats. *Asian-Australas. J. Anim. Sci.* **2017**. [CrossRef] [PubMed]
31. Foucquier, J.; Guedj, M. Analysis of drug combinations: current methodological landscape. *Pharmacol. Res. Perspect.* **2015**, *3*, e00149. [CrossRef] [PubMed]
32. Lehar, J.; Zimmermann, G.R.; Krueger, A.S.; Molnar, R.A.; Ledell, J.T.; Heilbut, A.M.; Short, G.F.; Giusti, L.C.; Nolan, G.P.; Magid, O.A.; et al. Chemical combination effects predict connectivity in biological systems. *Mol. Syst. Biol.* **2007**, *3*, 80. [CrossRef] [PubMed]
33. Zhao, W.; Sachsenmeier, K.; Zhang, L.; Sult, E.; Hollingsworth, R.E.; Yang, H. A new bliss independence model to analyze drug combination data. *J. Biomol. Screen.* **2014**, *19*, 817–821. [CrossRef] [PubMed]
34. Carrozzino, F.; Pugnale, P.; Feraille, E.; Montesano, R. Inhibition of basal p38 or JNK activity enhances epithelial barrier function through differential modulation of claudin expression. *Am. J. Physiol.-Cell Physiol.* **2009**, *297*, C775–C787. [CrossRef] [PubMed]
35. Oshima, T.; Sasaki, M.; Kataoka, H.; Miwa, H.; Takeuchi, T.; John, T. Wip1 protects hydrogen peroxide-induced colonic epithelial barrier dysfunction. *Cell. Mol. Life Sci.* **2007**, *64*, 3139–3147. [CrossRef] [PubMed]
36. Pinton, P.; Braicu, C.; Nougayrede, J.P.; Laffitte, J.; Taranu, I.; Oswald, I.P. Deoxynivalenol impairs porcine intestinal barrier function and decreases the protein expression of claudin-4 through a mitogen-activated protein kinase-dependent mechanism. *J. Nutr.* **2010**, *140*, 1956–1962. [CrossRef] [PubMed]
37. Bracarense, A.P.; Lucioli, J.; Grenier, B.; Drociunas Pacheco, G.; Moll, W.D.; Schatzmayr, G.; Oswald, I.P. Chronic ingestion of deoxynivalenol and fumonisin, alone or in interaction, induces morphological and immunological changes in the intestine of piglets. *Br. J. Nutr.* **2012**, *107*, 1776–1786. [CrossRef] [PubMed]
38. Grenier, B.; Bracarense, A.P.; Schwartz, H.E.; Lucioli, J.; Cossalter, A.M.; Moll, W.D.; Schatzmayr, G.; Oswald, I.P. Biotransformation approaches to alleviate the effects induced by fusarium mycotoxins in swine. *J. Agric. Food Chem.* **2013**, *61*, 6711–6719. [CrossRef] [PubMed]
39. Bouhet, S.; Oswald, I.P. The effects of mycotoxins, fungal food contaminants, on the intestinal epithelial cell-derived innate immune response. *Vet. Immunol. Immunopathol.* **2005**, *108*, 199–209. [CrossRef] [PubMed]
40. Gratz, S.; Wu, Q.K.; El-Nezami, H.; Juvonen, R.O.; Mykkanen, H.; Turner, P.C. Lactobacillus rhamnosus strain GG reduces aflatoxin B1 transport, metabolism, and toxicity in Caco-2 Cells. *Appl. Environ. Microbiol.* **2007**, *73*, 3958–3964. [CrossRef] [PubMed]
41. Mahfoud, R.; Maresca, M.; Garmy, N.; Fantini, J. The Mycotoxin Patulin Alters the Barrier Function of the Intestinal Epithelium: Mechanism of Action of the Toxin and Protective Effects of Glutathione. *Toxicol. Appl. Pharmacol.* **2002**, *181*, 209–218. [CrossRef] [PubMed]
42. McLaughlin, J.; Padfield, P.J.; Burt, J.P.; O'Neill, C.A. Ochratoxin A increases permeability through tight junctions by removal of specific claudin isoforms. *Am. J. Physiol.-Cell Physiol.* **2004**, *287*, C1412–C1417. [CrossRef] [PubMed]
43. Madara, J.L. Regulation of the movement of solutes across tight junctions. *Annu. Rev. Physiol.* **1998**, *60*, 143–159. [CrossRef] [PubMed]
44. Akbari, P.; Braber, S.; Gremmels, H.; Koelink, P.J.; Verheijden, K.A.; Garssen, J.; Fink-Gremmels, J. Deoxynivalenol: A trigger for intestinal integrity breakdown. *FASEB J.* **2014**, *28*, 2414–2429. [CrossRef] [PubMed]
45. Pinton, P.; Nougayrede, J.P.; Del Rio, J.C.; Moreno, C.; Marin, D.E.; Ferrier, L.; Bracarense, A.P.; Kolf-Clauw, M.; Oswald, I.P. The food contaminant deoxynivalenol, decreases intestinal barrier permeability and reduces claudin expression. *Toxicol. Appl. Pharmacol.* **2009**, *237*, 41–48. [CrossRef] [PubMed]

46. Zeissig, S.; Bojarski, C.; Buergel, N.; Mankertz, J.; Zeitz, M.; Fromm, M.; Schulzke, J. Downregulation of epithelial apoptosis and barrier repair in active Crohn's disease by tumour necrosis factor α antibody treatment. *Gut* **2004**, *53*, 1295–1302. [CrossRef] [PubMed]

47. Watari, A.; Hasegawa, M.; Yagi, K.; Kondoh, M. Homoharringtonine increases intestinal epithelial permeability by modulating specific claudin isoforms in Caco-2 cell monolayers. *Eur. J. Pharm. Biopharm.* **2015**, *89*, 232–238. [CrossRef] [PubMed]

48. Wu, H.L.; Gao, X.; Jiang, Z.D.; Duan, Z.T.; Wang, S.K.; He, B.S.; Zhang, Z.Y.; Xie, H.G. Attenuated expression of the tight junction proteins is involved in clopidogrel-induced gastric injury through p38 MAPK activation. *Toxicology* **2013**, *304*, 41–48. [CrossRef] [PubMed]

49. Jeong, C.H.; Seok, J.S.; Petriello, M.C.; Han, S.G. Arsenic downregulates tight junction claudin proteins through p38 and NF-kappaB in intestinal epithelial cell line, HT-29. *Toxicology* **2017**, *379*, 31–39. [CrossRef] [PubMed]

50. Balda, M.S.; Matter, K. Tight junctions as regulators of tissue remodelling. *Curr. Opin. Cell Biol.* **2016**, *42*, 94–101. [CrossRef] [PubMed]

51. Speijers, G.J.; Speijers, M.H. Combined toxic effects of mycotoxins. *Toxicol. Lett.* **2004**, *153*, 91–98. [CrossRef] [PubMed]

52. Pfohl-Leszkowicz, A.; Bartsch, H.; Azémar, B.; Mohr, U.; Estève, J.; Castegnaro, M. MESNA protects rats against nephrotoxicity but not carcinogenicity induced by ochratoxin A, implicating two separate pathways. *Facta Univ. Ser. Med. Biol.* **2002**, *9*, 57–63.

53. Tavares, A.M.; Alvito, P.; Loureiro, S.; Louro, H.; Silva, M.J. Multi-mycotoxin determination in baby foods andin vitrocombined cytotoxic effects of aflatoxin M1and ochratoxin A. *World Mycotoxin J.* **2013**, *6*, 375–388. [CrossRef]

54. Wild, C.; Turner, P. The toxicology of aflatoxins as a basis for public health decisions. *Mutagenesis* **2002**, *17*, 471–481. [CrossRef] [PubMed]

55. Faucet-Marquis, V.; Pont, F.; Størmer, F.C.; Rizk, T.; Castegnaro, M.; Pfohl-Leszkowicz, A. Evidence of a new dechlorinated ochratoxin A derivative formed in opossum kidney cell cultures after pretreatment by modulators of glutathione pathways: Correlation with DNA-adduct formation. *Mol. Nutr. Food Res.* **2006**, *50*, 530–542. [CrossRef] [PubMed]

56. Heidtmann-Bemvenuti, R.; Mendes, G.; Scaglioni, P.; Badiale-Furlong, E.; Souza Soares, L. Biochemistry and metabolism of mycotoxins: A review. *Afr. J. Food Sci.* **2011**, *5*, 861–869. [CrossRef]

57. Tozlovanu, M.; Canadas, D.; Pfohl-Leszkowicz, A.; Frenette, C.; Paugh, R.J.; Manderville, R.A. Glutathione conjugates of ochratoxin A as biomarkers of exposure. *Arch. Ind. Hyg. Toxicol.* **2012**, *63*, 417–427.

58. Ferrer, E.; Juan-Garcia, A.; Font, G.; Ruiz, M.J. Reactive oxygen species induced by beauvericin, patulin and zearalenone in CHO-K1 cells. *Toxicol. In Vitro* **2009**, *23*, 1504–1509. [CrossRef] [PubMed]

59. Paciolla, C.; Florio, A.; Mulè, G.; Logrieco, A.F. Combined effect of beauvericin and T-2 toxin on antioxidant defence systems in cherry tomato shoots. *World Mycotoxin J.* **2014**, *7*, 207–215. [CrossRef]

60. Weber, F.; Freudinger, R.; Schwerdt, G.; Gekle, M. A rapid screening method to test apoptotic synergisms of ochratoxin A with other nephrotoxic substances. *Toxicol. In Vitro* **2005**, *19*, 135–143. [CrossRef] [PubMed]

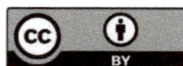

toxins

MDPI

Article

Dietary Deoxynivalenol (DON) May Impair the Epithelial Barrier and Modulate the Cytokine Signaling in the Intestine of Atlantic Salmon (*Salmo salar*)

Torfinn Moldal [1], Aksel Bernhoft [1], Grethe Rosenlund [2], Magne Kaldhusdal [1] and Erling Olaf Koppang [3,*

[1] Norwegian Veterinary Institute, Post box 750 Sentrum, 0106 Oslo, Norway; torfinn.moldal@vetinst.no (T.M.); aksel.bernhoft@vetinst.no (A.B.); magne.kaldhusdal@vetinst.no (M.K.)

[2] Skretting ARC, Post box 48, 4001 Stavanger, Norway; grethe.rosenlund@skretting.com

[3] Department of Basic Sciences and Aquatic Medicine, Norwegian University of Life Sciences, Post box 369 Sentrum, 0102 Oslo, Norway

* Correspondence: erling.o.koppang@nmbu.no

Received: 4 August 2018; Accepted: 12 September 2018; Published: 14 September 2018

Abstract: Impaired growth, immunity, and intestinal barrier in mammals, poultry, and carp have been attributed to the mycotoxin deoxynivalenol (DON). The increased use of plant ingredients in aquaculture feed implies a risk for contamination with mycotoxins. The effects of dietary DON were explored in 12-month-old Atlantic salmon (*Salmo salar*) (start weight of 58 g) that were offered a standard feed with non-detectable levels of mycotoxins (control group) or 5.5 mg DON/kg feed (DON group). Each group comprised two tanks with 25 fish per tank. Five fish from each tank were sampled eight weeks after the start of the feeding trial, when mean weights for the control and DON groups were 123.2 g and 80.2 g, respectively. The relative expression of markers for three tight junction proteins (claudin 25b, occludin, and tricellulin) were lower, whereas the relative expression of a marker for proliferating cell nuclear antigen was higher in both the mid-intestine and the distal intestine in fish fed DON compared with fish from the control group. The relative expression of markers for two suppressors of cytokine signaling (SOCS1 and SOCS2) were higher in the distal intestine in fish fed DON. There was no indication of inflammation attributed to the feed in any intestinal segments. Our findings suggest that dietary DON impaired the intestinal integrity, while an inflammatory response appeared to be mitigated by suppressors of cytokine signaling. A dysfunctional intestinal barrier may have contributed to the impaired production performance observed in the DON group.

Keywords: atlantic salmon; deoxynivalenol; feed; intestine; PCR; proliferating cell nuclear antigen; suppressor of cytokine signaling; tight junctions

Key Contribution: Dietary DON at a level of 5.5 mg/kg feed revealed lower expression of markers for tight junction proteins and higher expression of a marker for proliferating cell nuclear antigen in the intestine of Atlantic salmon. A dysfunctional intestinal barrier may have contributed to impaired production performance.

---

1. Introduction

Atlantic salmon (*Salmo salar*) is one of the most important species in aquaculture worldwide. Salmonids are carnivores by nature, but raw materials of vegetable origin are increasingly used in feed for farmed salmonids due to a limited supply of fish meal and fish oil [1–3]. The use of cereals in feeds for farmed fish implies a risk for contamination with mycotoxins that are metabolites of mold capable of having acute toxic, carcinogenic, mutagenic, teratogenic, immunotoxic, or hormonal effects in mammals [4]. Deoxynivalenol (DON) is one of the major mycotoxins produced by *Fusarium* spp. [5]. The current European Union (EU) legislation establishes 8000 µg/kg as a maximum guidance value for DON in cereals and cereal products (with an exception for maize by-products) intended for animal feed and 5000 µg/mg as a maximum guidance value for complementary and complete feeding stuffs [6,7]. The surveillance of feeds for salmonids in Norwegian aquaculture shows levels of mycotoxins far below the current guidance levels [8], but accidental intermixture may occur.

Mycotoxins do not appear to pose a hazard to the consumer, because carry-over is considered negligible in fillets from gilthead seabream (*Sparus aurata*) and Atlantic salmon experimentally exposed to dietary DON at levels up to 5.5 mg/kg feed [9,10]. However, adverse effects in fish ingesting feed contaminated by mycotoxins have been observed. In Atlantic salmon and rainbow trout (*Oncorhynchus mykiss*), there appears to be a linearity between increasing dietary levels of DON up to 5.5 mg/kg feed and 2.6 mg/kg feed, respectively, and decreasing weight gain and growth rate [11,12]. Furthermore, dose-related alterations in some blood parameters were shown in Atlantic salmon and rainbow trout [11,13], and pathological changes in the liver characterized by subcapsular hemorrhage and edema were observed in a number of DON-exposed rainbow trout [12]. In carp (*Cyprinus carpio*), the relative expression of markers for both pro- and anti-inflammatory cytokines as well as enzymes in different organs including the intestine were activated by feed-borne DON at a concentration of 953 µg/kg feed with an adaption over time [14].

The intestine is an important barrier for protection against pathogens in addition to its main task in digestion. Exposure of the intestine to mycotoxins, either via feed or gavage, may impair the intestinal integrity and consequently alter the absorption of nutrients as well as facilitate the invasion of microbes. In pigs exposed to dietary DON at levels from 0.9 to 3.5 mg/kg feed, the relative expression of markers for several tight junction proteins (TJs) and inflammatory markers in intestines were affected [15–17]. The relative expression of markers for certain cytokines was down-regulated in the intestines of broiler chickens on a diet contaminated with 10 mg DON/kg feed [18]. Furthermore, DON predisposes to the development of necrotic enteritis in broiler chickens at a contamination level of 3 to 4 mg/kg feed [19].

Dose-dependent up-regulation of pro-inflammatory cytokines, followed by up-regulation of suppressors of cytokine signaling and subsequent basal expression of the cytokines, has been demonstrated in several organs in mice orally exposed to DON over a dose range of 0.1–12.5 mg/kg body weight in short-time experiments [20]. Altered transcript levels as well as protein expression for TJs, decreased transepithelial electrical resistance, and increased permeability as a result of exposure to DON have been observed in several in vitro and in vivo models indicating functional effects [21].

So far, little is known about the impact of dietary mycotoxins on intestinal health of fish in general and of Atlantic salmon in particular. The aim of this study was to investigate in Atlantic salmon the long-term impact of dietary DON at a level of 5.5 mg/kg feed on parameters related to the epithelial barrier of the intestine (relative expression of markers for tight junction proteins and proliferating cell nuclear antigen as well as goblet cell density), cytokine-mediated inflammation (relative expression of a marker for interleukin 1β), and suppression of cytokine signaling (relative expression of markers for SOCS1 and SOCS2), as well as morphologic responses to intestinal insults. The chosen DON level was slightly higher than the maximum recommended level (5 mg DON/kg feed) established in the European Union's current legislation on animal feed.

2. Results

2.1. Gene Expression Analysis by Real-Time PCR

The relative expression of markers for the tight junction proteins claudin 25b, occludin, and tricellulin was significantly lower in both the mid-intestine and the distal intestine from fish fed DON compared with fish from the control group (see Table 1 and Figure 1). The relative expression of the marker for occludin was also lower in the pyloric ceca from fish fed DON compared with the controls.

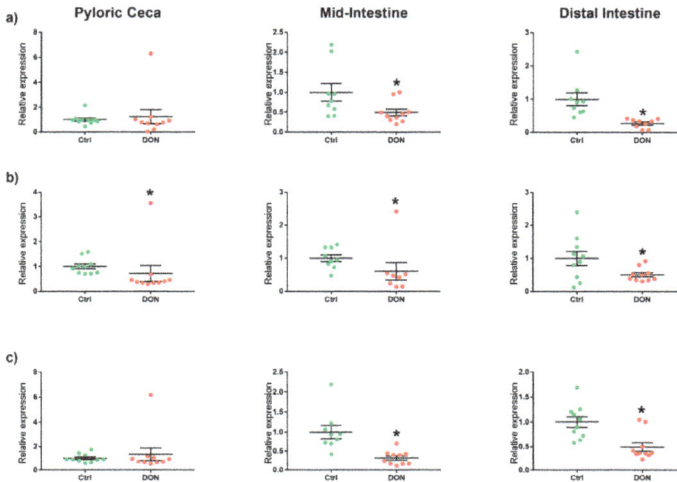

Figure 1. Relative expression of markers for tight junction proteins in the intestine of salmon fed deoxynivalenol (DON) (5.5 mg/kg feed) or no DON (controls) for eight weeks. * Significant differences (unpaired *t*-test or Mann–Whitney U test, *p* < 0.05) between the experimental groups in the same intestinal segment. The relative expression of markers for the tight junction proteins (**a**) claudin 25b, (**b**) occludin, and (**c**) tricellulin were significantly lower in both the mid-intestine and the distal intestine from fish fed DON compared with the controls. The relative expression of the marker for occludin was also significantly lower in the pyloric ceca from fish fed DON compared with the controls.

On the other hand, the relative expression of a marker for proliferating cell nuclear antigen (PCNA) was significantly higher in all intestinal segments in fish fed DON compared with the controls (see Table 1 and Figure 2).

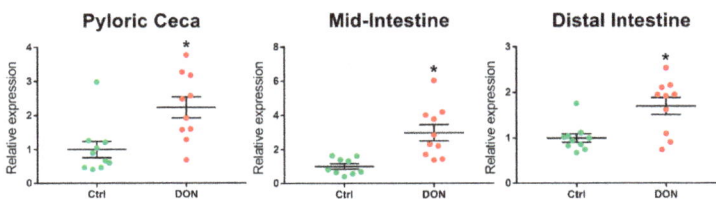

Figure 2. Relative expression of a marker for proliferating cell nuclear antigen (PCNA) in the intestine of salmon fed DON (5.5 mg/kg feed) or no DON (controls) for eight weeks. * Significant differences (unpaired *t*-test or Mann–Whitney U test, *p* < 0.05) between the experimental groups in the same intestinal segment. The relative expression of a marker for PCNA was significantly higher in all intestinal segments from fish fed DON compared with the controls.

The relative expression of markers for the suppressors of cytokine 1 and 2 (SOCS1 and SOCS2) was significantly higher in the distal intestine in fish fed DON compared with the controls. Further, the relative expression of the marker for SOCS1 was also significantly higher in the pyloric ceca in fish fed DON compared with the controls (see Table 1 and Figure 3).

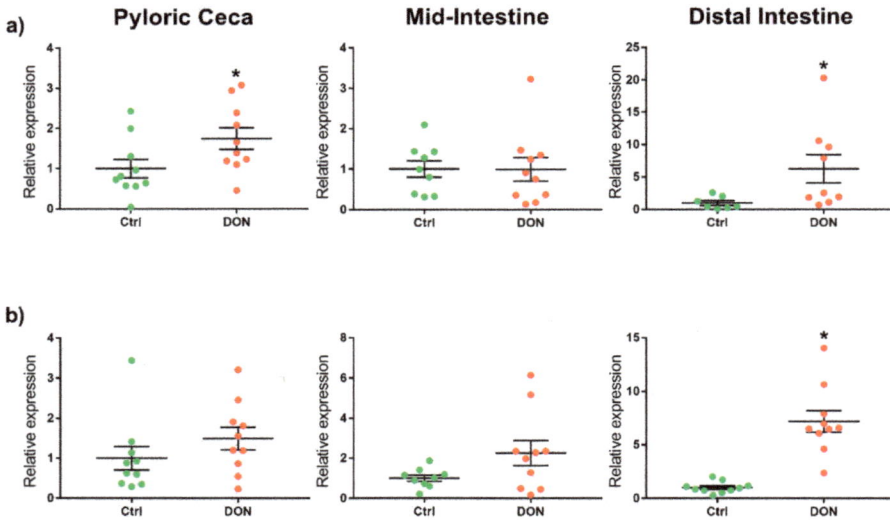

Figure 3. Relative expression of suppressors of cytokine signaling (SOCS) in the intestine of salmon fed DON (5.5 mg/kg feed) or no DON (controls) for eight weeks. * Significant differences (unpaired *t*-test or Mann–Whitney U test, $p < 0.05$) between the experimental groups in the same intestinal segment. The relative expression of markers for the suppressors of cytokine signaling (**a**) SOCS1 and (**b**) SOCS2 were significantly higher in the distal intestine from fish fed DON compared with the controls. The relative expression of the marker for SOCS1 was also significantly higher in the pyloric ceca from fish fed DON compared with the controls.

There was no significant difference between the dietary groups regarding the relative expression of a marker for the cytokine interleukin 1β in any of the intestinal segments (see Table 1).

Table 1. Relative transcription levels normalized to reference gene EF1AB in the intestine of salmon fed DON (5.5 mg/kg feed) or no DON (controls) for eight weeks.

	Pyloric Ceca		Mid-Intestine		Distal Intestine	
	Control	DON	Control	DON	Control	DON
IL-1β	1 ± 0.27 [a]	0.96 ± 0.40	1 ± 0.22 [a]	0.94 ± 0.13	1 ± 0.21 [a]	1.45 ± 0.25
SOCS1	1 ± 0.23	$\mathbf{1.74 \pm 0.27}$ *	1 ± 0.20 [a]	0.99 ± 0.29	1 ± 0.37 [c]	$\mathbf{6.24 \pm 2.17}$ *,[a]
SOCS2	1 ± 0.29	1.49 ± 0.28	1 ± 0.16 [a]	2.26 ± 0.63	1 ± 0.17	$\mathbf{7.19 \pm 1.01}$ *
Claudin 25b	1 ± 0.14	1.25 ± 0.57	1 ± 0.22 [a]	$\mathbf{0.49 \pm 0.09}$ *	1 ± 0.20 [a]	$\mathbf{0.27 \pm 0.05}$ *,[a]
Occludin	1 ± 0.10	$\mathbf{0.72 \pm 0.32}$ *	1 ± 0.10 [a]	$\mathbf{0.60 \pm 0.26}$ *,[b]	1 ± 0.22	$\mathbf{0.50 \pm 0.07}$ *
PCNA	1 ± 0.24	$\mathbf{2.23 \pm 0.31}$ *	1 ± 0.16 [a]	$\mathbf{2.98 \pm 0.47}$ *	1 ± 0.09	$\mathbf{1.70 \pm 0.19}$ *
Tricellulin	1 ± 0.12	1.34 ± 0.54	1 ± 0.17 [a]	$\mathbf{0.32 \pm 0.06}$ *	1 ± 0.11	$\mathbf{0.49 \pm 0.09}$ *

The data for the DON group are presented as mean $\pm$ standard error of the mean (SEM) relative to the mean $\pm$ SEM for the control group for the same intestinal segment; * Significant differences (unpaired *t*-test or Mann–Whitney U test, $p < 0.05$) between the experimental groups in the same intestinal segment. The values that differ significantly are highlighted in **bold** text. $n = 10$ for each group/gene/intestinal segment unless otherwise stated: [a]: $n = 9$, [b]: $n = 8$, and [c]: $n = 7$.

2.2. Histology and Immunohistochemistry

Histological examination did not reveal pathological changes in the intestines of any fish (see Figure 4a). The polarization of the enterocytes seemed non-affected, the density of goblet cells appeared similar in both dietary groups, while proliferating cells were mainly detected at the base of the intestinal folds with an equal pattern for both groups (see Figure 4b).

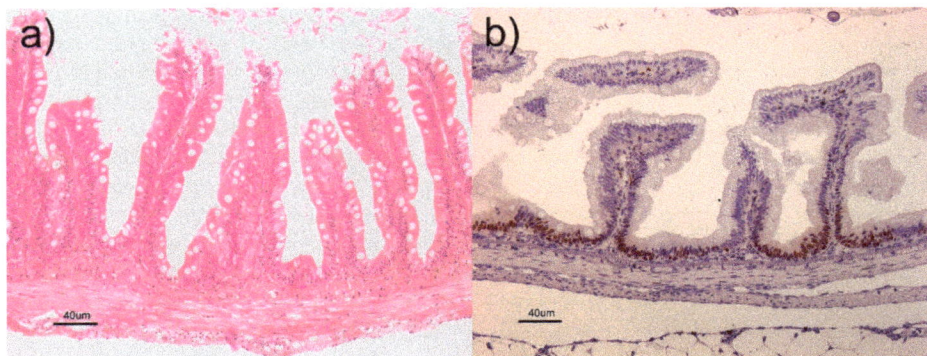

Figure 4. Micrographs of intestinal tissue. Following a histological evaluation, (**a**) pathological changes were not revealed in the intestines of any fish and (**b**) proliferating cells were detected mainly at the base of the folds with an equal pattern in the controls and the DON group.

3. Discussion

We found that 5.5 mg DON/kg feed was associated with reduced intestinal expression of markers for three tight junction proteins (claudin 25b, occludin, and tricellulin), suggesting insufficient expression of these proteins, which could lead to an epithelial barrier impairment with sequelae affecting both structure and function of the intestine. The effect was most prominent in the distal intestine. An assumed functional impairment was confirmed by the fact that feed intake and feed efficiency were significantly reduced by DON exposure [11], and the body weight gain of the DON group was only one third of the weight gain of the fish from the control group. It was therefore surprising that we did not detect indications of intestinal inflammation (expression of a marker for IL-1β and histological examination) or proliferation of goblet cells (tissue sections stained with Alcian Blue (AB) and Periodic acid–Schiff (PAS) in combination) and absorptive epithelial cells (tissue sections stained with an antibody toward proliferating cell nuclear antigen (PCNA)). However, other findings suggested a subtler mechanism behind the adverse impact of DON on production performance. We detected that the relative expression of markers for two suppressors of cytokine signaling proteins (SOCS1 and SOCS2) was increased. These increased levels may have contributed to the suppression of inflammatory cytokines and morphologic inflammatory responses. We also found that the intestinal level of an mRNA marker for PCNA was increased by DON, suggesting an attempt at increased proliferation of epithelial cells. However, for some unknown reason this gene transcription did not appear to translate into the appropriate protein.

To the best of our knowledge, this is the first study addressing the possible influence of any mycotoxin on certain parameters of the intestine of Atlantic salmon (*Salmo salar*). The relative expression of markers for three tight junction proteins (TJs) was significantly lower in both the mid-intestine and the distal intestine in fish experimentally exposed to dietary DON for eight weeks compared with fish fed a standard diet with non-detectable levels of mycotoxins. These findings suggest that the intestinal permeability was increased leading to a leakage of fluids and a suboptimal control of paracellular influx of macromolecules as undigested food particles, pathogens, and toxins. Possible consequences include reduced growth as observed in this trial [10,11] and a number of infections both locally and systemically. The relatively high expression of the marker for PCNA in all intestinal segments in fish exposed to DON compared with the controls may be interpreted as a local response aimed at regenerating intestinal integrity. In pigs experimentally exposed to DON in the feed, both the up- and down-regulation of markers for TJs have been reported [15,16]. This apparent response discrepancy might be attributed to different dosages and study periods.

In carp (*Cyprinus carpio*), the relative expression of markers for several cytokines was 2–3-fold higher in the intestine in fish on an experimental diet with DON at a level of 953 μg/kg feed compared with the controls at day 14 of the experiment, but the relative expression returned to basal levels at day 26 and day 56 [14]. In mice exposed to DON by oral gavage, both the relative expression of markers for tumor necrosis factor-α and interleukin 6 as well as the protein expression were rapidly induced in several organs and plasma, respectively, with a peak of 2 h after exposure and a subsequent decrease [20]. However, the relative expression of several suppressors of cytokine signaling (SOCS), a family of intracellular proteins that play critical roles in the regulation of innate and adaptive immune responses as well as growth and development through negative feedback on cytokine signaling, remained high for several hours with different kinetics for each SOCS and organ [22]. Functional conservation between teleosts and mammals for SOCS has been demonstrated [23], and the relatively high expression of markers for SOCS1 and SOCS2 in the distal intestine in Atlantic salmon exposed to dietary DON in our study, in combination with the absence of inflammation, suggest a successful and long-lasting response to DON in orchestrating the complex network of cytokines. Specifically, SOCS1 is central to the regulation of a number of cytokines including interferons (IFNs) and interleukins in mammals [22], and a strong and negative regulatory effect of salmon SOCS1 on type I and type II IFN-signaling has been demonstrated in cells originating from Atlantic salmon head kidney [23]. Salmon SOCS2 was only moderately affected by IFN responses in that study; however, given the analogy with SOCS2 in mammals [22], it can be assumed that in our study, SOCS2 has influenced growth hormone activity and thus contributed to the reduced growth in fish exposed to DON compared with the controls [10,11]. These findings underline the importance of taking into consideration the dynamics and complexity of cytokine signaling when designing studies and interpreting results.

The level of DON in the feed for the DON group was slightly higher than the maximum recommended level (5 mg DON/kg feed) established in the European Union's current legislation on animal feed. The surveillance of feeds for salmonids in Norwegian aquaculture shows in general low levels of mycotoxins [8], but a negative impact on certain biochemical parameters have already been observed in Atlantic salmon at 2 mg DON/kg feed [11].

Previous studies have produced findings suggesting that the distal intestine (also designated as the second segment of the mid-intestine and posterior intestine) is more vulnerable to disease and dysfunction and particularly important for the immunological defense of Atlantic salmon [24–26]. These works showed that the uptake of gold-labelled bovine serum albumin was restricted to the distal intestine and that the transcript levels of selected immune parameters in general were higher in this intestinal segment, where an inflammation associated with soy-bean meal also occurs in this species. Our results agree with the results from these studies as DON appeared to impair the epithelial barrier and modulate the cytokine signaling in the distal intestine to a larger degree than the other intestinal segments examined.

Studies applying real-time PCR have demonstrated that markers for several tight junction proteins, among these claudin 25b, occludin, and tricellulin, are expressed in the intestine of Atlantic salmon [27,28], and that the expression levels are elevated when juvenile Atlantic salmon are transferred to seawater, suggesting that they are involved in the reorganization of intestinal epithelium and have possibly changed the paracellular permeability. Studies on the protein expression of junctional proteins to reveal whether there is an association between gene expression and protein expression would be of great interest. Unfortunately, research in Atlantic salmon is hampered by the lack of relevant antibodies for performing immunohistochemistry or western blot. However, our findings demonstrate that DON-containing feed may influence certain parameters in the intestine in several ways that separately and in combination may have an adverse impact on fish growth and health. Because the increased use of raw materials of plant origin in aquaculture feed implies a risk for contamination of mycotoxins, the continued surveillance of feeds for the presence of mycotoxins as well as more research exploring the effects of mycotoxins on health and productivity are needed.

4. Materials and Methods

4.1. Animal Ethics and Rearing

The feed trial took place at the Skretting ARC Lerang Research Station that is approved by the Norwegian Animal Research Authority. The trial was approved by the responsible person for animal ethics at the facility on 12 April 2011 and carried out in accordance with the recommendations in the current animal welfare regulations in Norway (FOR-1996-01-15-23).

The trial is described in detail elsewhere [10,11]. Briefly, juvenile post-smolt Atlantic salmon (*Salmo salar*) (SalmoBreed, Bergen, Norway, 12 months old, both genders) with an average weight of approximately 58 g were randomly allocated into tanks supplied by flow-through seawater. All the fish were vaccinated intraperitonally against *Aeromonas salmonicidae* three weeks after the start of the experiment.

4.2. Study Design and Sampling

This experiment was designed with two treatment groups (see Figure 5): a control group fed a standard pelleted feed (Spirit 3 mm, Skretting, Stavanger, Norway) with non-detectable levels of mycotoxins and a group offered the same feed coated with pure deoxynivalenol (DON) (Biopure standard DON; lot #06221Z, degree of purity 99.4%, Romer Labs, Tulln, Austria) to a level of 5.5 mg DON/kg feed. Each group comprised two tanks with 25 fish per tank. Five fish from each tank were sampled eight weeks after the start of the feeding trial, when mean weights for the control and DON fish were 123.2 g and 80.2 g, respectively. Thus, the weight gain of the DON group was only one third of the weight gain in the control group. The feed efficiency was approximately 0.8 and 1.3, respectively [11].

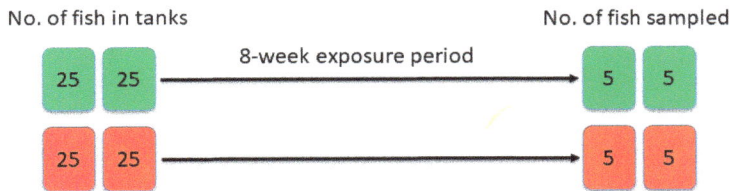

Figure 5. Design of the study on Atlantic salmon fed DON (5.5 mg/kg diet, red color) or no DON (controls, green color) for eight weeks. Five fish from each tank were sampled eight weeks after the start of the feeding trial.

Tissues from the pyloric ceca, the mid-intestine and distal intestine were collected on RNAlater and formalin (Figure 6). Tissues on RNAlater were stored cool for 24–48 h and then at −20 °C until further processing, while formalin-fixed tissues were routinely processed and embedded in paraffin after 24–48 h.

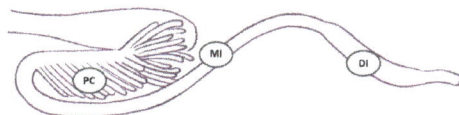

Figure 6. Sampling of intestinal tissues. Tissues from the pyloric ceca (PC), the mid-intestine (MI) and the distal intestine (DI) were collected on RNAlater and formalin. The drawing is a courtesy of Professor emeritus Inge Bjerkås, NMBU, Oslo, Norway.

4.3. Gene Expression Analysis by Real-Time PCR

Nucleic acids from all intestinal tissues were extracted automatically on easyMag (bioMérieux, Marcy l'Etoile, France) using the generic protocol. The RNA concentration and purity were determined using a NanoDrop™ 2000 spectrophotometer (Thermo Scientific, Wilmington, DE, USA). Purity was assessed by determining the ratio of absorbance at 260 and 280 nm (A260/A280). All samples had a ratio between 1.80 and 2.08. The RNA was diluted to 50 ng/μL. The elimination of genomic DNA and the synthesis of cDNA from 500 ng RNA were performed with the QuantiTect Reverse Transcription Kit (QIAGEN, Hilden, Germany) according to the manufacturer's recommendations using the included RT Primer Mix with an optimized blend of oligo-dT and random primers dissolved in water.

Real-time PCR was carried out using SsoAdvanced Universal SYBR Green Supermix (Bio-Rad, Hercules, CA, USA) with cDNA template corresponding to ~5 ng RNA in each reaction in a CFX384 Touch™ Real-Time PCR Detection System (Bio-Rad, Herkules, CA, USA) according to the producer's instructions with 60 °C as annealing temperature and running 40 cycles.

The expression of markers for the following genes was analyzed by real-time PCR: claudin 25b, interleukin 1β (IL-1β), occludin, proliferating cell nuclear antigen (PCNA), suppressor of cytokine signaling 1 and 2 (SOCS1 and SOCS2), tricellulin, and finally elongation factor 1AB (EF1AB) as the reference gene [29] (see Table 2). All analyses were performed in triplicate, and a control lacking template for each master mix was always included in the experiments.

Table 2. Primers for gene expression analyses.

Target	Gene Sequence 5→3′	Reference
Claudin 25b	F-CCTGTAAGAGGGGTCCATCA R-TGACACATGTTCTGCCCTGT	[27]
IL-1β	F-GCTGGAGAGTGCTGTGGAAGA R-TGCTTCCCTCCTGCTCGTAG	[30]
Occludin	F-GACAGTGAGTTCCCCACCAT R-ATCTCTCCCTGCAGGTCCTT	[28]
PCNA	F-TGAGCTCGTCGGGTATCTCT R-GTCCTCATTCCCAGCACACT	[31]
SOCS1	F-TTCTTGATCCGGGATAGTCG R-TGTTTCCTGCACAGTTCCTG	[23]
SOCS2	F-CACTGCCAACGAAGCCAAAGAGAT R-CAAACTGCTTCAGCTTGGGCTTGA	[23]
Tricellulin	F-GGATGCCATGATGGGTAAAC R-AGGAAGGCTGGGTCACTCTT	[28]
EF1AB	F-TGCCCCTCCAGGATGTCTAC R-CACGGCCCACAGGTACTG	[32]

4.4. Histology and Immunohistochemistry

Sections from all intestinal tissues were cut at 3 μm and stained with hematoxylin and eosin (HE) or Alcian Blue (AB) and Periodic acid–Schiff (PAS) in combination, whereas proliferating cells were detected using a monoclonal mouse antibody against proliferating cell nuclear antigen (PCNA; M0879, Dako, Glostrup, Denmark) previously used in fish [33]. After deparaffinization, antigen retrieval, and inhibition as described elsewhere [34], the sections were incubated with horse serum diluted 1:100 in 5% bovine serum albumin (BSA) in a tris-buffer solution (TBS) for 20 min to prevent non-specific binding. The antibody against PCNA was diluted 1:5000 in 1% BSA/TBS before incubation for 60 min. The secondary antibody, horseradish peroxidase-labelled polymer conjugated to horse anti-mouse Ig, was diluted 1:100 in 1% BSA/TBS before incubation for 30 min, followed by incubation with Vectastain® Elite ABC Reagent (PK-7100, Vector Laboratories, Burlingame, CA, USA) for 30 min and ImmPACT™ AEC (SK-4205, Vector Laboratories, Burlingame, CA, USA) for 5 min. The sections were thoroughly rinsed between each step except after the incubation with horse serum, counterstained with hematoxylin for 15 s and mounted with VectaMount™ AQ Aqueous Mounting Medium (H-5501, Vector Laboratories, Burlingame, CA, USA). Micrographs were captured with ACT-1 software (Nikon, Tokyo, Japan) using a digital camera D×1200 configured with a Leica DM4000 microscope.

4.5. Calculations and Statistical Analysis

Databases for the results from real-time PCR were established in Excel®for Windows, and statistical calculations and graphical presentation of gene expression were performed using Prism 7.0 software (GraphPad Software, La Jolla, CA, USA). Data were given as mean $\pm$ standard error of the mean (SEM) unless otherwise stated. The data for gene expression were analyzed for normality using the Shapiro–Wilk test. Data with normal distributions were further analyzed using the unpaired *t*-test, whereas non-normal data were analyzed using the Mann–Whitney U test. The significance level was set to 0.05.

Author Contributions: Conceptualization, A.B., E.O.K., G.R., M.K., and T.M.; Validation, T.M.; Formal Analysis, T.M.; Investigation, T.M.; Resources, G.R.; Data Curation, T.M.; Writing–Original Draft Preparation, T.M.; Writing–Review and Editing, A.B., E.O.K., G.R., and M.K.; Visualization, T.M.; Supervision, A.B., E.O.K, G.R., and M.K.; Project Administration, A.B.; Funding Acquisition, A.B.

Funding: The feed trial was funded by the Research Council of Norway through the project "Safe feed, safe and healthy seafood" (Project Number 199626) and Skretting ARC, whereas the laboratory work was funded by a basic grant from the Research Council of Norway to the Norwegian Veterinary Institute.

Acknowledgments: The authors would like to thank Randi Terland and Britt Saure for cutting sections and stainings; Inger Böckerman and Lone Engerdahl for the extraction of nucleic acids and the synthesis of cDNA; Maria Dahle, Søren Grove, Hilde Sindre, and Monika Hjortaas for scientific discussions; and Karen Bækken Soleim and Alexandra Bodura Göksu for their kind advice in the laboratory.

Conflicts of Interest: The authors declare no conflict of interest. The funders had no role in the design of the study; in the collection, analyses, or interpretation of data; in the writing of the manuscript; and in the decision to publish the results.

References

1. Powell, K. Eat your veg. *Nature* **2003**, *426*, 378–379. [CrossRef] [PubMed]
2. Liland, N.S.; Rosenlund, G.; Berntssen, M.H.G.; Brattelid, T.; Madsen, L.; Torstensen, B.E. Net production of Atlantic salmon (FIFO; Fish in Fish out < 1) with dietary plant proteins and vegetable oils. *Aquac. Nutr.* **2013**, *19*, 289–300.
3. Waagbø, R.; Berntssen, M.H.G.; Danielsen, T.; Helberg, H.; Kleppa, A.L.; Lea, T.B.; Rosenlund, G.; Tvenning, L.; Susort, S.; Vikesa, V.; et al. Feeding Atlantic salmon diets with plant ingredients during the seawater phase—A full-scale net production of marine protein with focus on biological performance, welfare, product quality and safety. *Aquac. Nutr.* **2013**, *19*, 598–618. [CrossRef]
4. Antonissen, G.; Martel, A.; Pasmans, F.; Ducatelle, R.; Verbrugghe, E.; Vandenbroucke, V.; Li, S.; Haesebrouck, F.; Van Immerseel, F.; Croubels, S. The impact of Fusarium mycotoxins on human and animal host susceptibility to infectious diseases. *Toxins* **2014**, *6*, 430–452. [CrossRef] [PubMed]
5. Nesic, K.; Ivanovic, S.; Nesic, V. Fusarial Toxins: Secondary Metabolites of *Fusarium* Fungi. In *Reviews of Environmental Contamination and Toxicology*; Whitacre, D., Ed.; Springer: Cham, Switzerland, 2014; Volume 228, pp. 101–120. ISBN 978-3-319-01619-1.
6. Cheli, F.; Battaglia, D.; Gallo, R.; Dell'Orto, V. EU legislation on cereal safety: An update with a focus on mycotoxins. *Food Control* **2014**, *37*, 315–325. [CrossRef]
7. Pinotti, L.; Ottoboni, M.; Giromini, C.; Dell'Orto, V.; Cheli, F. Mycotoxin Contamination in the EU Feed Supply Chain: A Focus on Cereal Byproducts. *Toxins* **2016**, *8*, 45. [CrossRef] [PubMed]
8. Sanden, M.; Hemre, G.; Måge, A.; Lunestad, B.; Espe, M.; Lie, K.; Lundebye, A.K.; Amlund, H.; Waagbø, R.; Ørnsrud, R. *Program for Overvåking av Fiskefôr*; Nasjonalt Institutt for Ernærings- og Sjømatforskning: Bergen, Norway, 2017; ISBN 978-82-91065-46-5.
9. Nacher-Mestre, J.; Serrano, R.; Beltran, E.; Perez-Sanchez, J.; Silva, J.; Karalazos, V.; Hernandez, F.; Berntssen, M.H.G. Occurrence and potential transfer of mycotoxins in gilthead sea bream and Atlantic salmon by use of novel alternative feed ingredients. *Chemosphere* **2015**, *128*, 314–320. [CrossRef] [PubMed]
10. Bernhoft, A.; Høgåsen, H.R.; Rosenlund, G.; Ivanova, L.; Berntssen, M.H.G.; Alexander, J.; Eriksen, G.S.; Fæste, C.K. Tissue distribution and elimination of deoxynivalenol and ochratoxin A in dietary-exposed Atlantic salmon (*Salmo salar*). *Food Addit. Contam. Part A Chem. Anal. Control Expo. Risk Assess.* **2017**, *34*, 1211–1224. [CrossRef] [PubMed]

11. Bernhoft, A.; Høgåsen, H.R.; Rosenlund, G.; Moldal, T.; Grove, S.; Berntssen, M.H.G.; Thoresen, S.I.; Alexander, J. Effects of dietary deoxynivalenol or ochratoxin A on performance and selected health indices in Atlantic salmon (*Salmo salar*). *Food Chem. Toxicol.* **2018**. [CrossRef] [PubMed]

12. Hooft, J.M.; Elmor, H.I.; Encarnacao, P.; Bureau, D.P. Rainbow trout (*Oncorhynchus mykiss*) is extremely sensitive to the feed-borne Fusarium mycotoxin deoxynivalenol (DON). *Aquaculture* **2011**, *311*, 224–232. [CrossRef]

13. Matejova, I.; Modra, H.; Blahova, J.; Franc, A.; Fictum, P.; Sevcikova, M.; Svobodova, Z. The effect of mycotoxin deoxynivalenol on haematological and biochemical indicators and histopathological changes in rainbow trout (*Oncorhynchus mykiss*). *Biomed. Res. Int.* **2014**, *2014*, 310680. [CrossRef] [PubMed]

14. Pietsch, C.; Katzenback, B.A.; Garcia-Garcia, E.; Schulz, C.; Belosevic, M.; Burkhardt-Holm, P. Acute and subchronic effects on immune responses of carp (*Cyprinus carpio* L.) after exposure to deoxynivalenol (DON) in feed. *Mycotoxin Res.* **2015**, *31*, 151–164. [CrossRef] [PubMed]

15. Alizadeh, A.; Braber, S.; Akbari, P.; Garssen, J.; Fink-Gremmels, J. Deoxynivalenol impairs weight gain and affects markers of gut health after low-dose, short-term exposure of growing pigs. *Toxins* **2015**, *7*, 2071–2095. [CrossRef] [PubMed]

16. Lessard, M.; Savard, C.; Deschene, K.; Lauzon, K.; Pinilla, V.A.; Gagnon, C.A.; Lapointe, J.; Guay, F.; Chorfi, Y. Impact of deoxynivalenol (DON) contaminated feed on intestinal integrity and immune response in swine. *Food Chem. Toxicol.* **2015**, *80*, 7–16. [CrossRef] [PubMed]

17. Bracarense, A.P.; Lucioli, J.; Grenier, B.; Drociunas Pacheco, G.; Moll, W.D.; Schatzmayr, G.; Oswald, I.P. Chronic ingestion of deoxynivalenol and fumonisin, alone or in interaction, induces morphological and immunological changes in the intestine of piglets. *Br. J. Nutr.* **2012**, *107*, 1776–1786. [CrossRef] [PubMed]

18. Ghareeb, K.; Awad, W.A.; Soodoi, C.; Sasgary, S.; Strasser, A.; Böhm, J. Effects of feed contaminant deoxynivalenol on plasma cytokines and mRNA expression of immune genes in the intestine of broiler chickens. *PLoS ONE* **2013**, *8*, e71492. [CrossRef] [PubMed]

19. Antonissen, G.; Van Immerseel, F.; Pasmans, F.; Ducatelle, R.; Haesebrouck, F.; Timbermont, L.; Verlinden, M.; Janssens, G.P.; Eeckhaut, V.; Eeckhout, M.; et al. The mycotoxin deoxynivalenol predisposes for the development of *Clostridium perfringens*-induced necrotic enteritis in broiler chickens. *PLoS ONE* **2014**, *9*, e108775. [CrossRef] [PubMed]

20. Amuzie, C.J.; Shinozuka, J.; Pestka, J.J. Induction of suppressors of cytokine signaling by the trichothecene deoxynivalenol in the mouse. *Toxicol. Sci.* **2009**, *111*, 277–287. [CrossRef] [PubMed]

21. Akbari, P.; Braber, S.; Varasteh, S.; Alizadeh, A.; Garssen, J.; Fink-Gremmels, J. The intestinal barrier as an emerging target in the toxicological assessment of mycotoxins. *Arch. Toxicol* **2017**, *91*, 1007–1029. [CrossRef] [PubMed]

22. Linossi, E.M.; Babon, J.J.; Hilton, D.J.; Nicholson, S.E. Suppression of cytokine signaling: The SOCS perspective. *Cytokine Growth Factor Rev.* **2013**, *24*, 241–248. [CrossRef] [PubMed]

23. Skjesol, A.; Liebe, T.; Iliev, D.B.; Thomassen, E.I.; Tollersrud, L.G.; Sobhkhez, M.; Lindenskov Joensen, L.; Secombes, C.J.; Jørgensen, J.B. Functional conservation of suppressors of cytokine signaling proteins between teleosts and mammals: Atlantic salmon SOCS1 binds to JAK/STAT family members and suppresses type I and II IFN signaling. *Dev. Comp. Immunol.* **2014**, *45*, 177–189. [CrossRef] [PubMed]

24. Fuglem, B.; Jirillo, E.; Bjerkås, I.; Kiyono, H.; Nochi, T.; Yuki, Y.; Raida, M.; Fischer, U.; Koppang, E.O. Antigen-sampling cells in the salmonid intestinal epithelium. *Dev. Comp. Immunol.* **2010**, *34*, 768–774. [CrossRef] [PubMed]

25. Løkka, G.; Austbø, L.; Falk, K.; Bromage, E.; Fjelldal, P.G.; Hansen, T.; Hordvik, I.; Koppang, E.O. Immune parameters in the intestine of wild and reared unvaccinated and vaccinated Atlantic salmon (*Salmo salar* L.). *Dev. Comp. Immunol.* **2014**, *47*, 6–16. [CrossRef] [PubMed]

26. Bæverfjord, G.; Krogdahl, Å. Development and regression of soybean meal induced enteritis in Atlantic salmon (*Salmo salar* L.) distal intestine. A comparison with the intestines of fasted fish. *J. Fish Dis.* **1996**, *19*, 375–387. [CrossRef]

27. Tipsmark, C.K.; Sørensen, K.J.; Hulgard, K.; Madsen, S.S. Claudin-15 and -25b expression in the intestinal tract of Atlantic salmon in response to seawater acclimation, smoltification and hormone treatment. *Comp. Biochem. Physiol. A Mol. Integr. Physiol.* **2010**, *155*, 361–370. [CrossRef] [PubMed]

28. Tipsmark, C.K.; Madsen, S.S. Tricellulin, occludin and claudin-3 expression in salmon intestine and kidney during salinity adaptation. *Comp. Biochem. Physiol. A Mol. Integr. Physiol.* **2012**, *162*, 378–385. [CrossRef] [PubMed]

29. Olsvik, P.A.; Lie, K.K.; Jordal, A.E.O.; Nilsen, T.O.; Hordvik, I. Evaluation of potential reference genes in real-time RT-PCR studies of Atlantic salmon. *BMC Mol. Biol.* **2005**, *6*, 21. [CrossRef] [PubMed]

30. Marjara, I.S.; Chikwati, E.M.; Valen, E.C.; Krogdahl, A.; Bakke, A.M. Transcriptional regulation of IL-17A and other inflammatory markers during the development of soybean meal-induced enteropathy in the distal intestine of Atlantic salmon (*Salmo salar* L.). *Cytokine* **2012**, *60*, 186–196. [CrossRef] [PubMed]

31. Kortner, T.M.; Gu, J.; Krogdahl, Å.; Bakke, A.M. Transcriptional regulation of cholesterol and bile acid metabolism after dietary soyabean meal treatment in Atlantic salmon (*Salmo salar* L.). *Br. J. Nutr.* **2013**, *109*, 593–604. [CrossRef] [PubMed]

32. Løvoll, M.; Austbø, L.; Jørgensen, J.B.; Rimstad, E.; Frost, P. Transcription of reference genes used for quantitative RT-PCR in Atlantic salmon is affected by viral infection. *Vet. Res.* **2011**, *42*, 8. [CrossRef] [PubMed]

33. Løkka, G.; Austbø, L.; Falk, K.; Bjerkås, I.; Koppang, E.O. Intestinal morphology of the wild Atlantic salmon (*Salmo salar*). *J. Morphol.* **2013**, *274*, 859–876. [CrossRef] [PubMed]

34. Moldal, T.; Løkka, G.; Wiik-Nielsen, J.; Austbø, L.; Torstensen, B.E.; Rosenlund, G.; Dale, O.B.; Kaldhusdal, M.; Koppang, E.O. Substitution of dietary fish oil with plant oils is associated with shortened mid intestinal folds in Atlantic salmon (*Salmo salar*). *BMC Vet. Res.* **2014**, *10*, 60. [CrossRef] [PubMed]

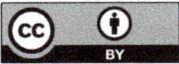

![toxins logo] *toxins*

MDPI

Article

Molecular and Physiological Effects on the Small Intestine of Weaner Pigs Following Feeding with Deoxynivalenol-Contaminated Feed

J. Alex Pasternak [1], Vaishnavi Iyer Aka Aiyer [2], Glenn Hamonic [1], A. Denise Beaulieu [3,†], Daniel A. Columbus [2,†] and Heather L. Wilson [1,*]

[1] Vaccine and Infectious Disease Organization-International Vaccine Centre (VIDO-InterVac), University of Saskatchewan, Saskatoon, SK S7N 5E3, Canada; alex.pasternak@usask.ca (J.A.P.); glenn.hamonic@usask.ca (G.H.)

[2] Prairie Swine Centre, Inc., Saskatoon, SK S7N 5E3, Canada; vaishiyer95@gmail.com (V.I.A.A.); dan.columbus@usask.ca (D.A.C.)

[3] Department of Animal and Poultry Science, University of Saskatchewan, Saskatoon, SK S7N 5E3, Canada; denise.beaulieu@usask.ca

* Correspondence: heather.wilson@usask.ca; Tel.: +1-(306)-966-1537; Fax: +1-(306)-966-7478

† These authors contributed equally to this work.

Received: 23 November 2017; Accepted: 9 January 2018; Published: 12 January 2018

Abstract: We intended to assess how exposure of piglets to deoxynivalenol (DON)-contaminated feed impacted their growth, immune response and gut development. Piglets were fed traditional Phase I, Phase II and Phase III diets with the control group receiving 0.20–0.40 ppm DON (referred to as the Control group) and treatment group receiving much higher level of DON-contaminated wheat (3.30–3.80 ppm; referred to as DON-contaminated group). Feeding a DON-contaminated diet had no impact on average daily feed intake (ADFI) ($p < 0.08$) or average daily gain (ADG) ($p > 0.10$) but it did significantly reduce body weight over time relative to the control piglets ($p < 0.05$). Cytokine analysis after initial exposure to the DON-contaminated feed did not result in significant differences in serum interleukin (IL) IL1β, IL-8, IL-13, tumor necrosis factor (TNF)-α or interferon (IFN)-γ. After day 24, no obvious changes in jejunum or ileum gut morphology, histology or changes in gene expression for IL-1β, IL-6, IL-10, TNFα, or Toll-like receptor (TLR)-4 genes. IL-8 showed a trend towards increased expression in the ileum in DON-fed piglets. A significant increase in gene expression for claudin (CLDN) 7 gene expression and a trend towards increased CLDN 2-expression was observed in the ileum in piglets fed the highly DON-contaminated wheat. Because CLDN localization was not negatively affected, we believe that it is unlikely that gut permeability was affected. Exposure to DON-contaminated feed did not significantly impact weaner piglet performance or gut physiology.

Keywords: ileum; jejunum; deoxynivalenol; piglet; contaminated feed; tight junction

Key contribution: Relative to control piglets receiving 0.20–0.40 ppm deoxynivalenol (DON)-contaminated feed, weaner piglets fed 3.30–3.80 ppm DON for 24 d had significantly reduced body weight. However we observed no significant impact on average daily feed intake, average daily gain, serum or gut cytokine expression (with exception of elevated ileal Claudin-7), gut morpholoyg, or histology.

1. Introduction

Deoxynivalenol (DON), commonly known as vomitoxin, is a potent mycotoxin produced by the fungus *Fusarium graminearum*, and its presence in wheat, corn, and barley crops can lead to them being downgraded to livestock feed grade. Pigs, and in particular young piglets, are poorly tolerant to

DON contamination. Although extremely high doses of contamination in feed (20 mg/kg feed) will induce vomiting [1,2], swine will tolerate lower-level feed contamination to varying degrees in a sex- and dose-dependent manner [3]. Longer-term exposure to moderate contamination of feed at levels between 5 and 8 mg/kg will be tolerated but has been shown to considerably decrease daily feed intake and growth rate [4,5]. As a result, governmental guidelines from the Canadian Food Inspection Agency, United States Food and Drug Administration and the European Union recommend limiting dietary inclusion in swine feed to under 1 mg/kg [6], 1 mg/kg [7], and 0.9 mg/kg [8] respectively. However even at these recommended inclusion levels DON has been shown to significantly decrease average daily gain (ADG) and alter intestinal morphology [9]. The majority of research to date has focused on the local effect of DON on the intestine but doses, age of animal, and exposure times have varied which makes it difficult to compare results. In vivo studies have demonstrated that chronic exposure to 3 mg/kg DON-contaminated feed altered intestinal morphology including villus atrophy and reduced villi height, reduced jejunal and ileal goblet cells and lymphocytes counts, as well as reduced expression of junctional adheren protein E-cadherin and tight-junction protein occludin in the intestine [10]. Several studies show that piglets fed DON had altered cytokine production either in the duodenum, jejunum, or the ileum or the mesenteric lymph nodes [9,11,12] indicating that DON-contaminated feed can alter the innate immune response in a piglet's gut. With increased quantities of DON-contaminated grain entering the livestock sector, complete avoidance of DON may not be possible.

The intestinal tract is the first physical barrier to protect the body from food contaminants, chemicals and intestinal pathogens. A single layer of epithelial cells separates the apical and basolateral domains of the gut mucosa. Tight junctions (TJs) between adjacent cells are regulated by structural and functional proteins including Occluden, Junction Adhesion molecules and Claudin family members, which together regulate permeability through the intercellular space on epithelial sheets [13–17]. How DON reportedly affects barrier function and specifically the proteins involved in TJ formation is variable based on experimental design, age of animals, amount of DON present and duration of exposure [10,18]. It is, therefore, neccessary to better understand the physiological effects underlying the reduced performance by pigs consuming DON-contaminated diets in order to develop effective and economical strategies.

We sought to clarify how weaner piglets fed traditional Phase I, Phase II and Phase III diets with the control group receiving 0.30 ppm DON and treatment group receiving 3.30 ppm DON in Phase I, control group receiving 0.20 ppm DON and treatment group receiving 3.80 ppm DON in Phase II, and control group receiving 0.40 ppm DON and treatment group receiving 3.80 ppm DON in Phase III were affected. We measured ADG, average daily feed intake (ADFI), and gene expression profiles for innate immune response receptors and cytokines, as well as genes that play a role in intestinal barrier function. Immunohistofluorescence was performed to establish localization of several proteins that mediate TJ formation in the jejunum and the ileum. This research will help to establish whether homeostatic mechanisms compensate for DON exposure in vivo over the long term.

2. Results

2.1. Feed Intake and Growth Performance

No pigs showed any signs of vomiting throughout the trials. One pig from the control diet died during the study due to reasons unrelated to dietary treatments. Body weight (Table 1) was not different between groups ($p > 0.05$) up to day 24 of the study but final body weight was significantly reduced ($p < 0.05$) in pigs fed the DON diet.

Average daily gain and average daily feed intake were not affected (Table 2, $p > 0.05$) in the first three weeks of the study period. There was a trend ($p < 0.08$) for average daily feed intake to be reduced in pigs fed the DON diet in the final days of the study.

Table 1. Body weight (kg) of piglets assigned to receive either a low-DON control diet or a DON-contaminated diet for 24 days. Piglets were weaned at 21 days of age (experimental day 0).

Time	Control Diet (0.20 to 0.40 ppm DON)	DON-Contaminated Diet (3.30 to 3.80 ppm DON)
Day 0	5.80	5.79
Day 3	5.85	5.77
Day 7	6.09	5.82
Day 14	7.43	6.94
Day 21	9.96	9.28
Day 24	11.43 *	10.39 *

Data are LSMeans. Analysis by repeated measures, overall effect of treatment $p = 0.04$, SEM 0.144; treatment by day, $p = 0.003$, SEM 0.277. * Day 24, $p < 0.01$.

Table 2. Growth and feed intake of piglets assigned to receive either a low-DON control diet or a DON-contaminated diet for 24 days. Piglets were weaned at 21 days of age (experimental day 0).

Interval	Control Diet (0.20 to 0.40 ppm DON)	DON-Contaminated Diet (3.30 to 3.80 ppm DON)
Average daily gain (d/g)		
Day 3–7	63.3	6.4
Day 7–14	190.8	158.3
Day 14–21	358.9	331.6
Day 21–24	367.0	273.6 *
Average daily feed intake (g/d)		
Day 3–7	137.6	90.4
Day 7–14	236.9	202.4
Day 14–21	519.7	457.9
Day 21–24	700.8 *	602.3 *

Data are LSMeans. Analysis by repeated measures, ADG, overall effect of treatment, $p < 0.001$, SEM 14.95, treatment by day, $p = 0.19$, SEM 33.28; ADFI, overall effect of treatment $p < 0.05$, SEM 21.11, treatment by day, $p = 0.46$, SEM 33.14. * Day 21–24, ADG, $p < 0.05$; ADFI, $p < 0.10$.

2.2. Serum Cytokine Analysis in Acute Period after DON Exposure

Three and seven days after introduction of the Phase I diets, sera were collected and systemic cytokines levels were assessed (Figure 1). We did not identify a significant difference in serum IL-1β (Figure 1A), IL-8 (Figure 1B) IL-13 (Figure 1C), TNF-α (Figure 1D) or IFN-γ (Figure 1E) between animals fed the Control or DON-contaminated diets after 3 or 7 d. We also did not detect a significant change in any of the serum cytokines over time within each treatment group. These data indicate that under the current experimental conditions, DON-contaminated feed did not promote a systemic inflammatory immune response.

2.3. Jejunal and Ileal Immune Response Gene Profile after Exposure to DON

Next, we wanted to assess how DON exposure for 24 days affected piglet cytokine gene expression in the jejunum and the ileum. In the jejunum, we observed no significant difference in the expression of IL-1β (Figure 2A), IL-6 (Figure 2B), IL-8 (Figure 2C), IL-10 (Figure 2D), and TNFα (Figure 2E) genes in control or DON-fed piglets. These same cytokines also showed no change in expression in the ileal tissue between the Control and DON-fed piglets ($p > 0.10$), with the exception of IL-8, which showed a trend towards increased expression in the DON-treated tissues (Figure 2C; $p < 0.06$). Likewise, the gene for TLR4 that codes for a receptor that detects lipopolysaccharide from Gram negative bacteria was not differentially expressed between the Control and DON-fed piglets (Figure 2F).

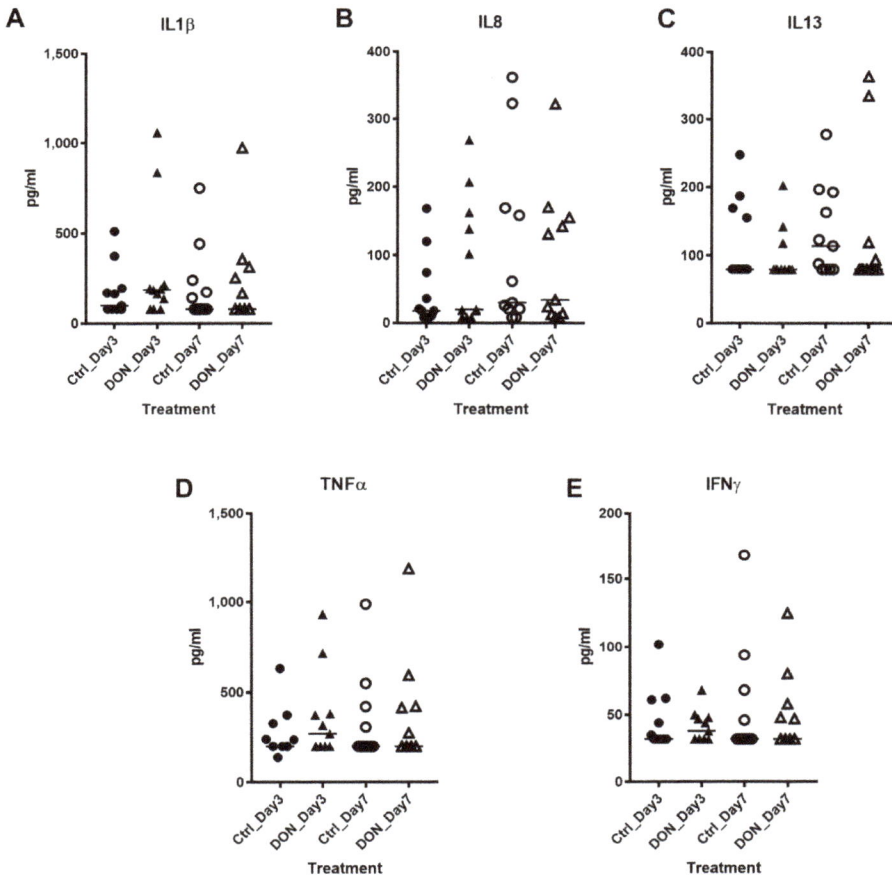

Figure 1. Acute but low-level exposure of DON-contaminated feed did not impact serum cytokine production. Sera were collected on Day 3 and Day 7 and subjected to BioPlex analysis to assess changes in (**A**) IL-1β, (**B**) IL-8, (**C**) IL-13, (**D**) TNF-α and (**E**) IFN-γ in response piglets fed DON-contaminated feed or Control feed after 3 and 7 days. Each data point represents a unique biological replicate and the horizontal line represents the median value for the group. Statistical analysis was performed with a nonparametric Kruskal-Wallis between DON and Control fed piglets on Day 3 and Day 7 as well as within each treatment group over time.

In recent years, occludens, junctional adhesion molecule proteins, claudin family members and others have been shown to be responsible for mediating TJ formation [19]. We investigated whether DON exposure could influence the expression profile of several genes, which encode TJ proteins including Claudins (CLDNs), Occluden (OCLN) and Zonula occludens-1 (ZO-1) in jejunal and ileal tissue. CLDN-1 expression (Figure 3A) was not significantly altered in response to DON but CLDN2 (Figure 3B; $p < 0.063$), CLDN-3 (Figure 3C; $p < 0.054$), and CLDN-4 (Figure 3D; $p < 0.063$) showed a trend towards upregulation in the ileum (but not the jejunum) in the DON-treated animals relative to age-matched Control-fed piglets. Expression of CLDN-7 was significantly induced in the ileal tissue from DON-treated animals (Figure 3F; $p < 0.031$) but no change in expression was observed in the jejunum relative to the Control-fed piglets. We observed no significant difference in gene expression for CLDN-10 (Figure 3G), CLDN-23 (Figure 3H), OCLN (Figure 3I) or ZO-1 (Figure 3J) in either tissue across treatment groups. Gene expression analysis for CLDN-8 and CLDN-14 were assessed however expression of these transcripts was below the threshold of detection (data not shown). DON-contaminated feed had no effect on expression patterns of the indicated genes in the jejunum and only modest effect on expression in the ileum.

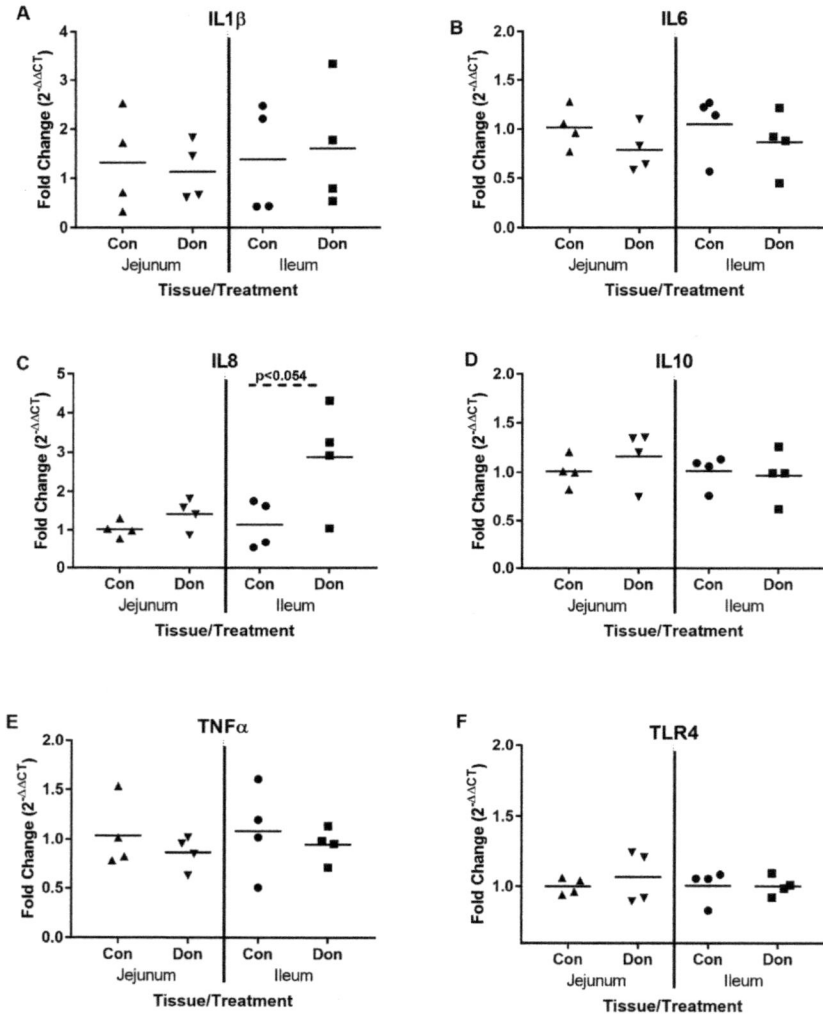

Figure 2. QPCR analysis of cytokines and TLR4 in jejunal and ileal gut tissue. After 24 days of exposure, jejunal and ileal gut samples from control and DON-fed piglets were investigated for relative expression of IL-1β (**A**), IL-6 (**B**), IL-8 (**C**), IL-10 (**D**), TNFα (**E**) and TLR4 (**F**) mRNA expression. The mRNA expression levels of each gene were normalized with the housekeeping genes and were calculated with $2^{-\Delta\Delta Ct}$ relative quantification. Each data point represents a unique biological replicate. Horizontal bars represent the median values.

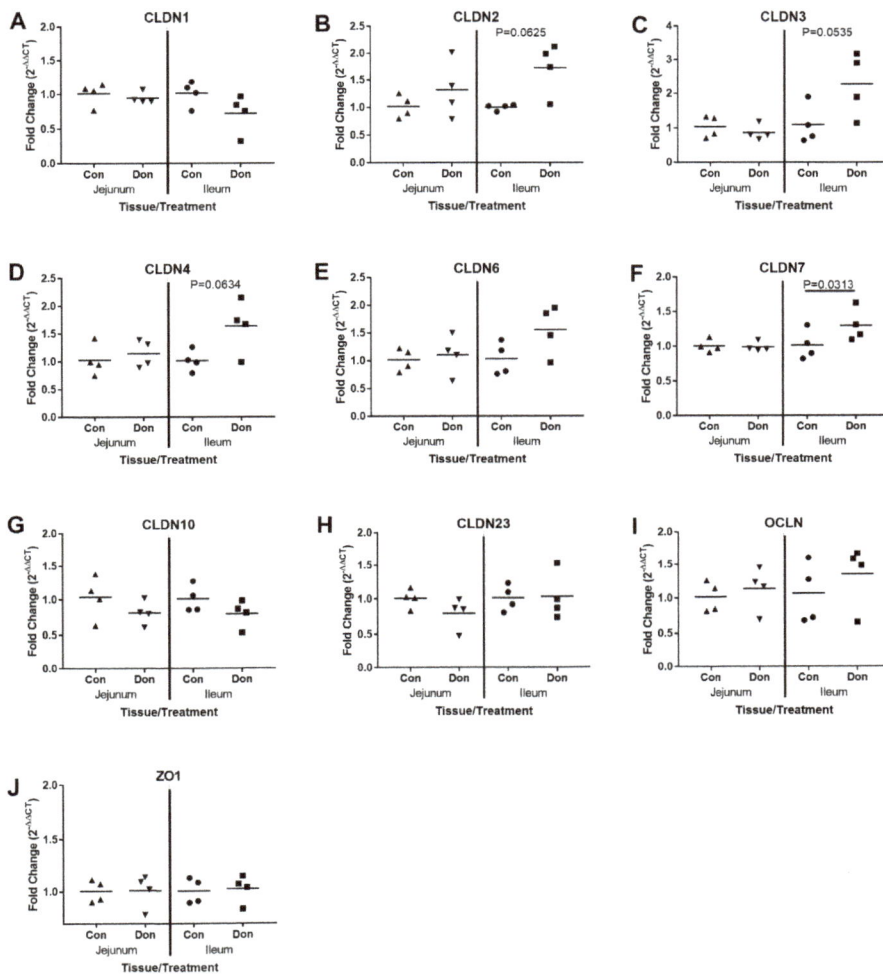

Figure 3. QPCR analysis of Claudins, Occluden and Zonodulin 1 in jejunal and ileal gut tissue. After 24 days of exposure, jejunal and ileal gut samples from control and DON-fed piglets were investigated for relative expression of Claudin (CLDN)-1 (**A**), (CLDN)-2 (**B**), (CLDN)-3 (**C**), (CLDN)-4 (**D**), (CLDN)-6 (**E**), (CLDN)-7 (**F**), (CLDN)-10 (**G**), (CLDN)-23 (**H**), Occluden (OCLN) (**I**), and Zonodulin-1 (ZO1) (**J**) mRNA expression. The mRNA expression levels of each gene were normalized with the housekeeping genes and were calculated with $2^{-\Delta\Delta Ct}$ relative quantification. Each data point represents a unique biological replicate. Horizontal bars represent the median values.

Next, we assessed whether DON-contaminated feed impacted villous or crypt morphology (using H & E staining) or surface localization of CLDN-1, CLDN-3, CLDN-4, CLDN-7 proteins in ileum villi (Figure 4A–H) and crypts (Figure 4I–P) and jejunal villi (Figure 5A–H) and crypts (Figure 5I–P) relative to control fed piglets using immunohistofluorescence. We observed no change in villous or crypt morphology per villi in piglets fed DON-contaminated or control feed (data not shown). In both regions of the gut, CLDN1 was localized to the full length of the pericellular junction within the crypts (Figure 4I,M and Figure 5I,M) where it was found more heavily localized to the apical aspect of the pericellular junction at the villus tip (Figure 4A,E and Figure 5A,E). CLDN1 was also expressed in intestinal endothelial cells (data not shown). CLDN3 stained the length of the pericellular junction at the villus tip (Figure 4B,F and Figure 5B,F) and within the crypts (Figure 4J,N and Figure 5J,N). CLDN4 staining at the villus tip was observed along the length of the pericellular junction (Figure 4C,G and Figure 5C,G) whereas it was found intracellularly localized in the epithelium of the crypt for both control fed and DON-fed piglets (Figure 4K,O and Figure 5K,O). CLDN7 stained along the length of the pericellular junction at both the villus tip (Figure 4D,H and Figure 5D,H) and within the crypts (Figure 4L,M and Figure 5L,M). The figures shown are representative of 4 biological replicates (Supplementary Figures S1–S8). We note that the IHF staining intensity was strongest for CLDN7 >>> CLDN3 > CLDN4 > CLDN1 which is not obvious from the figures because specific imaging protocols were used to evaluate each anti-CLDN antibody (data not shown). IHC analysis of this panel of CLDNs indicates that exposure of piglets to DON-contaminated feed did not negatively impact CLDN localization in jejunal and ileal villi or crypts relative to those fed control feed.

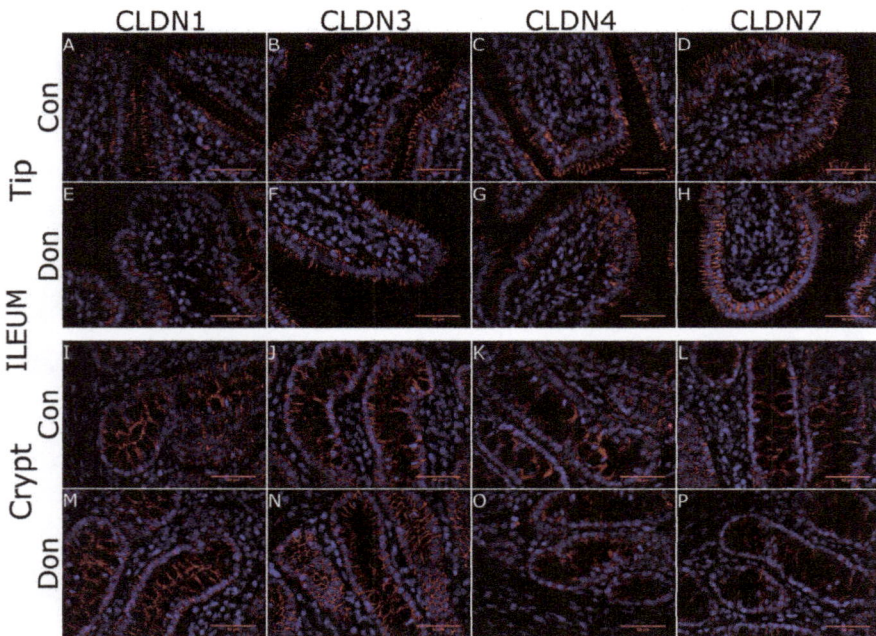

Figure 4. Claudin surface localization in piglet ileal villi and crypts in DON-fed and control fed piglets. Ileal tissue was obtained 24 days after DON-exposure to half of the piglets. CLDN1 was localized to the full length of the pericellular junction within the crypts where as it was found more heavily localized to the apical aspect of the pericellular junction at the villus tip (**A,E,I,M**). CLDN3 stained the length of the pericellular junction at the villus tip and within the crypts but was more abundant in the latter (**B,F,J,N**). CLDN4 stained the villous surface but was found intracellularly localized in the epithelium of the crypts (**C,G,K,O**). CLDN7 stained along the length of the pericellular junction at both the villus tip and within the crypts (**D,H,L,P**). Secondary antibody: Alexa555-conjugated goat α rabbit IgG (red) in incubation buffer for 4 h at room temperature. Nuclear stain: DAPI (blue). Scale bar represents 50 μm.

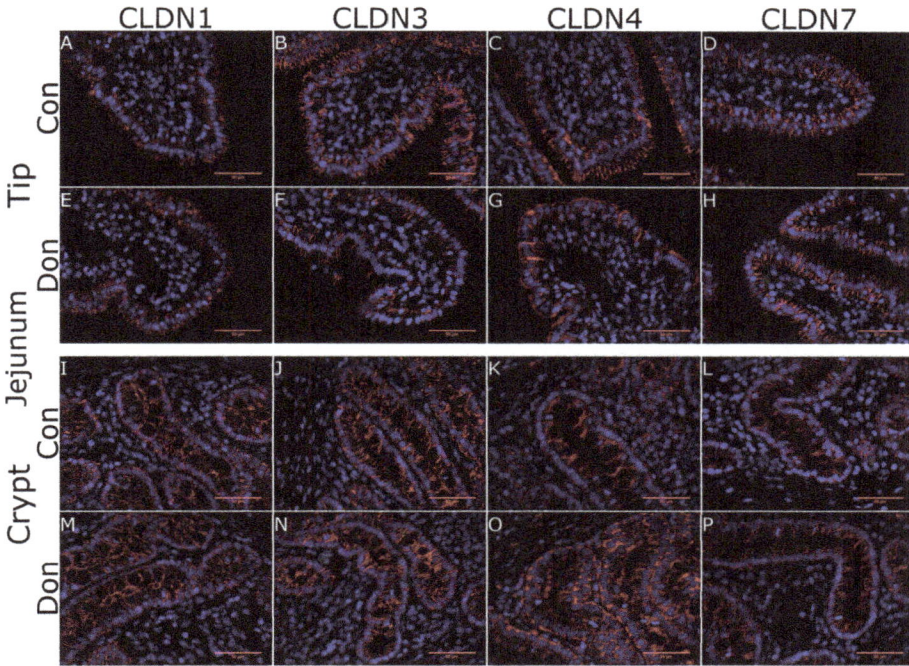

Figure 5. Claudin surface localization in piglet jejunal villi and crypts in DON-fed and control fed piglets. Jejunal tissue was obtained 24 days after DON-exposure to half of the piglets. CLDN1 was localized to the full length of the pericellular junction within the crypts where as it was found more heavily localized to the apical aspect of the pericellular junction at the villus tip (**A,E,I,M**). CLDN3 stained the length of the pericellular junction at the villus tip and within the crypts but was more abundant in the latter (**B,F,J,N**). CLDN4 stained the villous surface but was found intracellularly localized in the epithelium of the crypts (**C,G,K,O**). CLDN7 stained along the length of the pericellular junction at both the villus tip and within the crypts (**D,H,L,P**). Secondary antibody: Alexa555-conjugated goat α rabbit IgG (red) in incubation buffer for 4 h at room temperature. Nuclear stain: DAPI (blue). Scale bar represents 50 μm.

3. Discussion

The aim of this study was to determine whether the piglet gut can compensate for DON-contaminated feed by showing gut health and strong growth kinetics. Most studies show that piglets fed DON-contaminated feed have altered gut histology and reduced performance. For instance, jejunal explants from 4 to 5 week old piglets and 9–13 week old pigs exposed to 5 μM DON (corresponds to 1.5 mg/kg in diet) for 8 hours were shown to have shortened intestinal villi and lysed intestinal cells however the younger piglets were shown to have better morphological scores [20]. However, no effect on morphological scores was observed in 4–5 week old piglet gut explants exposed for 4 h to 1 μM DON (which corresponds to 0.3 mg DON/kg in diet) [20]. In vivo studies showed 0.9–2.29 mg/kg DON in feed resulted in shortening of villi and morphological effects [21]. In contrast, our results showed piglets fed up to 3.80 ppm DON-contaminated feed had reduced ADG and a tendency towards reduced ADFI relative to the control pigs that were exposed to up to 0.40 ppm DON, but only in the last days of the trial. The jejunum and ileum showed no significant changes in villous or crypt architecture between our control and DON-fed groups. We speculate that the low level DON contamination in the control diet may have had an impact on the gut, which makes it difficult to observe a difference between this diet and the treatment diet with 3.80 ppm DON.

How DON affects barrier function and specifically the proteins involved in TJ formation is unknown and results have been variable, possibly due to differences in experimental design, age of animals, amount of DON present, and duration of exposure. Using Ussing chambers to investigate jejunal tissues, it was determined that 2–3 month old pigs fed 4–8 mg/mL DON showed inhibited active transport of nutrient across the small intestinal wall [22]. Others [10] showed that 5-week old piglets fed 3 mg DON /kg feed for 35 days did not show significantly reduced weight but there was reduced adherent junction protein E-cadherin and the tight junction protein occludin in the intestine. Similarly, 4-week old piglets fed 0.9 mg DON/kg feed for 10 days showed reduced mRNA expression of occludin in the intestine [9]. Immunohistochemistry of the jejunum by Pinton et al. (2009) showed that 5 week old piglets fed 2.85 mg DON/kg feed had a 40% decrease of Claudin-4 expression (which was more pronounced in the villi) in samples from DON exposed animals when compared with controls animals [18]. Together, these studies suggest that DON exposure impacts expression of select TJ proteins and barrier function. Our research showed that piglets fed 3.80 ppm DON-contaminated feed starting at weaning for 24 days showed significantly reduced mRNA expression for only CLDN-7 in the ileum (but not for CLDN-1, -2, -3, -4, -6, -10, -23 or OCLN or ZO1) compared to piglets fed the control diet. However, the surface localization of CLDN-1, -3, -4 and -7 (as analyzed by immunohistofluorescence) did not show a difference in the villi or the crypts of jejunal or ileal tissues, regardless of the diet. Consequently, we speculate that any alteration in the intestinal architecture induced by both low level DON exposure (control diet) and higher-level DON exposure may be largely ameliorated over time.

The effect of DON on the piglet immune system in the gut is also unknown and variable results are described in the literature. An in vivo study showed that feeding 2.2–2.5 mg/kg DON-contaminated diet to pigs (starting weight approx. 11 kg) for 5 weeks had no notable effect on the mRNA expression of TGF-β, IFN-γ, IL-4 and IL-6 in the ileum [11]. In contrast, Becker et al showed that piglets (11.4 kg) fed 1.2 mg DON/kg for 41 days and then 2 mg DON/kg feed for 42 days responded with down-regulation in the expression of IL-1β, IL-8 and TNFα in the blood and down-regulation of IL-1β and IL-8 in the ileum [12]. This result again conflicts with another study where 4-week old piglets fed 0.9 mg/kg DON for 10 days had increased expression of IL-10 and IL-1β genes in the duodenum but expression was slightly down-regulated in the jejunum compared to piglets fed a control diet [9]. Others showed that 5-week old piglets fed a diet artificially contaminated with DON (3 mg/kg) for 35 days did not significantly modulate animal weight but they did result in significant upregulation of immune response genes IL-1β, IL-2, IL-6, IL-12p40 and MIP-1β in the jejunum and a significant induction of the expression of TNF-α, IL-1β and IL-6 in the ileum revealing the presence of active inflammation in the intestine [10]. Consistent with our results, Lessard et al., 2015 showed that 4-week-old piglets fed control diet or diet contaminated with 3.5 mg DON/kg did not show altered mRNA expression levels of proinflammatory cytokines IL1β, IL10, IL12β, and TNF-α in intestinal tissues [23]. In contrast to our study, they showed that pigs fed DON diet had significant up-regulated IFNγ and IL-8 in the ileum compared to control group [23] whereas our data shows that IL-8 showed a trend towards increased expression in DON-fed piglets in ileum after 7 days relative to the control diet fed piglets ($p < 0.0535$). IL-8 is a pro-inflammatory cytokine, which transmits the danger signals to the underlying local antigen-presenting cells and lymphocytes in the gut tissue. Together, these studies may suggest that the duration of DON exposure, as well as the dose and age of initial exposure, may significantly affect the modulation of genes regulating intestinal immune function.

4. Conclusions

This study indicates that feeding weaner piglets a diet with a high level of DON contamination (3.30 to 3.80 ppm) resulted in only modest effects on piglet gut health, immune response and body weight, compared to a diet with 0.20 to 0.40 ppm. With the exception of serum cytokine levels, the majority of the molecular analysis in the present study was performed on tissue collected at the end of a dietary treatment period, and as such the effect of DON on other molecular physiology in the acute period is not known. Our results do however suggest that if such an early effect occurred, subsequent compensatory mechanisms were capable of re-establishing intestinal homeostasis. It may, therefore be necessary to evaluate slow introduction of DON-contaminated feed to allow animal sufficient time to adapt without a negative impact on growth and performance.

5. Materials and Methods

5.1. Animal Care and Selection

All animals used in these experiments were cared for and monitored according to Prairie Swine Centre, Inc.'s (Saskatoon, SK, Canada) Standard Operating Procedures and the experiment was approved by the University of Saskatchewan Animal Research Ethics Board (Protocol #20130054) for adherence to guidelines outlined by the Canadian Council on Animal Care (2009). Date of approval: 8 March 2016.

A total of 24 newly weaned pigs (Camborough Plus x C3378; PIC Canada Ltd., Winnipeg, MB, Canada) were used for this experiment over 4 blocks (12 pigs/treatment). Piglets were weaned at 21 ± 2 (mean $\pm$ SD) days of age and 5.89 ± 0.33 kg body weight from sows consuming a commercial lactation diet (Prairie Swine Centre, Inc, Saskatoon, SK, Canada). Upon weaning pigs were placed on a common commercial starter diet for the first 3 d. The pigs were checked twice daily for any signs of ill health. On d 4 post-weaning, pigs were moved to metabolic crates (1.5×1.5 m) with plastic-coated, expanded metal floors, polyvinyl chloride walls (0.9 m high) and Plexiglas windows (0.3×0.3 m). Pigs were housed individually and remained in the metabolic crates for the duration of the study. Each pen had a bowl drinker and a single-spaced dry feeder providing *ad libitum* access to water and feed. Lights were on from 07:00 h to 19:00 h. The initial room temperature of 26 °C was decreased to 24 °C after 2 weeks and this temperature was maintained for the following 3 weeks.

5.2. Dietary Treatments and Preparation

Pigs were randomly assigned to 1 of the 2 dietary treatments within each block in a randomized complete block design. Diets were wheat and barley-based and were formulated based on a 3-phase feeding program to meet or exceed nutrient requirements according to NRC (2012). Pigs were fed a control diet formulated to contain 0 mg/kg DON or treatment diets formulated to contain 4 mg/kg DON (Table 3).

Phase I was fed for the first 4 days, phase II for the subsequent 2 weeks and phase III for 4 days. The DON-contaminated diet was produced by replacing clean wheat with an amount of DON-contaminated wheat to achieve a final concentration of 4 mg/kg feed. The DON-contaminated wheat was obtained from a single contaminated field in Saskatchewan, Canada. The DON content of the wheat was concentrated by sorting with a BoMill TriQ (BoMill AB, Vintrie, Sweden) NIR seed sorter which produces a wheat fraction with highly consistent level of DON contamination (Kautzman et al., 2015). DON content was determined using HPLC-tandem MS at Prairie Diagnostic Services (Saskatoon, SK, Canada). The mycotoxin composition of DON wheat used for the study is described in Table 4. Samples of each diet were obtained throughout the feeding trial and a composite sample was analyzed (Central Testing Laboratory in Winnipeg, Winnipeg, MB, Canada) for moisture (AOAC 930.15), dry matter, crude protein (AOAC 990.03), Ca (AOAC 968.08), P (AOAC 968.08), Na (AOAC 968.08), NDF (ANKOM) and DON (ELISA DON-V, Vicam, Nixa, MO, USA. 65714).

Table 3. Ingredient composition (%, as-fed) and calculated and analyzed nutrient content of experimental diets.

Ingredient	Phase I		Phase II		Phase III	
	Control Diet	DON-Contaminated Diet	Control Diet	DON-Contaminated Diet	Control Diet	DON-Contaminated Diet
Wheat (clean)	58.1	20.3	42.6	4.3	44.4	6.2
Wheat (DON)	-	34.8	-	34.8	-	34.8
Soybean meal	22.0	25.0	21.0	24.6	18.6	22.1
Barley	-	-	27.9	27.9	31.9	31.9
Whey	11.4	11.4	-	-	-	-
Fish meal	3.9	3.9	3.2	3.2	-	-
Canola oil	1.9	1.9	2.4	2.4	2.0	2.0
Limestone	1.05	1.05	1.30	1.30	1.55	1.55
Salt	0.40	0.40	0.40	0.40	0.40	0.40
L-Lys, HCl	0.615	0.568	0.573	0.508	0.637	0.575
DL-Met	0.125	0.180	0.105	0.105	0.050	0.050
L-Thr	0.180	0.125	0.175	0.175	0.130	0.130
L-Trp	0.057	0.057	0.004	0.004	0.021	0.021
Choline chloride	0.08	0.08	0.08	0.08	0.08	0.08
Copper sulfate	0.04	0.04	0.04	0.04	0.04	0.04
Vit/min premix [1]	0.20	0.20	0.20	0.20	0.20	0.20
Calculated nutrient content						
DM (%)	88.7	88.8	87.6	87.7	87.8	87.9
CP (%)	23.5	23.1	22.1	21.8	19.7	19.4
ME (kcal/kg)	3323	3323	3270	3273	3225	3228
Lys (% SID)	1.50	1.50	1.35	1.35	1.23	1.23
Ca (%)	0.73	0.74	0.72	0.73	0.66	0.67
P (%)	0.58	0.59	0.51	0.52	0.42	0.43
DON (ppm)	0.00	4.00	0.00	4.00	0.00	4.00
Analyzed nutrient content						
DM (%)	89.2	89.2	89.5	89.2	89.1	89.4
CP (%)	22.4	23.4	21.8	22.7	19.6	20.8
Ca (%)	0.80	0.88	0.82	1.00	0.86	0.94
P (%)	0.61	0.61	0.53	0.51	0.45	0.46
DON (ppm)	0.30	3.30	0.20	3.80	0.40	3.80

DM, dry matter; ME, metabolizable energy; CP, crude protein. [1] Provided per kg of complete diet: Vitamin A, 12,000 IU/kg; Vitamin D 1500 IU/kg; Vitamin E, 70 IU/kg); menadione, 5 mg/kg; Vitamin B12, 0.04 mg/kg; thiamine, 2 mg/kg; biotin, 0.2 mg/kg; niacin, 40 mg/kg; riboflavin, 8 mg/kg; pantothenate, 24 mg/kg; folic acid, 1 mg/kg; pyridoxine, 10 mg/kg; Fe, 150 mg/kg, Zn, 150 mg/kg; Mg, 40 mg/kg; Cu, 20 mg/kg; Se, 0.3 mg/kg; I, 1 mg/kg.

Table 4. Mycotoxin content of DON-contaminated wheat [1].

Mycotoxin	Level (ppb) [2]
Deoxynivalenol	11,470
3-acetyl-deoxynivalenol	763.9
15-acetyl-deoxynivalenol	<25.0
α-zearalenol	<66.0
Diacetoxyscirpenol	<25.0
HT-2 toxin	107
Nivalenol	59.2
Ochratoxin A	<25.0
T-2 toxin	<25.0
β-zearalenol	<66.0
Zeralenone	<25.0
Aflatoxin B1	<25.0

[1] Analyzed by HPLC/MS (Prairie Diagnostic Services, Inc., Saskatoon, SK, Canada). [2] Values of <25.0 and <66.0 indicates mycotoxin was below limit of detection.

Analyzed DON concentrations were 0.3, 0.2 and 0.4 mg/kg for the control diets for Phase I, II and III, and 3.3, 3.8 and 3.8 for the contaminated diets for Phase I, II and III, respectively. This level of variation among diets is typically observed in trials similar to this and attributed to sampling.

5.3. Animal Sampling and Weight Calculations

Body weight and feed intake (adjusted for wastage) were determined on day 0, 4, 7, 14, 21, and 24 of the study for the calculation of ADG and ADFI. Blood samples were obtained via jugular venipuncture on d 3, 7, 14, 21, and 25 for the determination of serum cytokine levels (IFN-γ, TNF-α, IL-1β, Il-6, IL-8, IL-10, IL-13) as a measure of overall immune status. On d 25, pigs were euthanized via non-penetrating captive bolt followed by exsanguination. Tissues were obtained from the small intestine (jejunum and ileum). Jejunum was defined as the mid-point of the small intestine and the ileum was defined as 1 m from the ileo-caecal junction.

5.4. Histology and Immunohistoflourescence

Two samples of gut tissue were obtained per site and stored in 10% neutral buffered formalin or snap frozen in dry ice and stored at $-20\,^\circ$C until further analysis. Tissue sections were fixed in 10% neutral buffered formalin for 36 h prior to processing and paraffin embedding. Samples were sectioned at 0.4 μm and mounted on slides (Superfrost Plus, ThermoFisher Scientific, Burlington, ON, Canada), deparaffinized in xylene and rehydrated to distilled water through decreasing concentrations of ethanol.

For histology, tissues were stained with hematoxylin and eosin following standard procedures. Villous height and width were measured and crypt depth was recorded for representative images (data not shown).

For immunohistofluorescence, heat-induced antigen retrieval was carried out in Tris-EDTA buffer (10 mM Tris, 1 mM EDTA Solution, 0.05% Tween 20, pH 9.0) for 30 min at 90 $^\circ$C prior to blocking in 5% (*w/v*) skim milk in PBS for 3hrs at room temperature. Immunohistofluorescent staining was carried out on two non-concurrent tissue sections from each sample with either 1:100 rabbit αCLDN1 (ab15098), 1:200 rabbit αCLDN3 (ab15102), 1:400 dilution of rabbit αCLDN4 (ab53156) or 1 in 200 rabbit αCLDN7 (ab27487). Primary antibodies were diluted in an incubation buffer consisting of 1% *w/v* BSA, 1% *v/v* Donkey Serum, 0.5% *v/v* triton X-100 in PBS and samples stained over night at 4 $^\circ$C. Slides were then washed three times in PBS and incubated in a 1:400 dilution of Alexa555-conjugated goat α rabbit IgG (ab150082) in incubation buffer for 4 hrs at room temperature. Slides were again washed before counter staining in 0.5 μg/mL DAPI in methanol for 10 min at room temperature prior to cover slipping with Mowiol. Imaging was carried out on an Axiovert 200 M with a 63X neoFluor objective (Zeiss, Oberkochen, Germany) under oil immersion, with a minimum of 4 representative images captured of both the intestinal villi and crypt. Fluorescent images had their background fluorescence subtracted using ImageJ [24].

5.5. Bioplex Cytokine Assays

Bioplex bead coupling was performed as per the manufacturer's instructions. The reagents are listed in Table 5. The multiplex assay was carried out in a 96 well Grenier Bio-One Fluotrac 200 96F black (VWR, #82050-754), which allows washing and retention of the Luminex beads. The 5 beadsets conjugated with the capture antibodies were vortexed for 30 s followed by sonication for another 30 s to ensure total bead dispersal. Bead density was 1200 beads per μl in PBS-BN (1x PBSA pH 7.4 + 1% BSA (Sigma-Aldrich A7030) + 0.05% sodium azide (Sigma-Aldrich, Oakville, ON, Canada). One μL of each beadset was added to 45 μL of diluent (PBSA + 1% New Zealand Pig Serum (Sigma-Aldrich P3484) + 0.05% sodium azide), which was added to each well. The plate was then washed using the Bio-Plex Pro II Wash Station (BioRad, Mississauga, ON, Canada; wash 2 X 100 μL PBST). The porcine IL1β, porcine IL8, porcine IL13, porcine TNFα and porcine IFNγ protein standards were added to the wells at 50 μL per well at a starting concentration of 5000 pg/mL, 200 pg/mL, 5000 pg/mL, 5000 pg/mL and 5000 pg/mL respectively with 2.5 fold dilutions done to produce the standard curve. Sera were pre-diluted 1:4 in diluent and added to the wells at 50 μL per well.

Table 5. Bio-Plex cytokine information for detection of pig proinflammatory cytokines in sera.

Cytokine	Capture Antibody; Supplier	Detection Antibody; Supplier; Dilution	Standard; Supplier; Initial Concentration	Bead; Supplier
IL1β	MAb anti porc IL1β/IF2; R & D MAB6811	Goat anti porc IL1β/IF2 biotin; R & D BAF681; 0.5 µg/mL	recombinant porc IL1β/IF2; R & D 681-PI-10; 5000 pg/mL	Region 26; BioRad MC10026-01
IL8	MAb anti sheep IL8 (86.9% homology); AbD Serotec MCA1660	MAb anti porc CXCL8/IL8; R & D MAB5351; biotinylated in house; 1/400 dilution	Recombinant porc IL-8; Kingfisher RP0109S-005; 200 pg/mL	Region 27; BioRad MC10027-01
IL13	Goat anti swine IL-13; Kingfisher PB0094S-100	Goat anti swine IL-13 biotin; Kingfisher PBB0096S-050; 0.5 µg/mL	Recombinant swine IL-13; Kingfisher RP0007S-005; 5000 pg/mL	Region 52 ; BioRad MC10052-01
TNFα	MAb anti porcine TNFα; R&D MAB6902	Goat anti porcine TNF α biotin; R & D BAF690; 0.5 µg/mL	Recombinant porcine TNFα; R & D 690-PT-025; 5000 pg/mL	Region 34; BioRad MC10034-01
IFNγ	MAb anti-porcine IFNγ; Fisher ENMP700	MAb anti-porc IFNγ; Fisher ENPP700; biotinylated in-house; 1/400 dilution	Recombinant porcine IFNγ; Ceiba Geigy (gift); 2000 pg/mL	Region 43; BioRad MC10043-01

The plate was sealed with plate sealer (ThermoFisher Scientific, #12565491) and covered with a foil lid. The plate was agitated at 800 rpm for 1 h at room temperature. After 1 h incubation with serum, the plate was washed (3 × 150 µL PBST). Fifty µl of a biotin cocktail consisting of commercially purchased biotins each at 0.5 µg/mL, in house biotinylated anti IL8 at 1/500 and in house biotinylated anti IFNγ at 1/400 was added to each well. The plate was again sealed, covered and agitated at 800 rpm for 30 min at room temperature then washed again as indicated above. Fifty µL of Streptavidin RPE (ProZyme (Cedarlane) PJRS20, Burlington, ON, Canada); diluted to 5 µg/mL) was added to each well. The plate was again sealed, covered and agitated at 800 rpm for 30 min at room temperature and washed as indicated above. A 100 µL of 1x Tris-EDTA was added to each well and then the plate was vortexed for 5 min before reading on the BioRad BioPlex 2000 instrument following the manufacturer's instructions as described in (Anderson et al., 2011). The instrument was configured to read beadsets in regions 26, 27, 34, 43, and 52 for IL1β, IL8, TNFα, IFNγ and IL13, respectively. A minimum of 60 events per beadset were read and the median value obtained for each reaction event per beadset. For all samples the multiplex assay MFI data was corrected by subtracting the background levels. The lower limit of detection for each cytokine was 32 pg/mL for IFNγ, 80 pg/mL for IL1β and IL-13, 8 pg/mL for IL-8 and 200 pg/mL for TNFα.

5.6. Quantitative Gene Expression Analysis

We reduced the number of animals used in the molecular portion of this experiment to allow a greater number of targets to be assessed with both qPCR and by IHF. Animals used for molecular assessment were selected randomly from each of the 4 experimental batches. Jejunal and Ileal tissues samples were ground with mortar and pestle to a fine powder under liquid nitrogen. Total RNA was then extracted using Trizol (Life Technologies, Carlsbad, CA, USA) as per the manufacturer's directions. DNA contamination was removed using the TURBO DNA-free kit (Life Technologies) before RNA quantity was determined on a NanoDrop spectrophotometer ND-1000 (NanoDrop, Wilmington, DE, USA). RNA integrity was then evaluated on a 1.2% (*w/v*) denaturing agarose gel to verify a clear ribosomal RNA banding pattern. Reverse transcription (RT) was done on 2 µg of total RNA using the High Capacity cDNA Reverse Transcription Kit (Life Technologies) before diluting to a final concentration of 10 ng/µL equivalent cDNA. Quantitative real-time polymerase chain reaction (qPCR) was then carried out, in duplicate, using 20 ng of equivalent cDNA, Kappa SYBR fast mastermix (Kapa Biosystems, Wilmington, MA USA) and a primer concentration of 0.75 µM on a Step-One-Plus real time system (Life Technologies, (ThermoFisher Scientific)). Real time primer sets for each gene of interest were designed against RefSeq data obtained from NCBI (Table 6). Where possible, primers were designed to span exon-exon junctions as identified by BLAST Like Alignment Tool (BLAT) comparison with SusScrofa10.2 genomic build. The PCR efficiency for each primer probe set was evaluated against a serial dilution of pooled samples, and found to be greater than 95% for targets. Finally, the data was normalized to the geometric mean of four stable housekeeping genes (ACTB, B2MI, HPRT and RPL19). Data are presented in the form of fold change ($2^{-\Delta\Delta Ct}$) relative to the control group within tissue.

5.7. Statistics

Growth performance data was analyzed using the MIXED procedure of the SAS statistical program (SAS 9.4, SAS Institute Inc., Cary, NC, USA). Treatment and block were included as fixed effects, pig was included as a random effect, and data were analyzed as repeated measures. The optimal variance structure was determined using the fit statistics within SAS. Differences were between means were determined using the Tukey test and considered statistically significant at $p \leq 0.05$. A trend towards significant was considered at $p < 0.10$. Statistical analysis of gene expression and serum cytokine results was carried out with a nonparametric Kruskal-Wallis examining preselected comparison of means of the treatment vs. control within tissue or sera or across time.

Table 6. Target, source and primer-specific information for qPCR analysis in piglet gut tissue.

Target	Source	Forward Primer	Reverse Primer	Amplicon Length (bp)	Annealing Temp (°C)
Actin B	Nygard et al., 2007	5′-CACGCCATCCTGCGTCTGGA-3′	5′-AGCACCGTGTTGGCGTAGAG-3′	100	63
ALOX5	XM_001927671.3	5′-TGGCTTCCCCTTGAGTATTG-3′	5′-CAGGTTCTCCATCGCTTTTG-3′	118	62
ALOX5AP	NM_001164001.1	5′-TCGAGCACGAAAGCAAGAC-3′	5′-CACAGTTCTGTTGGCAGTG-3′	93	60
B2MI	Nygard et al., 2007	5′-CAAGATAGTTAAGTGGGATCG-AGAC-3′	5′-TCGTAACATCAATACGATTI-CTGA-3′	161	58
CLDN1	NM_001244539.1	5′-TCCTTGCTGAATCTGAACACC-3′	5′-ACACTTCATGCCAACAGTGG-3′	108	60
CLDN2	NM_001161638.1	5′-CGTTGCGTGGAATCTTCAT-3′	5′-GGGAGAACACGGAGGAAATG-3′	119	60
CLDN3	NM_001160075.1	5′-GCCAAAGCCAAGATCCTCTAC-3′	5′-AGCATCTGGGTGGACTGGT-3′	190	60
CLDN4	NM_001161637.1	5′-CAACTCGTGGATGATGAGA-3′	5′-CCAGGCGGATTGTAGAAGTCG-3′	140	62
CLDN6	NM_001161645.1	5′-CTTCATCGGCAACAGCATC-3′	5′-CAGCAGCGAGTCATACACCT-3′	112	60
CLDN7	NM_001160076.1	5′-ATCGTGGCAGGTCTTTGTG-3′	5′-CTCACTCCCAGGACAAGAGC-3′	192	60
CLDN8	NM_001161646.1	5′-GGAGTGCTCTTCGTCCTCAC-3′	5′-CTGCCGTCCAGCCTATGTA-3′	148	62
CLDN10	NM_001243444.1	5′-GCCCTGTTTGGAATGAAATG-3′	5′-AGCACAGCCCTGCACGTATG-3′	103	62
CLDN14	NM_001161642.1	5′-ACGCCTACAAGGACAATCG-3′	5′-AATGAACTCGGTGTGGGAAC-3′	168	62
CLDN23	NM_001159778.1	5′-TGTCTGGCTGAAGGACTCG-3′	5′-CCACAGGAAAGAAGGTCAC-3′	112	60
IL1b	NM_001005149	5′-AGAAGAGCCCATCGTCCTTG-3′	5′-GAGAGCCTTCAGCTCATGTG-3′	139	62
IL6	NM_214399	5′-ATCAGGAGACCTGCTTGATG-3′	5′-TGGTGGCTTTGTCTGGATTC-3′	177	60
IL8	NM_213867	5′-TCCTGCTTTCTGCAGCTCTC-3′	5′-GGGTGGAAAGGTGTGGAATG-3′	100	62
IL10	NM_214041	5′-GGTTGCCAAGCCTTGTCAG-3′	5′-AGGCACTCTTCACCTCCTC-3′	202	60
LTA4H	NM_001185132.1	5′-CTGGGAAGGAACACCCCTAT-3′	5′-GGGACAGACACCTCTGCACT-3′	118	60
LTC4S	XM_0031236454.4	5′-CTACCGAGCCCAAGTAAACTG-3′	5′-GCGTGCGTACAGGTAGATGA-3′	124	60
OCCLN	NM_001163647.2	5′-GAGTACATCGCTCGCTGCTGA-3′	5′-TTTGCTCTTCAACTGCTTGC-3′	102	62
TLR2	NM_213761	5′-ACGGACTGTGGTGCATGAAG-3′	5′-GGACACGAAAGCGTCATAGC-3′	101	62
TLR4	NM_001113039	5′-TGTGCCGTGTGAACACCAGAC-3′	5′-AGGTGCCGTTCCTGAAACTC-3′	136	60
TNFa	NM_214022	5′-CCAATGGCAGAGTGGGTATG-3′	5′-TGAAGAGGACCTGGGAGTAG-3′	116	60
ZO1	XM_003353439.2	5′-ACGGCGAAGGTAATTCAGTG-3′	5′-CTTCTCGGTTTGGTGTCTCTG-3′	111	62
GAPDH	AF017079	5′-CTTCACGACCATGGAGAAGG-3′	5′-CCAAGCAGTTGGTGGTACAG-3′	170	63
HPRT	Nygard et al., 2007	5′-GGACTTGAATCATGTTTGTG-3′	5′-CAGATGTTTCCAAACTCAAC-3′	91	60
RPL19	AF_435591	5′-AACTCCCGTCAGCAGATCC-3′	5′-AGTACCCTTCCGCTTACCG-3′	147	60
SDHA	Nygard et al., 2007	5′-CTACAAGGCGCAGGTTCTGA-3′	5′-AAGACAACGAGGTCCAGGAG-3′	141	58

Supplementary Materials: The following are available online at www.mdpi.com/2072-6651/10/1/40/s1, Figure S1: Claudin-1 surface localization in piglet ileal villi and crypts in DON-fed and control fed piglets, Figure S2: Claudin-3 surface localization in piglet ileal villi and crypts in DON-fed and control fed piglets, Figure S3: Claudin-4 surface localization in piglet ileal villi and crypts in DON-fed and control fed piglets, Figure S4: Claudin-7 surface localization in piglet ileal villi and crypts in DON-fed and control fed piglets, Figure S5: Claudin-1 surface localization in piglet jejunal villi and crypts in DON-fed and control fed piglets, Figure S6: Claudin-3 surface localization in piglet jejunal villi and crypts in DON-fed and control fed piglets, Figure S7: Claudin-4 surface localization in piglet jejunal villi and crypts in DON-fed and control fed piglets, Figure S8: Claudin-7 surface localization in piglet jejunal villi and crypts in DON-fed and control fed piglets.

Acknowledgments: The authors acknowledge and thank the skill and support of animal care staff at the Prairie Swine Center. Heather L. Wilson is an adjunct professor at the Department of Veterinary Microbiology in the Western College of Veterinary Medicine as well as the School of Public Health at the University of Saskatchewan. Daniel A. Columbus is an adjunct professor and A. Denise Beaulieu is an assistant professor in the Department of Animal and Poultry Science, the College of Agriculture and Bioresources at the University of Saskatchewan. This paper is published with the permission of the Director of VIDO as journal series No. 827. Sources of financial support: J. Alex Pasternak is supported by fellowships from the Natural Sciences and Engineering Research Council of Canada (NSERC) and the Saskatchewan Health Research Foundation (3632). The authors gratefully acknowledge the financial support from the Saskatchewan Agriculture Development Fund (20130162; Saskatchewan Ministry of Agriculture and the Canada-Saskatchewan Growing Forward bilateral agreement) to A. Denise Beaulieu and an NSERC Discovery Grant (RGPIN 06437-2015) to Heather L. Wilson.

Author Contributions: J.A.P. performed the extensive histology, immunohistofluorescence, and PCR analysis, assisted in the collection of animal tissues and contributed to the first draft of the manuscript. V.I.A.A., D.A.C. and A.D.B. performed the study and the performance analysis, G.H. performed the Bioplex analysis, A.D.B. and D.A.C. conceived of the study and directed the nutritional analysis, and H.L.W. wrote the manuscript. All authors edited the later draft of the manuscript.

Conflicts of Interest: The authors have no conflict of interest to report.

References

1. Pierron, A.; Alassane-Kpembi, I.; Oswald, I.P. Impact of two mycotoxins deoxynivalenol and fumonisin on pig intestinal health. *Porcine Health Manag.* **2016**, *2*, 21. [CrossRef] [PubMed]

2. Prelusky, D.B. A study on the effect of deoxynivalenol on serotonin receptor binding in pig brain membranes. *J. Environ. Sci. Health B* **1996**, *31*, 1103–1117. [CrossRef] [PubMed]

3. House, J.D.; Abramson, D.; Crow, G.H.; Nyachoti, C.M. Feed intake, growth and carcass parameters of swine consuming diets containing low levels of deoxynivalenol from naturally contaminated barley. *Can. J. Anim. Sci.* **2002**, *82*, 559–565. [CrossRef]

4. Goyarts, T.; Dänicke, S. Effects of deoxynivalenol (DON) on growth performance, nutrient digestibility and DON metabolism in pigs. *Mycotoxin Res.* **2005**, *21*, 139–142. [CrossRef] [PubMed]

5. Swamy, H.V.; Smith, T.K.; MacDonald, E.J.; Boermans, H.J.; Squires, E.J. Effects of feeding a blend of grains naturally contaminated with *Fusarium* mycotoxins on swine performance, brain regional neurochemistry, and serum chemistry and the efficacy of a polymeric glucomannan mycotoxin adsorbent. *J. Anim. Sci.* **2002**, *80*, 3257–3267. [CrossRef] [PubMed]

6. Charmley, L.L.; Trenholme, H.L. RG-8 Regulatory Guidance: Contaminants in Feed. Canadian Food Inspection Agency. Available online: http://www.inspection.gc.ca/animals/feeds/regulatory-guidance/rg-8/eng/1347383943203/1347384015909 (accessed on 8 January 2018).

7. FDA. Guidance for Industry and FDAi Advisory Levels for Deoxynivalenol (DON) in Finished Wheat Products for Human Consumption and Grains and Grain By-Products Used for Animal Feed. 2010. Available online: http://www.fda.gov/downloads/Food/GuidanceRegulation/UCM217558.pdf (accessed on 8 January 2018).

8. Commission_Recommendation. On the presence of deoxynivalenol, zearalenone, ochratoxin A, T-2 and HT-2 and fumonisins in products intended for animal feeding (2006/576/EC). *J. Eur. Union* **2006**. Available online: http://eur-lex.europa.eu/legal-content/EN/TXT/?uri=CELEX%3A32006H0576 (accessed on 8 January 2018).

9. Alizadeh, A.; Braber, S.; Akbari, P.; Garssen, J.; Fink-Gremmels, J. Deoxynivalenol Impairs Weight Gain and Affects Markers of Gut Health after Low-Dose, Short-Term Exposure of Growing Pigs. *Toxins* **2015**, *7*, 2071–2095. [CrossRef] [PubMed]

10. Bracarense, A.-P.F.L.; Lucioli, J.; Grenier, B.; Drociunas Pacheco, G.; Moll, W.-D.; Schatzmayr, G.; Oswald, I.P. Chronic ingestion of deoxynivalenol and fumonisin, alone or in interaction, induces morphological and immunological changes in the intestine of piglets. *Br. J. Nutr.* **2012**, *107*, 1776–1786. [CrossRef] [PubMed]

11. Pinton, P.; Accensi, F.; Beauchamp, E.; Cossalter, A.-M.; Callu, P.; Grosjean, F.; Oswald, I.P. Ingestion of deoxynivalenol (DON) contaminated feed alters the pig vaccinal immune responses. *Toxicol. Lett.* **2008**, *177*, 215–222. [CrossRef] [PubMed]

12. Becker, C.; Reiter, M.; Pfaffl, M.W.; Meyer, H.H.D.; Bauer, J.; Meyer, K.H.D. Expression of immune relevant genes in pigs under the influence of low doses of deoxynivalenol (DON). *Mycotoxin Res.* **2011**, *27*, 287–293. [CrossRef] [PubMed]

13. Anderson, J.M.; Van Itallie, C.M. Tight junctions and the molecular basis for regulation of paracellular permeability. *Am. J. Physiol.* **1995**, *269 Pt 1*, G467–G475. [CrossRef] [PubMed]

14. Schneeberger, E.E.; Lynch, R.D. The tight junction: A multifunctional complex. *Am. J. Physiol. Cell Physiol.* **2004**, *286*, C1213–C1228. [CrossRef] [PubMed]

15. Tsukita, S.; Furuse, M.; Itoh, M. Multifunctional strands in tight junctions. *Nat. Rev. Mol. Cell Biol.* **2001**, *2*, 285–293. [CrossRef] [PubMed]

16. Berkes, J.; Viswanathan, V.K.; Savkovic, S.D.; Hecht, G. Intestinal epithelial responses to enteric pathogens: Effects on the tight junction barrier, ion transport, and inflammation. *Gut* **2003**, *52*, 439–451. [CrossRef] [PubMed]

17. Furuse, M.; Fujita, K.; Hiiragi, T.; Fujimoto, K.; Tsukita, S. Claudin-1 and -2: Novel integral membrane proteins localizing at tight junctions with no sequence similarity to occludin. *J. Cell Biol.* **1998**, *141*, 1539–1550. [CrossRef] [PubMed]

18. Pinton, P.; Nougayrede, J.P.; Del Rio, J.C.; Moreno, C.; Marin, D.E.; Ferrier, L.; Bracarense, A.P.; Kolf-Clauw, M.; Oswald, I.P. The food contaminant deoxynivalenol, decreases intestinal barrier permeability and reduces claudin expression. *Toxicol. Appl. Pharmacol.* **2009**, *237*, 41–48. [CrossRef] [PubMed]

19. Rodriguez-Lagunas, M.J.; Storniolo, C.E.; Ferrer, R.; Moreno, J.J. 5-Hydroxyeicosatetraenoic acid and leukotriene D4 increase intestinal epithelial paracellular permeability. *Int. J. Biochem. Cell Biol.* **2013**, *45*, 1318–1326. [CrossRef] [PubMed]

20. Kolf-Clauw, M.; Castellote, J.; Joly, B.; Bourges-Abella, N.; Raymond-Letron, I.; Pinton, P.; Oswald, I.P. Development of a pig jejunal explant culture for studying the gastrointestinal toxicity of the mycotoxin deoxynivalenol: Histopathological analysis. *Toxicol. In Vitro* **2009**, *23*, 1580–1584. [CrossRef] [PubMed]

21. Pinton, P.; Tsybulskyy, D.; Lucioli, J.; Laffitte, J.; Callu, P.; Lyazhri, F.; Grosjean, F.; Bracarense, A.P.; Kolf-Clauw, M.; Oswald, I.P. Toxicity of deoxynivalenol and its acetylated derivatives on the intestine: differential effects on morphology, barrier function, tight junction proteins, and mitogen-activated protein kinases. *Toxicol. Sci.* **2012**, *130*, 180–190. [CrossRef] [PubMed]

22. Halawa, A.; Danicke, S.; Kersten, S.; Breves, G. Effects of deoxynivalenol and lipopolysaccharide on electrophysiological parameters in growing pigs. *Mycotoxin Res.* **2012**, *28*, 243–252. [CrossRef] [PubMed]

23. Lessard, M.; Savard, C.; Deschene, K.; Lauzon, K.; Pinilla, V.A.; Gagnon, C.A.; Lapointe, J.; Guay, F.; Chorfi, Y. Impact of deoxynivalenol (DON) contaminated feed on intestinal integrity and immune response in swine. *Food Chem. Toxicol.* **2015**, *80*, 7–16. [CrossRef] [PubMed]

24. Schneider, C.A.; Rasband, W.S.; Eliceiri, K.W. NIH Image to ImageJ: 25 years of image analysis. *Nat. Methods* **2012**, *9*, 671–675. [CrossRef] [PubMed]

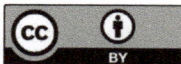

toxins

MDPI

Article

The Effects of Deoxynivalenol and Zearalenone on the Pig Large Intestine. A Light and Electron Microscopy Study

**Barbara Przybylska-Gornowicz [1],*, Bogdan Lewczuk [1], Magdalena Prusik [1],
Maria Hanuszewska [1], Marcela Petrusewicz-Kosińska [1], Magdalena Gajęcka [2],
Łukasz Zielonka [2] and Maciej Gajęcki [2]**

[1] Department of Histology and Embryology, Faculty of Veterinary Medicine, University of Warmia and Mazury in Olsztyn, Oczapowskiego 13, 10-719 Olsztyn, Poland; lewczukb@uwm.edu.pl (B.L.); mprusik@gmail.com (M.P.); marysia-h@wp.pl (M.H.); marcelapetrusewicz@wp.pl (M.P.-K.)

[2] Department of Veterinary Prevention and Feed Hygiene, Faculty of Veterinary Medicine, University of Warmia and Mazury in Olsztyn, Oczapowskiego 13, 10-719 Olsztyn, Poland; mgaja@uwm.edu.pl (M.G.); lukaszz@uwm.edu.pl (Ł.Z.); gajecki@uwm.edu.pl (M.G.)

* Correspondence: przybyl@uwm.edu.pl; Tel.: +48-89-523-39-49; Fax: +48-89-523-34-40

Received: 28 February 2018; Accepted: 2 April 2018; Published: 4 April 2018

Abstract: The contamination of feed with mycotoxins results in reduced growth, feed refusal, immunosuppression, and health problems. Deoxynivalenol (DON) and zearalenone (ZEN) are among the most important mycotoxins. The aim of the study was to examine the effects of low doses of these mycotoxins on the histological structure and ultrastructure of the large intestine in the pig. The study was performed on 36 immature gilts of mixed breed (White Polish Big × Polish White Earhanging), which were divided into four groups administrated per os with ZEN at 40 µg/kg BW, DON at 12 µg/kg BW, a mixture of ZEN (40 µg/kg BW) and DON (12 µg/kg BW) or a placebo. The pigs were killed by intravenous overdose of pentobarbital after one, three, and six weeks of treatment. The cecum, ascending and descending colon samples were prepared for light and electron microscopy. Administration of toxins did not influence the architecture of the mucosa and submucosa in the large intestine. ZEN and ZEN + DON significantly decreased the number of goblet cells in the cecum and descending colon. The mycotoxins changed the number of lymphocytes and plasma cells in the large intestine, which usually increased in number. However, this effect differed between the intestine segments and toxins. Mycotoxins induced some changes in the ultrastructure of the mucosal epithelium. They did not affect the expression of proliferative cell nuclear antigen and the intestinal barrier permeability. The obtained results indicate that mycotoxins especially ZEN may influence the defense mechanisms of the large intestine.

Keywords: mycotoxins; zearalenone; deoxynivalenol; histology; ultrastructure; large intestine; pig

Key contribution: Administration of mycotoxins decreases the amount of goblet cells and increases the number of lymphocytes and plasma cells in the large intestine. The large intestine should be considered as a place of mycotoxin action.

1. Introduction

Zearalenone (ZEN) and deoxynivalenol (DON) are mycotoxins produced by *Fusarium* fungi. Their wide distribution in nature and negative effects of consumption of food and feed contaminated with ZEN and DON for human and animal health mean that they have become a subject of extensive research [1]. The toxic outcome of these mycotoxins includes feed refusal, reduced growth, gastrointestinal lesions, immunosuppression, and reproductive disorders [2]. At the cellular level, ZEN and DON can negatively affect numerous pathways and processes. Many aspects of mycotoxins impacting on humans and animals especially in the case of mixed mycotoxicosis are still not fully recognized. Animal species show differential sensitivity to mycotoxins.

Deoxynivalenol (DON, IUPAC name: $(3\alpha,7\alpha)$-3,7,15-trihydroxy-12,13-epoxytrichothec-9-en-8-one) belongs to type B trichothecene mycotoxins and is the most commonly detected toxin of this group. DON in acute and moderate to low doses induces toxic and immuno-toxic effects in a variety of cell systems and animal species [3]. The differential susceptibility to DON in animal species evaluated to date presumably depends on differences in metabolism, absorption, distribution, and elimination of DON among animal species [4]. Pig is the most sensitive livestock species to DON. Absorption of DON in pigs is rapid and the toxin reaches peak plasma concentrations within 30 min of oral administration [5]. Results of Dänicke et al. [6] showed that, in pigs, a majority of the ingested DON is absorbed in the proximal part of the small intestine. In the large intestine, de-epoxidation takes place, which does not contribute much to detoxification. DON is primarily excreted in urine in free and conjugated forms and much smaller amounts of the toxin are excreted in feces as de-epoxidase and free forms [6,7]. Research provides evidence that the chronic ingestion of DON, also in low doses, alters the small intestine morphology affecting the mucosal epithelial cells and the villi [8–10]. DON modulates the immune responsiveness of the intestinal mucosa, the cytokine production, and the cross-talk between epithelial cells and the intestinal immune cells [11]. DON reduces the expression of the adherent junction protein and the tight junction protein in the small intestine [12]. In the large intestine, DON in a dosage of 1008 µg/kg of feed modified the local immune response by changing the expression of toll-like receptors [13].

Zearalenone (ZEN, IUPAC name: (3S,11E)-14,16-dihydroxy-3-methyl-3,4,5,6,9,10-hexahydro-1H-2-benzoxacyclotetradecine-1,7(8H)-dione) and its metabolites have estrogenic activity and compete with endogenous hormones for the binding sites of estrogen receptors [14]. ZEN also influences the activities of enzymes involved in steroid metabolism: 3-β-hydroxysteroid dehydrogenase type 1, cytochrome P450 side-chain cleavage enzyme, and P450 aromatase. Treatment with ZEN leads to precocious puberty, reproductive disorders, and hyperestrogenizm [15]. ZEN and its derivatives impair the inflammatory response and, therefore, may affect the capacity of organisms to both eradicate injurious stimuli and initiate the healing process [16]. The small intestine absorbs ZEN first so it is exposed to a high concentration of the toxin, which has the deleterious effect on its morphology even in the case of low doses [17,18]. In pig, the total biological recovery of ZEN in feces is about 34% ± 3% [19] and taking into account the slow passage of digestion in the large intestine ZEN can influence the structure and function of this part of the gastrointestinal tract as well. However, this aspect of ZEN intoxication has not been investigated.

The toxicity of mycotoxins needs to be addressed in the context of mycotoxins mixtures to assess health risks [20], however the effects of mycotoxin combination are poorly known. Existing data indicate that the type of interaction depends on the type of toxins, the ratio between toxins, and the concentration of the toxin mixture at a constant ratio [20,21].

In many cases, a diet contains DON and ZEN together [22]. However, the effects of concurrent exposition to these mycotoxins are still poorly recognized and difficult to predict [8,23]. So far, both additive and non-additive effects were found when DON and ZEN were administrated together [24]. DON + ZEN in combination were toxic on swine jejunal epithelial cells at concentrations nontoxic when administrated individually [20,24]. On the other hand, no additive effects of these toxins on the height of villi and the percentage of goblet cells in crypts of the pig jejunum were observed [18].

The intestinal tract is the main barrier to ingested feed contaminants. The intestine possesses three basic protective mechanisms—physical, chemical, and immunological. Several reports have demonstrated that mycotoxins are able to compromise these mechanisms. Most of the studies concern the small intestine, but very little is known about the effect of mycotoxins on the large intestine. On the other hand, the presence of DON and ZEN derivatives and non-metabolized mycotoxins in digesta of the large intestine along with the slow passage of content through this part of the gastrointestinal tract result in a long-time of mucosa exposure to the toxins [25].

The aim of the present study was to determine the effects of DON (12 μg/kg BW) and ZEN (40 μg/kg BW) when fed, individually and in combination, to the pigs for one, three, or six weeks on the cecum and colon histology and ultrastructure. Moreover, the effect of mycotoxins on the permeability of the intestinal epithelial barrier was studied using the lanthanum method. Additionally, immunocytochemical study of proliferative cell nuclear antigen (PCNA) was performed to assess the effect of toxins on the proliferation of the intestinal epithelial cell.

The selection of doses used in our experiment was previously widely discussed [17,18,26]. Briefly, the dosage of DON used in our study, 12 μg/kg BW, was much lower than No Observed Adverse Effect Level (NOAEL) proposed for pigs [27]. The dose of ZEN used in this study, 40 μg/kg BW, was the same as the NOAEL established by—The joint FAO/WHO Expert Committee on Food Additives for pigs [28].

2. Results and Discussion

2.1. Light Microscopy Study

2.1.1. Architecture of the Mucosa

The cecum, colon ascending and descending of the control pigs were characterized by numerous, well-developed mucosal crypts that span the depth of the lamina propria. The columnar epithelium lining the crypts and covering the luminal surface comprised primarily goblet cells and absorptive cells. The lamina propria consisted of the stromal elements and cells of the immune system. The well-developed muscularis mucosa separated the mucosa from the tunica submucosa, which had loose arrangement and contained numerous adipocytes. The muscularis and the serosa were typical for these segments of the large intestine in pigs. No noticeable qualitative differences were observed in the architecture of the cecum and both colon regions between the control group and the groups of pigs treated with mycotoxins.

Morphometric analysis demonstrated no significant differences in the thickness of mucosa and submucosa between the investigated groups of pigs (see Figure 1).

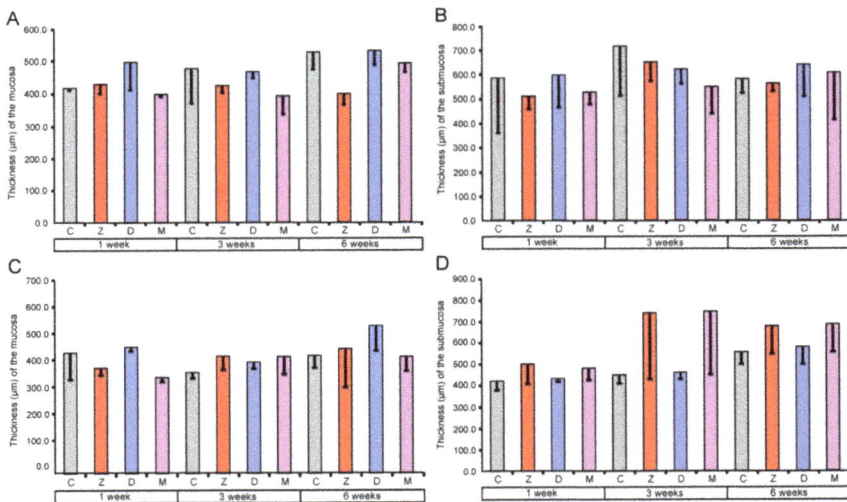

Figure 1. *Cont.*

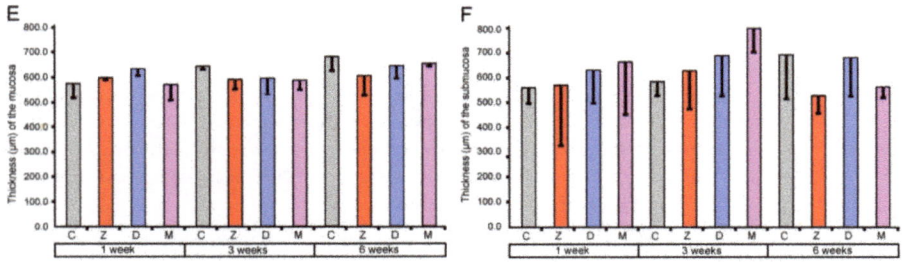

Figure 1. Morphometric characteristic of the mucosa and submucosa of the large intestine segments. Thickness of the cecum mucosa (**A**) and submucosa (**B**), ascending colon mucosa (**C**) and submucosa (**D**), and descending colon mucosa (**E**) and submucosa (**F**). Values presented are means and the standard errors of the mean (SEM). The capital letters under horizontal axis, C—control group, Z—group treated with zearalenone (ZEN), D—group treated with deoxynivalenol (DON), and M—group treated with ZEN + DON.

The obtained data showed that ZEN and DON as well as ZEN + DON had no effect on the qualitative and quantitative characteristics of the mucosa and submucosa in all regions of the large intestine investigated. Previous studies indicated that the dosages of mycotoxin used in our experiment affected histology of the small intestine. However, the significant quantitative changes were noted exclusively after six weeks of the treatment [17,18]. The thickness of the duodenum submucosa was significantly higher in the pigs receiving DON + ZEN for six weeks than in the control pigs [17]. In the jejunum, the thickness of the mucosa was affected in the groups treated by DON and ZEN + DON for six weeks [18]. So far, there has been no research regarding the effects of ZEN and DON on the large intestine architecture.

2.1.2. Goblet Cells

The percentage of goblet cells after ZEN treatment for one, three, and six weeks in the cecum along with one and three weeks in the descending colon were significantly decreased (see Figure 2). The effect of DON was significant only in the descending colon after one and three weeks of treatment. Administration of ZEN + DON also resulted in a decrease in the percentage of goblet cells. The statistically significant effects were observed in the descending colon after one, three, and six weeks of the experiment.

Our results demonstrate that the mycotoxins used in the experiment especially ZEN decrease the number of goblet cells in the large intestine. It should be noted that mycotoxins have the most adverse influence on goblet cells in the descending colon. However, results indicate the complexity of this action and its dependence on many factors.

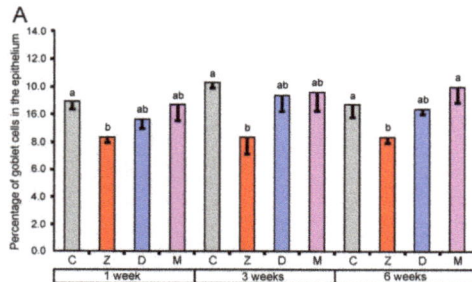

Figure 2. *Cont.*

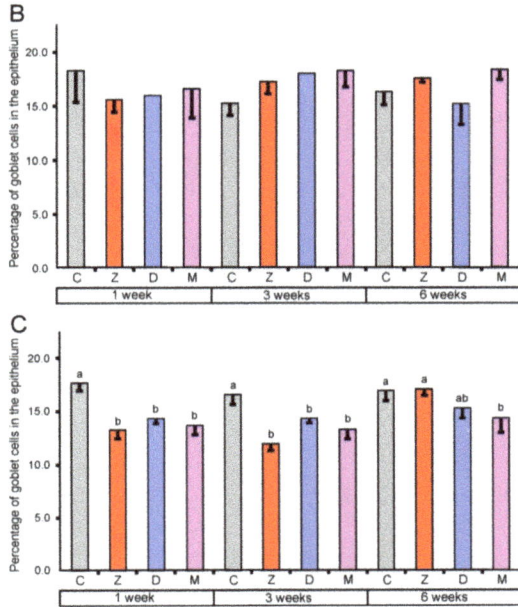

Figure 2. The percentage of goblet cells in the mucosal epithelium of the cecum (**A**), ascending colon (**B**), and descending colon (**C**). Values presented are means and SEM. Means annotated with different lower case letters above the bars are significantly different at $p \leq 0.05$. For other explanations, see Figure 1.

Goblet cells are mucin-secreting cells forming the mucus layer that protects the mucosal surface. This layer is a result of the dynamic balance between the secretion of mucin by goblet cells and the degradation of mucin. Reduction in the goblet cell number is associated with disorders of intestinal protection [29,30]. The number of goblet cells changes under various factors [31]. Dietary components modulate the function of goblet cells and affect composition of mucin [30,31].

There are no data concerning the influence of mycotoxins on goblet cells in the epithelium of the large intestine. In the small intestine epithelium, the ingestion of the DON contaminated diets induced a significant decrease in the number of goblet cells in the pig jejunum and ileum [9,10,12]. On the other hand, more numerous goblet cells were found after administration of a diet containing ZEN [32]. Our previous results concerning the small intestine in the pigs treated with the same doses of ZEN and DON demonstrated that the effect of toxins is dependent on the part of the intestine and the duration of treatment [17,18]. No changes in goblet cells were found in the duodenum including the villus epithelium and the crypt epithelium [17]. However, in the jejunum, the percentage of goblet cells was transiently increased in the villus epithelium, but not in the crypt epithelium [18]. The differences between these two parts of the small intestine could be explained by the fact that large amounts of mucous are produced in the duodenum by Brunner's glands. These glands showed hypertrophy after administration of DON + ZEN for six weeks [18]. It should be noted that the mucous system differs substantially between the small and large intestine and these differences concern both goblet cells and regulation of their secretion [33].

The decrease in the number of goblet cells observed in the present study suggests some discrepancy in mucous secretion and, as a consequence, the depletion in the protective mechanism in the large intestine was a result of mycotoxin treatment. The recent discoveries placed goblet cells at the center position of our understanding of mucosal biology and the immunology of the intestinal tract [33].

The mucous layer is stratified and organized as a filter that physically separates the bacteria from the epithelial cell [34]. Several studies lead to the conclusion that goblet cells form the major line of defense at the intestinal mucosa. However, this is far from a full understanding of the phenomenon [33,35,36].

2.1.3. Lymphocytes and Plasma Cells

The effect of mycotoxins on the number of lymphocytes in the epithelium covering lumen and crypts of the large intestine, and in the lamina propria showed regional differences.

In the cecum, quantitative analysis revealed a significant increase (compared to the corresponding control groups) in the number of lymphocytes in the epithelium after the treatment with ZEN for one, three, and six weeks. However, the administration of DON and ZEN + DON did not cause significant changes (see Figure 3). In the lamina propria of the cecum, significantly higher counts of lymphocytes were found after treatment with ZEN for one and three weeks, DON for one and six weeks, and ZEN + DON for three and six weeks. The plasma cell number was also influenced by mycotoxins in the cecum (see Figure 4). The significant increase in their number in the lamina propria was noted after treatment with ZEN for three weeks, with DON for one, three, and six weeks, and with ZEN + DON for one and three weeks (see Figure 4).

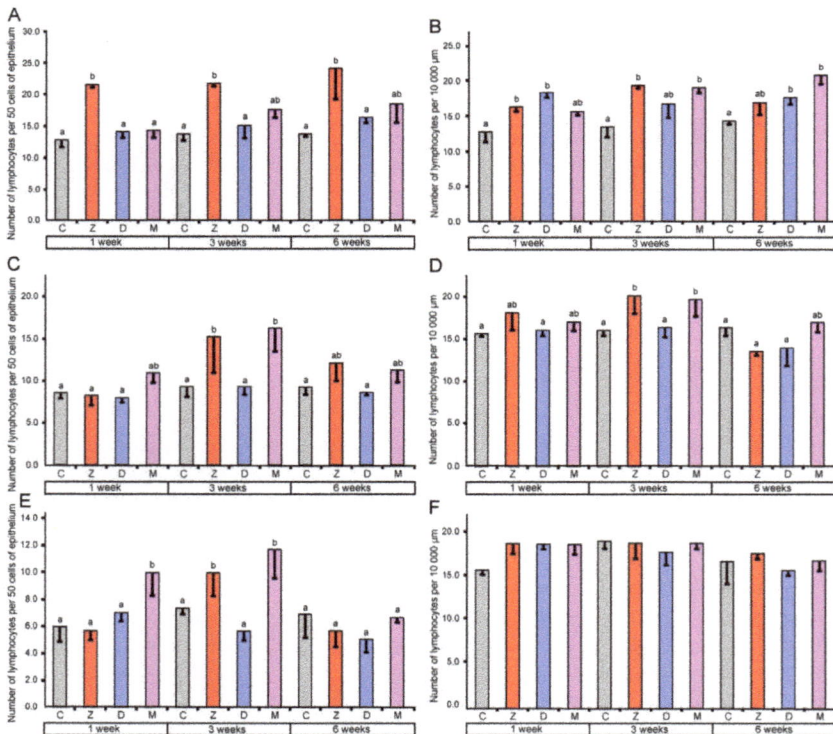

Figure 3. Number of lymphocytes in the mucosal epithelium (**A**) and in the lamina propria (**B**) of the cecum, in the mucosal epithelium (**C**) and in the lamina propria (**D**) of the ascending colon, in the mucosal epithelium (**E**) and in the lamina propria (**F**) of the descending colon. Number of lymphocytes in the mucosal epithelium was expressed per 50 epithelial cells and in the lamina propria was expressed per 10,000 μm^2. Values presented are means and SEM. Means annotated with different lower case letters above the bars are significantly different at $p \leq 0.05$. For other explanations, see Figure 1.

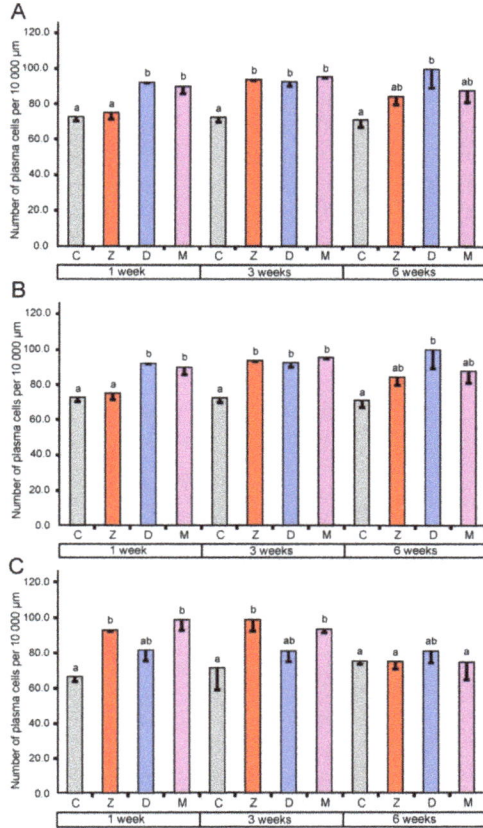

Figure 4. Number of plasma cells per 10,000 μm in the lamina propria of the cecum (**A**), the ascending colon (**B**), and the descending colon (**C**). Values presented are the means and SEM. Means annotated with different lower case letters above the bars are significantly different at $p \leq 0.05$. For other explanations, see Figure 1.

In the ascending colon, the relative number of lymphocytes in the mucosal epithelium showed a significant increase after three weeks of the treatment with ZEN and ZEN + DON (see Figure 3). Similarly, a significant increase in the number of lymphocytes was observed after ZEN and ZEN + DON treatment for three weeks in the lamina propria of the ascending colon (see Figure 3). Surprisingly, the number of plasma cells in the lamina propria of the ascending colon was lower than in the control pigs after three and six weeks of ZEN + DON administration (see Figure 4).

The administration of ZEN for three weeks and ZEN + DON for one week and three weeks resulted in a significant increase in the relative number of lymphocytes in the mucosal epithelium of the descending colon (see Figure 3). No significant changes were noted in the number of lymphocytes in the lamina propria of the descending colon (see Figure 3). In contrast, the number of plasma cells was significantly elevated in this part of the large intestine after one and three weeks of ZEN and ZEN + DON treatments (see Figure 4).

Based on the obtained results, it could be stated that ZEN stimulates the local immune system in the large intestine as indicated by the increase in the lymphocyte number in the mucosal epithelium as well as lymphocytes and plasma cells numbers in the lamina propria. The response of the intestinal immune system was unambiguous and clear in the cecum while more variable and sometimes difficult-to-interpret results were obtained in the ascending colon and the descending colon. It is a well-known phenomenon that the response of the immune system including the local subsystems to immunomodulators is dependent on several factors. Such variability was also reported in a case of mycotoxin effects on intestinal immune response in vivo and in vitro [37,38].

Mechanism of ZEN action on the intestinal immune system is poorly understood. ZEN in vivo and in vitro could activate the ROS-mediated NLRP3 inflammasome and, in turn, contribute to the caspase-1-dependent activation of the inflammatory cytokines Il-1β and IL-18 [39]. The direct effect of ZEN on lymphocytes by estrogen receptors presented in these cells was also postulated [16,40]. The studies concerning the effect of ZEN on the intestinal immune system were concentrated almost exclusively on the small intestine [18,41]. ZEN at the daily dose of 40 μg/kg BW caused increase in lymphocyte number in the villus epithelium of the jejunum after one week of treatment [18]. On the other hand, the toxin had no effect on lymphocytes in the villus epithelium after three and six weeks of the treatment. The same results were found in the lamina propria. In the duodenum, no effects of ZEN on lymphocytes in the epithelium covering the villi were observed. However, the toxin caused an increase in the lymphocyte number in the lamina propria [17]. The most recent histological study revealed inflammatory cell infiltration and tissue damage in the colon of mice fed by gavage with ZEN [39].

The results of quantitative analyses revealed that DON has no effect on the number of lymphocytes in the epithelium of the examined parts of the large intestine. However, the treatment with DON increased the number of lymphocytes and plasma cells in the lamina propria of the cecum and the ascending colon. This effect was dependent on the duration of treatment. Previous studies demonstrate the modulatory effects of DON on the mucosal immune response [3,42]. DON has been found to stimulate the production of mucosal antibodies [43] and IgA by Peyer's patches lymphocytes [44]. The mechanism of the DON-induced increase in the lymphocyte number in the epithelium and the lamina propria as well as plasma cells in the lamina propria is likely related to the activation of cytokine synthesis by this mycotoxin [8,11,45]. In porcine jejunal explants, DON (10 μM) caused a significant increase in expression of mRNA encoding for Il-8, Il-1α, Il-1β, and TNF-α [11]. A phenomenon that DON induces an increase in the number of lymphocytes may also be related to the reduction of claudin and occludin production by this toxin, which enhanced permeability of the epithelial barrier [8,12]. In vitro, DON (0.5–1 μg/mL) contributed to the increase in permeability of *Salmonella Typhimurium* through the intestinal epithelium [46]. On the other hand, in our previous in vivo study, DON (12 μg/kg BW) did not disturb the intestinal barrier in the jejunum [18]. It was observed that DON causes changes in the basal membrane composition that facilitate the migration of lymphocytes from the lamina propria [47]. In some studies, the decrease of lymphocyte infiltration in the pig jejunum was found after DON administration (1.5–3 mg/kg feed) for four to five weeks.

When the experimental pigs received DON + ZEN, different types of interactions were noted depending on the segment of the large intestine and the duration of treatment. In the cecum, they were antagonistic in the case of lymphocytes in the mucosal epithelium or less than additive in the case of lymphocytes and plasma cells in the lamina propria. In the ascending colon, they were antagonistic-lymphocytes in the mucosal epithelium and plasma cells in the lamina propria or less than additive—lymphocytes in the lamina propria. In the descending colon, they were additive or less than additive-lymphocytes in the mucosal epithelium and plasma cells in the lamina propria.

From previous studies on the small intestine it appears that a co-contaminated diet can cause several types of interactions. Bracarense et al. [12] investigated the effect of food contaminated with low doses of DON + FB (fumonisin) on the small intestine (jejunum and ileum) and stated synergistic (immune cells), additive (cytokines and junction protein expression), less than additive (histological lesions and cytokine expression), antagonistic (immune cells and cytokine expression) interactions of these mycotoxins. The authors' [12] data provide strong evidence that chronic ingestion of low doses of mycotoxins alters the intestine and, therefore, may predispose animals to infections by enteric pathogens. Our results concerning the jejunum showed that the effect of ZEN and DON administered in combination is antagonistic on plasma cells after one, three, and six weeks of treatment, and on lymphocytes in the villus epithelium and the lamina propria after one week of treatment as well as less than additive on lymphocytes in the villus epithelium and in the lamina propria after three and six weeks of treatment [18]. In the duodenum, distinct effects were noted including additive on lymphocytes in the villus epithelium after one week of treatment, less than additive on lymphocytes in the epithelium and the lamina propria after three and six weeks, and on plasma cells in the lamina propria after six weeks, and antagonistic on lymphocytes (after one week) and plasma cells (after one and three weeks) in the lamina propria [17].

2.1.4. Expression of the Proliferating Cell Nuclear Antigen (PCNA) in the Mucosa Epithelium

PCNA positive cells were observed in the mucosal epithelium and in the lamina propria in all samples (see Figure 5A). The quantitative study performed on the samples taken at the end of the experiment did not show significant differences in the percentage of PCNA-positive cells in the mucosal epithelium between the control pigs and the animals treated with mycotoxins (see Figure 5B).

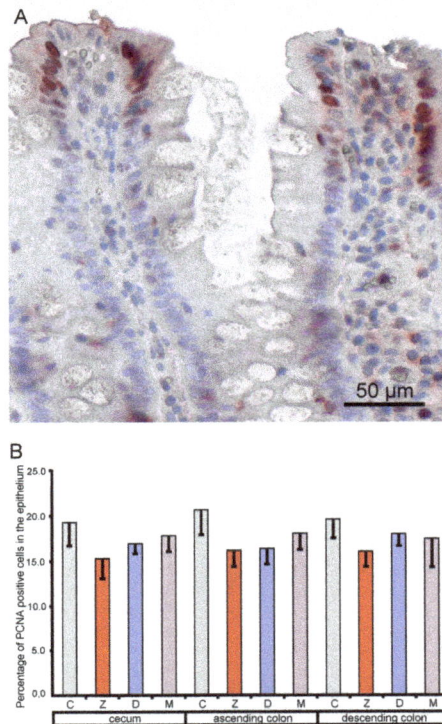

Figure 5. Effects of toxins on the proliferating cell nuclear antigen labeling index in the mucosal epithelium of the cecum, ascending colon, and descending colon in pigs after six weeks of treatment. (**A**) Immunopositive cells. (**B**) Percentage of proliferating cell nuclear antigen (PCNA) positive cells in the cecum, ascending colon, and descending colon. Values presented are means and SEM. For other explanations, see Figure 1.

The PCNA index is generally considered a valid measure of cell proliferation. Mycotoxins show an anti-proliferative effect on different cells. A significant decrease in expression of the proliferation marker PCNA was noted as effects of beta-zearalenol and DON on porcine endometrial cells in vitro [48]. DON in vitro inhibited the proliferation of human intestinal Caco-2 cells in a dose dependent manner with a significant effect appearing at 0.2 µg/mL [49]. The PCNA indexes for the jejunum and ileum in the piglets receiving DON (basal diet + 4 mg/kg of toxin) were significantly lower ($p < 0.05$) than those in the piglets that received the basal diet only [50]. In the present study, no negative effects of DON and ZEN on the PCNA labeling index were observed.

2.2. Electron Microscopy Study

2.2.1. Ultrastructure of the Mucosa

In the control pigs, the mucosal epithelium of the cecum, ascending colon, and descending colon comprised mainly absorptive cells and goblet cells. Enteroendocrine cells and regenerative cells were less frequently observed. Lymphocytes were present between epithelial cells. The absorptive cells were columnar with a basally situated, oval nucleus. Their cytoplasm contained numerous ribosomes, profiles of rough and smooth endoplasmic reticulum, mitochondria, the moderately-developed Golgi apparatus, and a network of microtubules and filaments. Some of these cells comprised small, round granules with a content of variable electron density located in the upper part of the cell. The absorptive cells formed microvilli on the apical surface, whose number varied from cell to cell. The goblet cells were more or less elongated with a cup-shaped upper part, which was filled with large granules showing moderate electron density. The tall, lower part of these cells contained a cell nucleus, numerous cisterns of rough endoplasmic reticulum, the well-developed Golgi apparatus, mitochondria, and some secretory granules. The absorptive cells and goblet cells created junctional complexes in their upper parts. The intercellular spaces were frequently dilated beneath the junctional complexes and cells formed numerous irregular processes. Usually, the epithelium was covered with a layer of mucous. The lamina propria and the muscularis mucosae showed typical organization. Abundant lymphocytes, plasma cells, and macrophages were observed in the lamina propria.

In the pigs treated with mycotoxins, the ultrastructure of mucosal epithelium showed some differences in comparison with the control animals. The most prominent changes concerned the goblet cell in the cecum and the descending colon of pigs receiving ZEN and ZEN + DON for one, three, or six weeks. In these pigs when compared to the control pigs, the goblet cells frequently contained much fewer granules in their apical parts (see Figure 6) and did not show a goblet-like shape. Our ultrastructural studies were only qualitative, however, it should be noted that the goblet cells were less frequently found in the group of pigs treated with ZEN and ZEN + DON than in two other investigated groups.

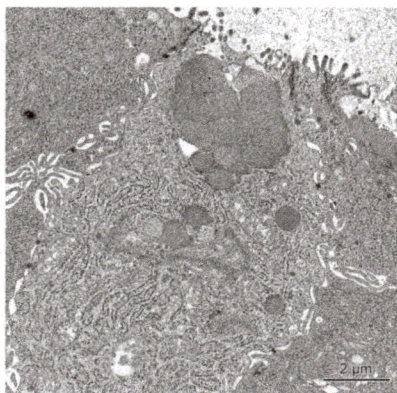

Figure 6. Goblet cell in the cecum of a pig receiving ZEN + DON for six weeks. Note the presence of sparse secretory granules in the apical part of the cell.

The alternations were also observed in the absorptive cells in the pigs treated with ZEN and ZEN + DON for one, three, and six weeks. As in the case of the goblet cells, they were most prominent in the cecum and descending colon. The apical surface of the absorptive cells of these pigs frequently formed only sparse microvilli, which usually were short and irregular (see Figure 7). Moreover, numerous small granules with moderate to high electron density were found in the upper parts of many absorptive cells (see Figure 7). In the group receiving ZEN + DON, some absorptive cells contained numerous electron dense bodies (see Figure 8).

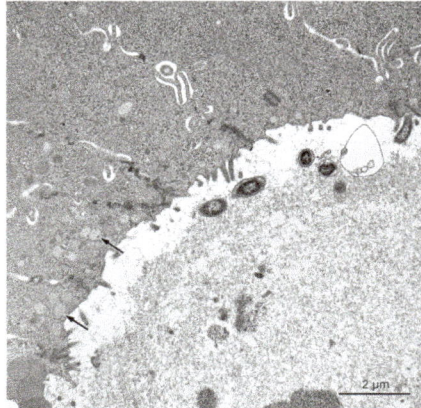

Figure 7. The transverse section through the intestinal crypt in the descending colon in a pig treated with ZEN + DON for three weeks. The apical surfaces of absorptive cells contain only single microvilli. Note the presence of numerous round granules in some absorptive cells (arrows).

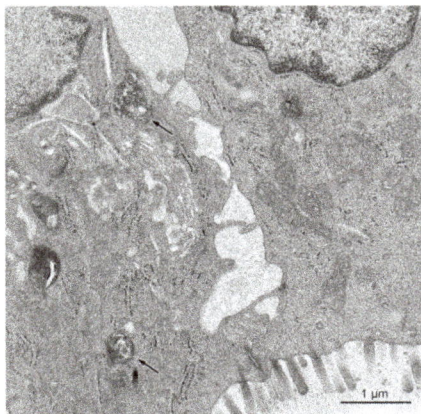

Figure 8. Dilated intercellular spaces between the epithelial cells in a pig treated with ZEN + DON for six weeks (ascending colon). Note presence of electron dense bodies in cytoplasm of the absorptive cell (arrows).

The intercellular spaces between the epithelial cells were frequently largely dilated in pigs treated with DON and ZEN + DON for three and six weeks in the ascending and descending colon (see Figure 7). The damaged or dead epithelial cells were noted in all studied groups, but they were more frequently found in pigs treated with ZEN + DON for three and six weeks. The lamina propria of the large intestine in the animals treated with ZEN + DON for three and six weeks contained numerous macrophages, which were much less frequently observed in other groups of pigs.

Summing up, the results obtained in ultrastructural studies showed that ZEN and ZEN + DON affected mainly goblet cells, which often contained fewer secretory granules than in the control animals. Further studies are needed to determine if the synthesis of granules is decreased or the release of their content is increased. Both toxins also induced some changes in absorptive cells.

The literature data about effects of mycotoxins on the intestine ultrastructure are sparse and concerned almost exclusively with the small intestine. The administration of ZEN, DON, and ZEN + DON in the same dosages and according to the same schedule as in the present study did not cause changes in the ultrastructure of the mucosa of the jejunum with exception for adsorptive cells with drop-like protrusions of apical cytoplasm in the pigs receiving ZEN and DON + ZEN [17]. The treatment of gilts with ZEN at doses of 200 and 400 µg/kg BW for seven days had no effect on the ultrastructure of the jejunal epithelium [10]. In in vitro studies, incubation of jejunal explants with 10 µM DON resulted in an increase in intercellular spaces, a decrease in the size and number of microvilli, and a loss of junction complexes [51].

2.2.2. Permeability of the Intestinal Barrier: Studies Using Lanthanum Ions

For evaluation of the effect of studied mycotoxins on the permeability of the epithelial barrier, we applied the lanthanum technique, which is commonly used in examining tight junctions at the ultrastructural level [52,53]. In the investigated material, electron dense lanthanum particles were observed on the surface of intestine epithelium between the microvilli and in intercellular spaces higher up in the tight junctions. The presence of deposits was never observed in intercellular spaces beneath the tight junctions (see Figure 9).

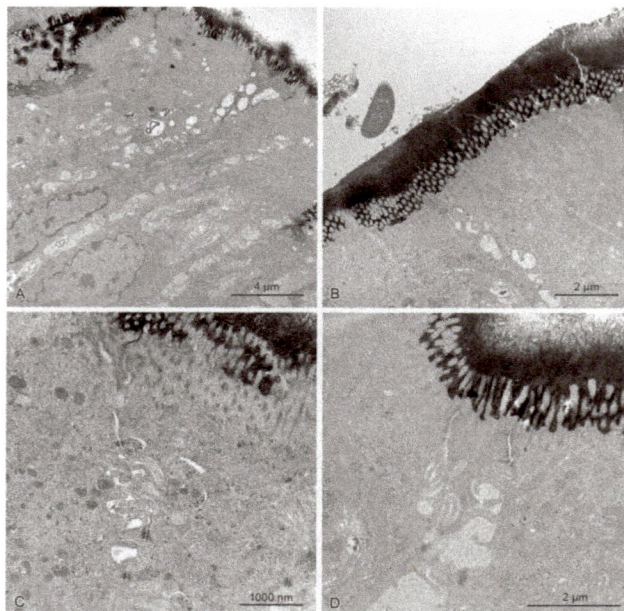

Figure 9. The mucosal epithelium in the samples of the descending colon in control pigs (**A**) and pigs treated with ZEN (**B**), DON (**C**), ZEN + DON (**D**) for six weeks. Note numerous precipitates on the epithelium surface and their lack beneath the tight junctions. The intercellular spaces did not contain any precipitates.

The obtained results demonstrated that the treatment of DON, ZEN, and ZEN + DON did not change the permeability of epithelium in the examined segments of the large intestine. The lack of junction complexes on enterocytes exposed to mycotoxins was reported by Basso et al. [51]. Pinton et al. [54] associated alterations of barrier function in the pig jejunum after treatment with DON with a specific reduction in the expression of claudin. It should be stressed that the doses of toxins used in our study had no effects on the epithelial barrier in the jejunum [18].

3. Experimental Section

3.1. Toxins, Animals, and Experimental Design

Deoxynivalenol and zearalenon were synthesized and standardized at the Department of Chemistry, Faculty of Wood Technology, Poznań University of Life Sciences, Poland. Assessment of toxin purity was made using mass spectrometry (UPLC/TQD, Waters, Milford, MA, USA). The analytical purity of ZEN and DON were higher than 99.9%.

The study was performed on 36 clinically healthy gilts of mixed breed (White Polish Big × Polish White Earhanging) with body weights of 25 ± 2 kg at the beginning of the experiment. The animals were purchased from a farm where they received feed without detectable amounts of ZEN, DON, α-zearalenol, aflatoxin, and ochratoxin. The serological test excluded the presence of Auyeski's disease, mycoplasmosis, parvovirosis, actinobacillosis, and porcine reproductive-respiratory syndrome. The pigs were fed twice daily and had free access to water. The tests for the presence of mycotoxins in feed were performed as described previously [55].

The animals were divided into four experimental groups (Z, D, and M; $n = 9$ in each group) and a control group (C; $n = 9$). The animals of the group Z received ZEN at a dose of 40 µg/kg BW per day, the animals of the group D—DON at a dose of 12 µg/kg BW per day, and the animals of group M— a mixture of ZEN and DON (40 µg ZEN/kg BW + 12 µg DON/kg BW per day). The mycotoxins were administrated per os during the morning feeding in water-soluble capsules containing oat bran as a vehicle. The gilts were weighed every week to establish the amount of DON and ZEN given for each animal. The animals of group C received capsules without mycotoxins.

Three animals from each experimental group were killed by intravenous (marginal vein of the ear) administration of sodium pentobarbital (Vetbutal, Biowet, Poland) at a dose of 140–150 mg/kg and exsanguination after 1, 3, and 6 weeks of the experiment. The tissue samples were taken 3 min after cardiac arrest.

All procedures were carried out in compliance with Polish legal regulations, which determine the terms and methods for performing experiments on animals, and the European Community Directive for the ethical use of experimental animals. The protocol was approved by the Local Ethical Council in Olsztyn (opinion No. 88/N of 16 December 2009).

3.2. Histological Examinations

The tissue samples (approximately 1×0.5 cm) were cut from the middle parts of the cecum and the ascending and descending colon. They were flushed in saline and fixed in 4% paraformaldehyde in 0.1 M phosphate buffer (pH 7.4) for 48 h, dehydrated in ethanol (TP 1020, Leica, Wetzlar, Germany), and embedded in paraffin (EG1150, Leica, Wetzlar, Germany). The 4-µm-thick sections were prepared with the use of HM 340E microtome (Microm, Lugo, Spain) and stained with the hematoxylin and eosin method (HE), periodic acid Schiff method (PAS), and methyl green-pyronine method (MGP) using automated multistainer ST 5020 (Leica, Wetzlar, Germany). The slides were signed in a way that prevented the people involved in their microscopic analysis from knowing the kind and duration of the animal treatment. The specimens were analyzed and photographed in an Axioimager light microscope equipped with an AxioCam MRc5 camera (Carl Zeiss, Oberkochen, Germany).

For morphometrical evaluations, the sections were scanned in a Mirax Desk scanner (Carl Zeiss, Oberkochen, Germany). The following parameters were determined: the thickness of mucosa and submucosa, the percentage of goblet cells in the surface epithelium covering the mucosa, the number of lymphocytes per 50 epithelial cells, the number of lymphocytes, and the number of plasma cells per 10,000 μm^2 of the lamina propria. Goblet cells were counted in PAS-stained sections and plasma cells in MPG stained sections. All other measurements were performed on HE-stained sections. The linear measurements were repeated 20 times per animal. The percentage of lymphocytes and goblet cells were determined by counting their number per 50 epithelial cells in 10 randomly selected areas and the density of lymphocytes and plasma cells in the lamina propria were measured by counting the cells in 10 randomly selected areas of 6000 to 12,000 μm^2 each. The measurements were performed using Pannoramic Viewer software (Version 1.15.3 RTM, 3D-Histech, Budapest, Hungary, 2012) and AxioVision software (Version 4.6.3, Carl Zeiss, Oberkochen, Germany, 2007).

3.3. Immunohistochemical Staining

The staining was performed on paraffin sections mounted on Superfrost Plus slides prepared from the tissue samples taken for histological examinations after 6 weeks of the treatment. After dewaxing in xylene and rehydration in graded alcohols (96%, 70%, 50%), tissue sections were subjected to heat antigen retrieval in a microwave oven (600 W, 15 min) in 0.01 mol·L^{-1} 0.03% H_2O_2. Then slices were washed in phosphate buffered saline (PBS) and incubated for 20 min with 10% normal goat serum. The sections were then incubated overnight with primary antibodies anti-PCNA (clone PC10, M0879, Dako Agilent Technologies, Santa Clara, CA, USA) at a dilution 1:200 in a humidified chamber. Next, they were incubated with secondary antibodies for 30 min at a room temperature (EnVision System-HRP/AEC, Dako K4004, Santa Clara, CA, USA). For visualization of antigen-antibody complexes, the sections were immersed in 3-amino-9-ethyl-carbazole substrate-chromogenic (EnVision System-HRP/AEC, Dako K4004, Santa Clara, CA, USA) for 20 min. Afterwards, they were counterstained with Mayer's hematoxyline (Sigma-Aldrich, St. Louis, MO, USA) and mounted using Mounting Glycergel (C0563, Dako Agilent Technologies, Santa Clara, CA, USA). The specimens were analyzed and photographed in a motorized Axioimager light microscope equipped with an AxioCamMRc5 camera (Carl Zeiss, Oberkochen, Germany). The PCNA labeling index (LI) was expressed as the ratio of cell positively stained for PCNA to all epithelial cells in at least 5 areas randomly selected for counting. The positive cell nuclei were counted on the images with AxioVision software (Version 4.6.3, Carl Zeiss, Oberkochen, Germany, 2007).

3.4. Ultrastructural Examinations

The samples of the mucous membrane from the cecum, ascending colon, and descending colon were collected from sites adjacent to the sites of sampling for histological examination. The tissues were immersion-fixed in a mixture of 1% paraformaldehyde and 2.5% glutaraldehyde in 0.2 M phosphate buffer (pH 7.4) for 2 h at 4 °C, washed, and post-fixed in 2% osmium tetroxide for 2 h. After dehydration, the samples were embedded in Epon 812. Semithin sections were cut from each block of tissue, stained with 1% toluidine blue, and examined under a light microscope in order to choose the sites for preparing ultrathin sections. Ultrathin sections contrasted with uranyl acetate and lead citrate were examined with a Tecnai 12 Spirit G2 BioTwin transmission electron microscope (FEI, Hillsboro, OR, USA) equipped with two digital cameras: Veleta (Olympus, Tokyo, Japan) and Eage 4k (FEI, Hillsboro, OR, USA).

3.5. Lanthanum Procedure

The mucosal specimens were fixed for 2 h in a freshly prepared mixture of 2.5% glutaraldehyde and 1% lanthanum nitrate, La(NO$_3$)·6H$_2$O, in cacodylate buffer (pH 7.2). Next, the samples were rinsed for 30 min in the cacodylate buffer containing 1% lanthanum nitrate and postfixed for 2 h in a freshly prepared mixture of 1% osmium tetroxide and 1% of lanthanum nitrate in the cacodylate buffer. Then, the tissues were dehydrated and embedded in Epon 812. Unstained, ultrathin sections were examined with a Tecnai 12 Spirit G2 BioTwin transmission electron microscope (FEI, Hillsboro, OR, USA).

3.6. Statistical Analysis

The data were analyzed using two-way or one-way ANOVA with the Duncan test as a post-hoc procedure. Statistical analyses were performed by using Statistica software (Version 10.0 PL, StatSoft, Tulsa, OK, USA, 2011).

4. Conclusions

Taken together, the obtained data provide evidence that administration of low doses of DON and ZEN as well as a mixture of both toxins does not affect the architecture of the mucosa and submucosa in the large intestine of the pig. However, the treatment with toxins alters the system of goblet cells and the amount of lymphocytes and plasma cells in the mucosa. Modifications caused by mycotoxins vary depending on the duration of intoxication, the toxin, and the part of the large intestine. ZEN and ZEN + DEN significantly decrease the number and modify the ultrastructure of goblet cells. Taking into consideration the position of goblet cells in the mucosal biology especially in the mucosal protective mechanisms, the observed changes should be considered unfavorable for large intestine homeostasis. The results concerning lymphocytes and plasma cells are not unequivocal. However, they point to the influence of toxins on immune processes in the large intestine and pay attention to their complexity. Examinations of the PCNA labeling index and permeability of the intestinal epithelium show no significant effects of the examined mycotoxins on these parameters. The obtained results indicate that mycotoxins especially ZEN may influence the defense mechanisms of the large intestine.

Acknowledgments: The study was supported by research grant No. NR12-0080-10 from the Polish National Center for Research and Development. Publication cost was covered by KNOW (Leading National Research Center) Scientific Consortium "Healthy Animal-Safe Food", decision of Ministry of Science and Higher Education No. 05-1/KNOW2/2015.

Author Contributions: Maciej Gajęcki and Magdalena Gajęcka conceived and designed the study. Łukasz Zielonka and Magdalena Gajęcka performed the animal experiment. Barbara Przybylska-Gornowicz, Marcela Petrusewicz-Kosińska, and Magdalena Prusik conducted the histological studies. Bogdan Lewczuk and Maria Hanuszewska performed the ultrastructural studies. Barbara Przybylska-Gornowicz, Bogdan Lewczuk, Magdalena Gajęcka, Magdalena Prusik, and Łukasz Zielonka analyzed and interpreted the data. Barbara Przybylska-Gornowicz and Bogdan Lewczuk wrote the paper. Maciej Gajęcki and Magdalena Prusik discussed the manuscript.

Conflicts of Interest: The authors declare no conflict of interest.

References

1. Shephard, G.S. Determination of mycotoxin in human foods. *Chem. Soc. Rev.* **2008**, *37*, 2468–2477. [CrossRef] [PubMed]
2. Oswald, I.P.; Comera, C. Immunotoxicity of mycotoxins. *Rev. Med. Vet.* **1998**, *149*, 585–590.
3. Rotter, B.A.; Prelusky, D.B.; Pestka, J.J. Toxicology of deoxynivalenol (vomitoxin). *J. Toxicol. Environ. Health* **1996**, *48*, 1–34. [CrossRef] [PubMed]
4. Pestka, J.J. Deoxynivalenol: Toxicity, mechanisms and animal health risks. *Anim. Feed Sci. Technol.* **2007**, *137*, 283–298. [CrossRef]
5. Prelusky, D.B.; Hartin, K.E.; Trenholm, H.L.; Miller, J.D. Pharmacokinetic fate of ^{14}C-labeled deoxynivalenol in swine. *Toxicol. Sci.* **1988**, *10*, 276–286. [CrossRef]
6. Dänicke, S.; Valenta, S.; Döll, S. On the toxicokinetics and the metabolism of deoxynivalenol (DON) in the pig. *Arch. Anim. Nutr.* **2004**, *58*, 169–180. [CrossRef] [PubMed]
7. Eriksen, G.S.; Pettersson, H.; Lindberg, J.E. Absorption, metabolism and excretion of 3-acetyl DON in pigs. *Arch. Tierernahr.* **2003**, *57*, 335–345. [CrossRef] [PubMed]
8. Pinton, P.; Oswald, I.P. Effects of deoxynivalenol and other Type B trichothecenes on the intestine: A review. *Toxins* **2014**, *6*, 1615–1643. [CrossRef] [PubMed]
9. Gerez, J.R.; Pinton, P.; Callu, P.; Grosjean, F.; Oswald, I.P.; Bracarense, A.P. Deoxynivalenol alone or in combination with nivalenol and zearalenone induce systemic histological changes in pigs. *Exp. Toxicol. Pathol.* **2015**, *67*, 89–98. [CrossRef] [PubMed]

10. Obremski, K.; Zielonka, L.; Gajęcka, M.; Jakimiuk, E.; Bakuła, T.; Baranowski, M.; Gajecki, M. Histological estimation of the small intestine wall after administration of feed containing deoxynivalenol, T-2 toxin and zearalenone in the pig. *Pol. J. Vet. Sci.* **2008**, *4*, 339–345.

11. Cano, P.M.; Seeboth, J.; Meurens, F.; Cognie, J.; Abrami, R.; Oswald, I.P.; Guzylack-Piriou, L. Deoxynivalenol as a new factor in the persistence of intestinal inflammatory diseases: An emerging hypothesis through possiblemodulation of Th-17 mediated response. *PLoS ONE* **2013**, *8*, e53647. [CrossRef] [PubMed]

12. Bracarense, A.P.; Lucioli, J.; Grenier, B.; Drociunas Pacheco, G.; Moll, W.D.; Schatzmayr, G.; Oswald, I.P. Chronic ingestion of deoxynivalenol and fumonisin, alone or in interaction, induces morphological and immunological changes in the intestine of piglets. *Br. J. Nutr.* **2012**, *107*, 1776–1786. [CrossRef] [PubMed]

13. Dąbrowski, M.; Jakimiuk, E.; Gajęcka, M.; Gajęcki, M.T.; Zielonka, Ł. Effect of deoxynivalenol on the levels of toll-like receptors 2 and 9 and their mRNA expression in enterocytes in the porcine large intestine: A preliminary study. *Pol. J. Vet. Sci.* **2017**, *20*, 213–220. [CrossRef] [PubMed]

14. Doll, S.; Danicke, S.; Ueberschsar, K.H.; Valenta, H.; Flachowsky, G. Fusarium toxin residues in physiological samples of piglets. *Mycotoxin Res.* **2003**, *19*, 171–175. [CrossRef] [PubMed]

15. Gajęcki, M. Zearalenone—Undesirable substances in feed. *Pol. J. Vet. Sci.* **2002**, *5*, 117–122. [PubMed]

16. Marin, D.E.; Taranu, I.; Burlacu, R.; Manda, G.; Motiu, M.; Neagoe, I.; Dragomir, C.; Stancu, M.; Calin, L. Effects of zearalenone and its derivatives on porcine immune response. *Toxicol. In Vitro* **2011**, *25*, 1981–1988. [CrossRef] [PubMed]

17. Lewczuk, B.; Przybylska-Gornowicz, B.; Gajęcka, M.; Targońska, K.; Ziółkowska, N.; Prusik, M.; Gajęcki, M. Histological structure of duodenum in gilts receiving low doses of zearalenone and deoxynivalenol in feed. *Exp. Toxicol. Pathol.* **2016**, *68*, 157–166. [CrossRef] [PubMed]

18. Przybylska-Gornowicz, B.; Tarasiuk, M.; Lewczuk, B.; Prusik, M.; Ziółkowska, N.; Zielonka, Ł.; Gajęcki, M.; Gajęcka, M. The effects of low doses of two Fusarium toxins, zearalenone and deoxynivalenol, on the pig jejunum. A light and electron microscopic study. *Toxins* **2015**, *7*, 4684–4705. [CrossRef] [PubMed]

19. Binder, S.B.; Schwartz-Zimmermann, H.E.; Varga, E.; Bichl, G.; Michlmayr, H.; Adam, G.; Berthiller, F. Metabolism of Zearalenone and Its Major Modified Forms in Pigs. *Toxins* **2017**, *9*, 56. [CrossRef] [PubMed]

20. Wan, L.Y.M.; Turner, P.C.; El-Nezami, H. Individual and combined cytotoxic effects of Fusarium toxins (deoxynivalenol, nivalenol, zearalenone and fumonisins B1) on swine jejunal epithelium cells. *Food Chem. Toxicol.* **2013**, *57*, 276–283. [CrossRef] [PubMed]

21. Alassane-Kpembi, I.; Kolf-Clauw, M.; Gauthier, T.; Abrami, R.; Abiola, F.A.; Oswald, P.; Puel, O. New insights into mycotoxin mixtures: The toxicity of low doses of Type B trichothecenes on intestinal epithelial cells is synergistic. *Toxicol. Appl. Pharmacol.* **2013**, *272*, 191–198. [CrossRef] [PubMed]

22. Streit, E.; Schatzmayr, G.; Tassis, P.; Tzika, E.; Marin, D.; Taranu, I.; Tabuc, C.; Nicolau, A.; Aprodu, I.; Puel, O.; et al. Current situation of mycotoxin contamination and co-occurrence in animal feed—Focus on Europe. *Toxins* **2012**, *4*, 788–809. [CrossRef] [PubMed]

23. Döll, S.; Dänicke, S. The Fusarium toxins deoxynivalenol (DON) and zearalenone (ZON) in animal feeding. *Prev. Vet. Med.* **2011**, *102*, 132–145. [CrossRef] [PubMed]

24. Maresca, M.; Fantini, J. Some food-associated mycotoxins as potential risk factors in humans predisposed to chronic intestinal inflammatory diseases. *Toxicon* **2010**, *56*, 282–294. [CrossRef] [PubMed]

25. Hecker, J.; Grovum, W.L. Rates of passage of digesta and water absorption along the large intestines of sheep, cows and pigs. *Aust. J. Biol. Sci.* **1975**, *28*, 161–167. [CrossRef] [PubMed]

26. Zielonka, Ł.; Waśkiewicz, A.; Beszterda, M.; Kostecki, M.; Dąbrowski, M.; Obremski, K.; Goliński, P.; Gajęcki, M. Zearalenone in the intestinal tissues of immature gilts exposed *per os* to mycotoxins. *Toxins* **2015**, *7*, 3210–3223. [CrossRef] [PubMed]

27. Candy, R.; Coker, R.; Rgan, S.; Krska, R.; Kuiper-Goodman, T.; Olsen, M.; Pestka, J.; Resnik, S.; Schlatter, J. *Safety Evaluation of Certein Mycotoxin in Food*; World Health Organization: Geneva, Switzerland, 2001; pp. 419–555.

28. Eriksen, G.S.; Pennington, J.; Schlatter, J.; Alexander, J.; Thuvander, A. Zearalenone. In *Safety Evaluation of Certein Food Additives and Contaminants*; World Health Organization: Geneva, Switzerland, 2000; pp. 393–482.

29. Gersemann, M.; Becker, S.; Kübler, I.; Koslowski, M.; Wang, G.; Herrlinger, K.R.; Griger, J.; Fritz, P.; Fellermann, K.; Schwab, M.; et al. Differences in goblet cell differentiation between Crohn's disease and ulcerative colitis. *Differentiation* **2009**, *77*, 84–94. [CrossRef] [PubMed]

30. Montagne, L.; Piel, C.; Lallès, J.P. Effect of diet on mucin kinetics and composition: Nutrition and health implications. *Nutr. Rev.* **2004**, *62*, 105–114. [CrossRef] [PubMed]

31. Castillo, M.; Martín-Orúe, S.M.; Nofrarías, M.; Manzanilla, E.G.; Gasa, J. Changes in caecal microbiota and mucosal morphology of weaned pigs. *Vet. Microbiol.* **2007**, *124*, 239–247. [CrossRef] [PubMed]

32. Obremski, K.; Gajęcka, M.; Zielonka, L.; Jakimiuk, E.; Gajęcki, M. Morphology and ultrastructure of small intestine mucosa in gilts with zearalenone mycotoxicosis. *Pol. J. Vet. Sci.* **2005**, *8*, 301–307. [PubMed]

33. Birchenough, G.M.H.; Johansson, M.E.W.; Gustafsson, J.K.; Bergström, J.H.; Hansson, G.C. New developments in goblet cell mucus secretion and function. *Mucosal Immunol.* **2015**, *8*, 712–719. [CrossRef] [PubMed]

34. Johansson, M.E.V.; Phillipson, M.; Petersson, J.; Holm, L.; Velcich, A.; Hansson, G.C. The inner of the two Muc2 mucin dependent mucus layers in colon is devoid of bacteria. *Proc. Natl. Acad. Sci. USA* **2008**, *105*, 15064–15069. [CrossRef] [PubMed]

35. Brown, P.J.; Miller, B.G.; Stokes, C.R.; Blazquez, N.B.; Bourne, F.J. Histochemistry of mucins of pig intestinal secretory epithelial cells before and after weaning. *J. Comp. Pathol.* **1988**, *98*, 313–323. [CrossRef]

36. Che, C.; Pang, X.; Hua, X.; Zhang, B.; Shen, J.; Zhu, J.; Wei, H.; Sun, L.; Chen, P.; Cui, L.; et al. Effects of human fecal flora on intestinal morphology and mucosal immunity in human flora-associated piglet. *Scand. J. Immunol.* **2009**, *69*, 223–233. [CrossRef] [PubMed]

37. Pierron, A.; Alassane-Kempi, I.; Oswald, I.P. Impact of two mycotoxins deoxynivalenol and fumisin on pig intestinal health. *Porcine Health Manag.* **2016**, *2*, 21. [CrossRef] [PubMed]

38. Marin, D.E.; Motiu, M.; Taranu, I. Food contaminant zearalenone and its metabolites affect cytokine synthesis and intestinal epithelial integrity of porcine cells. *Toxins* **2015**, *7*, 1979–1988. [CrossRef] [PubMed]

39. Fan, W.; Lv, Y.; Ren, S.; Shao, M.; Shen, T.; Huang, K.; Zhou, J.; Yan, L.; Song, S. Zearalenone (ZEA)-induced intestinal inflammation is mediated by the NLRP3 inflammasome. *Chemosphere* **2018**, *190*, 272–279. [CrossRef] [PubMed]

40. Törnwall, J.; Carey, A.B.; Fox, R.I.; Fox, H.S. Estrogen in autoimmunity: Expression of estrogen receptors in thymic and autoimmune T cells. *J. Gend. Specif. Med.* **1999**, *2*, 33–40. [PubMed]

41. Gajęcka, M.; Zielonka, Ł.; Gajęcki, M. Activity of Zearalenone in the Porcine Intestinal Tract. *Molecules* **2016**, *22*, 18. [CrossRef] [PubMed]

42. Ghareeb, K.; Awad, W.A.; Böhm, J.; Zebeli, Q. Impacts of the feed contaminant deoxynivalenol on the intestine of monogastric animals: Poultry and swine. *J. Appl. Toxicol.* **2015**, *35*, 327–337. [CrossRef] [PubMed]

43. Islam, M.R.; Roh, Y.S.; Kim, J.; Lim, C.W.; Kim, B. Differential immune modulation by deoxynivalenol (vomitoxin) in mice. *Toxicol. Lett.* **2013**, *221*, 152–163. [CrossRef] [PubMed]

44. Jia, Q.; Pestka, J.J. Role of cyclooxygenase-2 in deoxynivalenol-induced immunoglobulin a nephropathy. *Food Chem. Toxicol.* **2005**, *43*, 721–728. [CrossRef] [PubMed]

45. Pestka, J.J. Deoxynivalenol: Mechanisms of action, human exposure, and toxicological relevance. *Arch. Toxicol.* **2010**, *84*, 663–679. [CrossRef] [PubMed]

46. Vanderbroucke, V.; Croubels, S.; Martel, A.; Verbrughe, E.; Goossens, J.; Van Deun, K.; Boyen, F.; Thompson, A.; Shearer, N.; De Backer, P.; et al. The mycotoxins deoxynivalenol potentiates intestinal inflammation by *Salmonella typhimurium* in porcine ileal loops. *PLoS ONE* **2011**, *6*, e23871. [CrossRef]

47. Nossol, C.; Diesing, A.K.; Kahlert, S.; Kersten, S.; Kluess, J.; Ponsuksili, S.; Hartig, R.; Wimmers, K.; Dänicke, S.; Rothkötter, H.J. Deoxynivalenol affects the composition of the basement membrane proteins and influences en route the migration of CD16(+) cells into the intestinal epithelium. *Mycotoxin Res.* **2013**, *29*, 245–254. [CrossRef] [PubMed]

48. Tiemann, U.; Viergutz, T.; Jonas, L.; Schneider, F. Influence of the mycotoxins alpha- and beta-zearalenol and deoxynivalenol on the cell cycle of cultured porcine endometrial cells. *Reprod. Toxicol.* **2003**, *17*, 209–218. [CrossRef]

49. Sergent, T.; Parys, M.; Garsou, S.; Pussemier, L.; Schneider, Y.J.; Larondelle, Y. Deoxynivalenol transport across human intestinal CaCO$_2$ cells and its effects on cellular metabolism at realistic intestinal concentrations. *Toxicol. Lett.* **2006**, *164*, 167–176. [CrossRef] [PubMed]

50. Xiao, H.; Tan, B.E.; Wu, M.M.; Yin, Y.L.; Li, T.J.; Yuan, D.X.; Li, L. Effects of composite antimicrobial peptides in weanling piglets challenged with deoxynivalenol: II. Intestinal morphology and function. *J. Anim. Sci.* **2013**, *91*, 4750–4756. [CrossRef] [PubMed]

51. Basso, K.; Gomes, F.; Bracarense, A.P. Deoxynivanelol and fumonisin, alone or in combination, induce changes on intestinal junction complexesand in E-cadherin expression. *Toxins* **2013**, *5*, 2341–2352. [CrossRef] [PubMed]

52. De Souza, L.C.M.; Retmal, C.A.; Rocha, G.M.; Lopez, M.L. Morphological evidence for permeability barrier in the testis and spermatic duct of *Gymnotus carpo* (Teleostei: Gymnotidae). *Mol. Reprod. Dev.* **2015**, *82*, 663–678. [CrossRef] [PubMed]

53. Mazzon, E.; Sturniolo, G.C.; Puzzolo, D.; Frisina, N.; Fries, W. Effect of stress on the paracellular barrier in the rat ileum. *Gut* **2002**, *51*, 507–513. [CrossRef] [PubMed]

54. Pinton, P.; Nougayrede, J.P.; DelRio, J.C.; Moreno, C.; Ferrier, L.; Bracarense, A.P.; Kolf-Clauw, M.; Oswald, I.P. The good contaminant deoxynivalenol, decreases intestinal barrier permeability and reduces claudin expression. *Toxicol. Appl. Pharmacol.* **2009**, *237*, 41–48. [CrossRef] [PubMed]

55. Zwierzchowski, W.; Gajęcki, M.; Obremski, K.; Zielonka, Ł.; Baranowski, M. The occurence of zearalenone and its dervatives in standard and therapeutic feeds for companion animals. *Pol. J. Vet. Sci.* **2004**, *7*, 289–293. [PubMed]

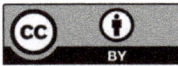

Article

Histopathological Injuries, Ultrastructural Changes, and Depressed TLR Expression in the Small Intestine of Broiler Chickens with Aflatoxin B$_1$

Fengyuan Wang [1,†], Zhicai Zuo [1,†], Kejie Chen [2,†], Caixia Gao [1,†], Zhuangzhi Yang [3], Song Zhao [1], Jianzhen Li [4], Hetao Song [1], Xi Peng [5,*], Jing Fang [1,*], Hengmin Cui [1], Ping Ouyang [1], Yi Zhou [6], Gang Shu [1] and Bo Jing [1]

1   College of Veterinary Medicine, Sichuan Agricultural University, Chengdu 611130, China; wfy_sccd@163.com (F.W.); zzcjl@126.com (Z.Z.); m15009661712@163.com (C.G.); bingozhaosong@163.com (S.Z.); sht854844223@sina.com (H.S.); cuihengmin2008@sina.com (H.C.); ouyang.ping@163.com (P.O.); dyysg2005@sicau.edu.cn (G.S.); jingbo@sicau.edu.cn (B.J.)
2   School of Public Health, Chengdu Medical College, Chengdu 610500, China; ckj930@126.com
3   Animal Research Institute, Chengdu Academy of Agriculture and Forestry Sciences, Chengdu 611130, China; yangzhuangzhi8@163.com
4   Department of Preventive Veterinary, Chengdu Agricultural College, Chengdu 611130, China; jianzhenli2006@163.com
5   College of Life Sciences, China West Normal University, Nanchong 637002, China
6   Life Science Department, Sichuan Agricultural University, Yaan 625014, China; 13981616210@139.com
*   Correspondence: pengxi197313@163.com (X.P.); fangjing4109@163.com (J.F.); Tel.: +86-139-0809-3903 (X.P.); +86-130-5657-7921 (J.F.)
†   These authors contributed equally to this work.

Received: 30 January 2018; Accepted: 18 March 2018; Published: 21 March 2018

Abstract: To explore AFB$_1$-induced damage of the small intestine, the changes in structure and expression of TLRs (Toll-like Receptors) in the small intestine of chickens were systematically investigated. Ninety healthy neonatal Cobb chickens were randomized into a control group (0 mg/kg AFB$_1$) and an AFB$_1$ group (0.6 mg/kg AFB$_1$). The crypt depth of the small intestine in the AFB$_1$ group was significantly increased in comparison to the control chickens, while the villus height and area were evidently decreased, as well as the villus:crypt ratio and epithelial thickness. The histopathological observations showed that the villi of the small intestine exposed to AFB$_1$ were obviously shedding. Based on ultrastructural observation, the absorptive cells of small intestine in the AFB$_1$ group exhibited fewer microvilli, mitochondrial vacuolation and the disappearance of mitochondrial cristae, and junctional complexes as well as terminal web. Moreover, the number of goblet cells in the small intestine in the AFB$_1$ group significantly decreased. Also, AFB$_1$ evidently decreased the mRNA expression of TLR2-2, TLR4, and TLR7 in the small intestine. Taken together, our study indicated that dietary 0.6 mg/kg AFB$_1$ could induce histopathological injuries and ultrastructural changes, and depress levels of TLR mRNA in the chicken small intestine.

Keywords: aflatoxin B$_1$; small intestine; histopathological lesions; ultrastructural changes; toll-like receptors

Key contribution: The aim of this paper is to comprehend the damaged innate immunity of small intestine induced by AFB1. The results could provide important insights for the future studies of AFB1 related to animals and humans.

---

1. Introduction

Aflatoxins, secondary metabolites produced by some *Aspergillus* species [1,2], are important mycotoxins since about 0.5 to 4.5 billion people are exposed to high levels of aflatoxins. [3,4]. Aflatoxin B_1 (AFB$_1$) is the main source and most toxic type of aflatoxins [5]. The liver is the main target organ for aflatoxins [6,7]. The negative effects of AFB$_1$ have also been well-documented, including reduced performance, decreased immune system function, and increased susceptibility to diseases in several animal species [8–10].

Conversion and absorption of food components mainly take place in the gastrointestinal tract. Normal nutrient supply is supported by several factors, including absorptive surfaces, residing microorganisms, and host-derived physiological processes [10]. Meanwhile, the intestinal mucosa is continually exposed to a series of antigens, especially the bacterial antigens. Intestinal epithelial cells (IECs) act as a defense system between the intestinal lumen and the lamina propria [11]. The entire structure and function of IECs, which possess tight junction and goblet cells producing mucus, prevent luminal antigens from translocating to the subepithelial tissue [12,13].

The immunotoxicity of AFB$_1$ to the intestine has drawn research attention. It has been reported that AFB$_1$ decreased the proportion of T-cell subset and number of IgA$^+$ cells in the small intestine of chickens [14,15]. The literature, however, is scanty and controversial as to the effects of AFB$_1$ on the morphology and histopathology of the gastrointestinal tract [10]. After exposure to 0.02 mg/kg or 0.7 mg/kg AFB$_1$ for three weeks, the density (weight/length) of the whole intestine in chickens was evidently decreased [16,17]. Grozeva et al. found that 0.5 mg/kg AFB$_1$ induced generalized hyperaemia and mononuclear cell infiltration in the small intestine of broilers within the 42 days of an experiment [18], but, at a higher level of 4 mg/kg diet, Ledoux et al. revealed no histological damage to male broilers' small intestine after a three-week exposure [19].

The pattern recognition receptors (PRRs) have been confirmed to be associated with immunity, inflammation, and cancer [20]. TLRs, one type of the PRRs, have been studied in different areas, including immunotoxicity, inflammation, oxidative stress and cell survival [21]. A few in vitro studies reported that mycotoxins affected TLRs' expression or TLRs-associated pathways. Mixed aflatoxins B and G up-regulated TLR2 and TLR4 transcript in human peripheral blood mononuclear cells [21], while deoxynivalenol led to the inhibition of TLR-MyD88 signaling in RAW264 cells [22].

The gastrointestinal tract is the first organ by which AFB$_1$ comes into the body of human and animals; thus, compared with other organs, this toxin should exert greater impacts on the small intestine. However, the effects of AFB$_1$ on the small intestine are often neglected and inconclusive [10]. And the doses and exposure time of AFB$_1$ to cause histopathological changes of the intestine were controversial in chickens [16–19]. Our team's research has shown that 0.15 mg/kg, 0.3 mg/kg and 0.6 mg/kg AFB$_1$ could cause obvious toxic effects on chichen immune organs with dose-response [9,23,24]. In our previous study, 0.3 mg/kg AFB$_1$ decreased jejunal villus height, villus height/crypt ratio, and induced shedding of epithelial cells on the tip of chicken jejunal villus from 7 to 21 days of age [25]. To observe whether 0.6 mg/kg AFB$_1$ would cause more serious damage to the whole small intestine in the same exposure time, we determined to use a higher dose (0.6 mg/kg AFB$_1$) to do the further systemic research. Furthermore, TLRs play vital roles in the innate immune system, and several studies on the effects of different mycotoxins on TLR gene expression were focused on TLR2, TLR4 and TLR7 [21,22,26–28]. Thus, these three TLRs were chosen for this research in order to compare the AFB$_1$-induced effects on TLR2, TLR4 and TLR7 with other mycotoxins.

Therefore, this research was conducted to systematically study the histopathological damages and TLR expression in the small intestine of chickens caused by dietary 0.6 mg/kg AFB$_1$ through multiple technologies, such as hematoxylin and eosin staining, histological chemistry, microscopic analyses of the villus, crypt depth and goblet cells, the mucosal epithelium observation by transmission electron microscope, and TLR2, TLR4, and TLR7 mRNA expression by qRT-PCR.

2. Results

2.1. Morphological Measurements in the Small Intestine

At three different time points, compared with the control group, the villus height of duodenum in the AFB_1 group was significantly decreased ($p < 0.05$ or $p < 0.01$), while the villus width was significantly increased ($p < 0.05$ or $p < 0.01$). Overall, the villus area of the duodenum in the AFB_1 group was evidently decreased ($p < 0.01$). Although the crypt depth of duodenum in the AFB_1 group was significantly increased ($p < 0.01$), the villus:crypt ratio in the AFB_1 group dropped significantly ($p < 0.01$). Moreover, the epithelial thickness of duodenum in the AFB_1 group significantly declined ($p < 0.05$) (Figure 1).

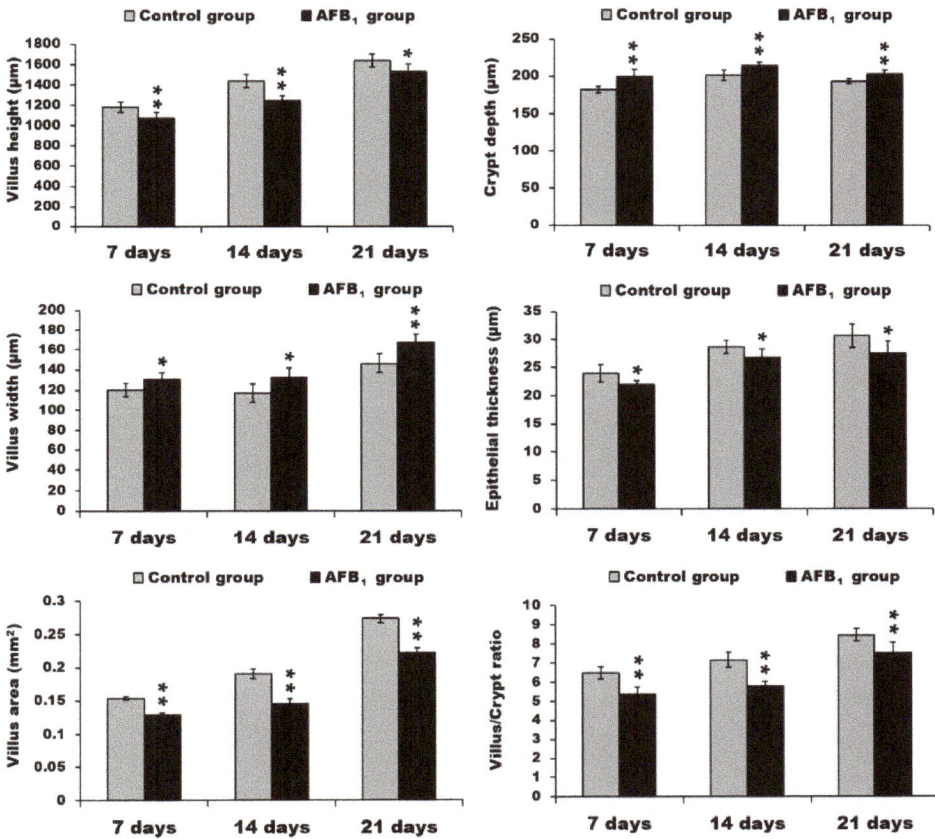

Figure 1. The data of villus height, crypt depth, villus width, epithelial thickness, villus area, and villus/crypt ratio in the duodenum. * $p < 0.05$, ** $p < 0.01$.

Compared with the control group, the jejunum of the AFB_1 group exhibited lower villus height, width, and area ($p < 0.05$ or $p < 0.01$). The jejunal crypt depth in the AFB_1 group, moreover, was significantly increased ($p < 0.05$ or $p < 0.01$), in addition, the villus:crypt ratio was evidently lower ($p < 0.01$). At all three time points, the epithelial thickness of jejunum in the AFB_1 group was significantly decreased ($p < 0.05$ or $p < 0.01$) (Figure 2).

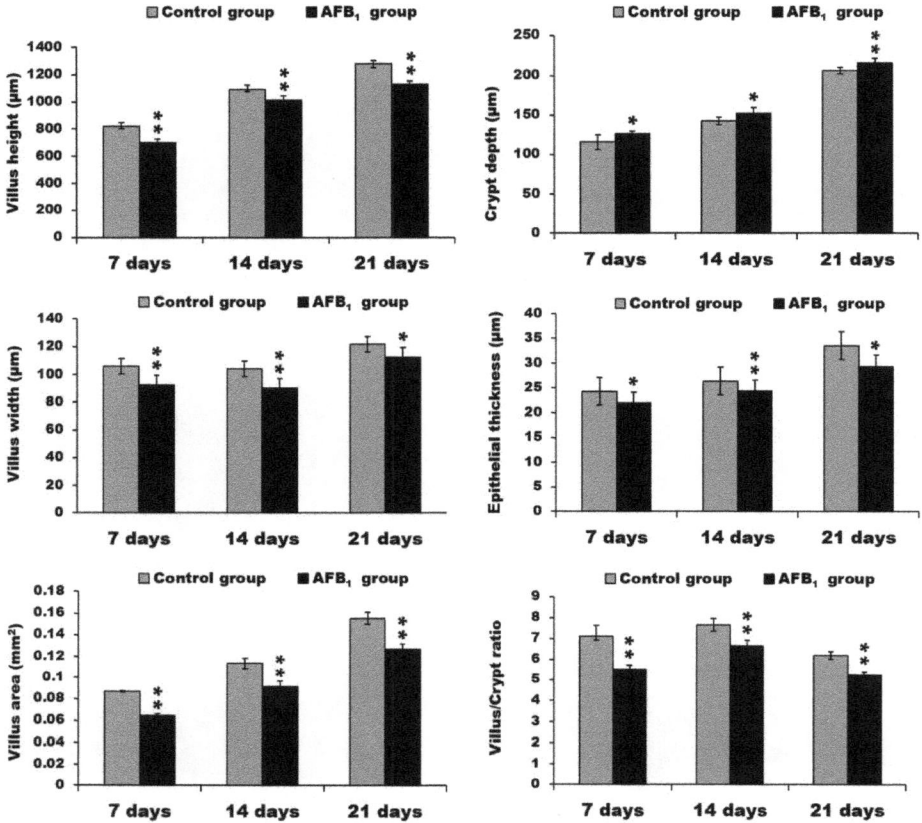

Figure 2. The data of villus height, crypt depth, villus width, epithelial thickness, villus area, and villus/crypt ratio in the jejunum. * $p < 0.05$, ** $p < 0.01$.

Compared with the control group, the ileum of broilers exposed to AFB_1 showed lower villus height, width, and area ($p < 0.05$ or $p < 0.01$). The ileac crypt depth in the AFB_1 group, moreover, was significantly increased ($p < 0.05$ or $p < 0.01$), and the villus:crypt ratio had evidently dropped ($p < 0.01$). On day 14, the epithelial thickness of the ileum in the AFB_1 group was significantly decreased ($p < 0.05$) (Figure 3).

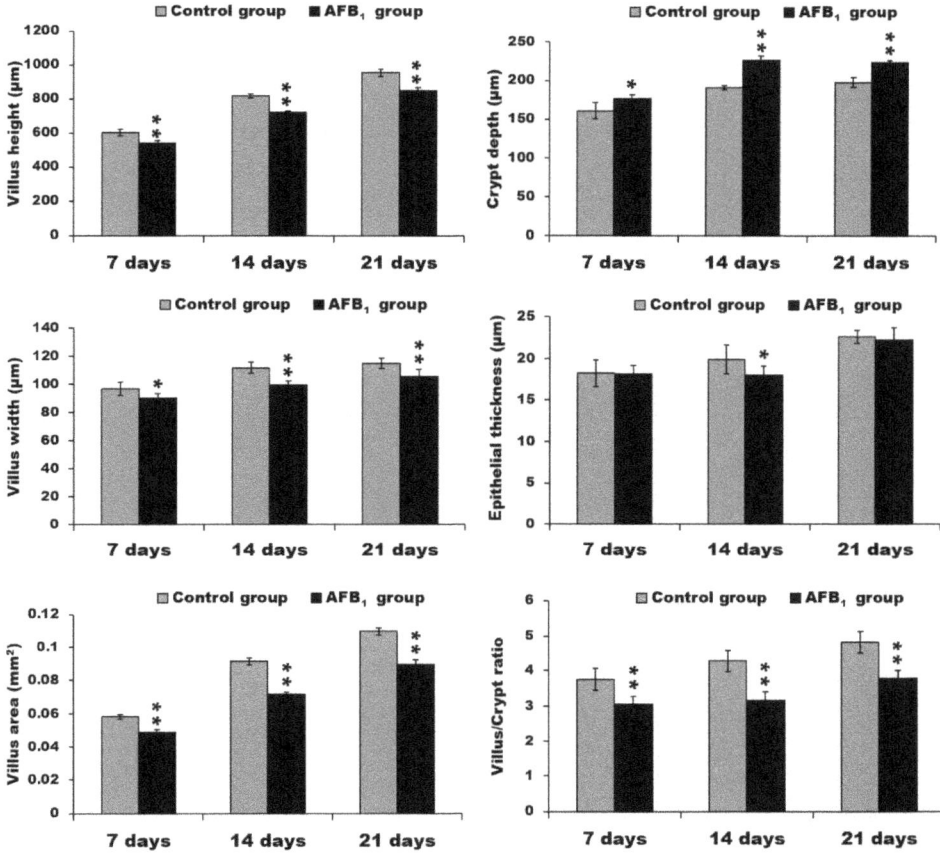

Figure 3. The data of villus height, crypt depth, villus width, epithelial thickness, villus area, and villus/crypt ratio in the ileum. * $p < 0.05$, ** $p < 0.01$.

2.2. Histopathological Analysis

The apical epithelia of villi in the small intestine in the AFB$_1$ group were shedding (Figure 4). No other obvious pathological damage to the chicken intestine in the AFB$_1$ group was observed.

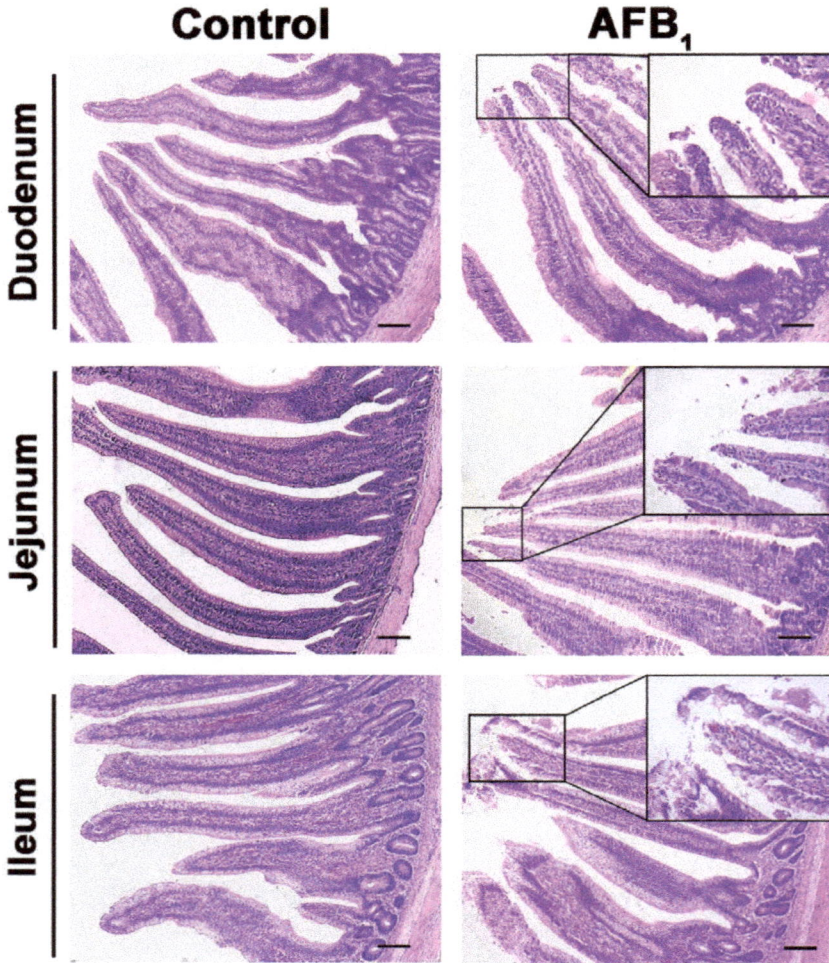

Figure 4. The representative microstructure of intestinal villi at 21 days of age. Note: The enlarged box shows the shedding of epithelial cells; H.E. stain, scale bar = 200 μm.

2.3. Ultrastructure Changes

The mucosal epithelium of the small intestine consists predominately of absorptive cells and goblet cells (Figure 5). In the duodenum, jejunum, and ileum of the control group on day 21 of the experiment, there are closely packed microvilli in the apical border of absorptive cell. Also, abundant mitochondria with normal ultra-structure were located in the apical cytoplasm of this cell. Junctional complexes including tight junction, intermediate junction, and desmosome were distributed between the epithelial cells at the luminal surface. A terminal web containing many micro-filaments was well organized under the microvilli.

In the duodenum of the AFB_1 group on day 21, reduced mitochondrial cristae and mitochondrial vacuolation and lysis of mitochondrial contents in the apical portion of some absorptive cells were the most obvious ultrastructural pathological changes (Figure 5).

In the jejunum of the AFB$_1$ group, the microvilli on the surface of some absorptive cells were completely shed, and the junctional complexes and terminal web were partly or completely disappeared. In addition, the number of mitochondria had evidently decreased (Figure 5).

Also, the microvilli of some ileac absorptive cells in the AFB$_1$ group on day 21 were fewer or shorter, or even completely shed, and the junctional complexes and terminal web had partially or entirely disappeared. Finally, fewer mitochondria, a decreased electron density, and lysis contents of apical cytoplasm were observed (Figure 5).

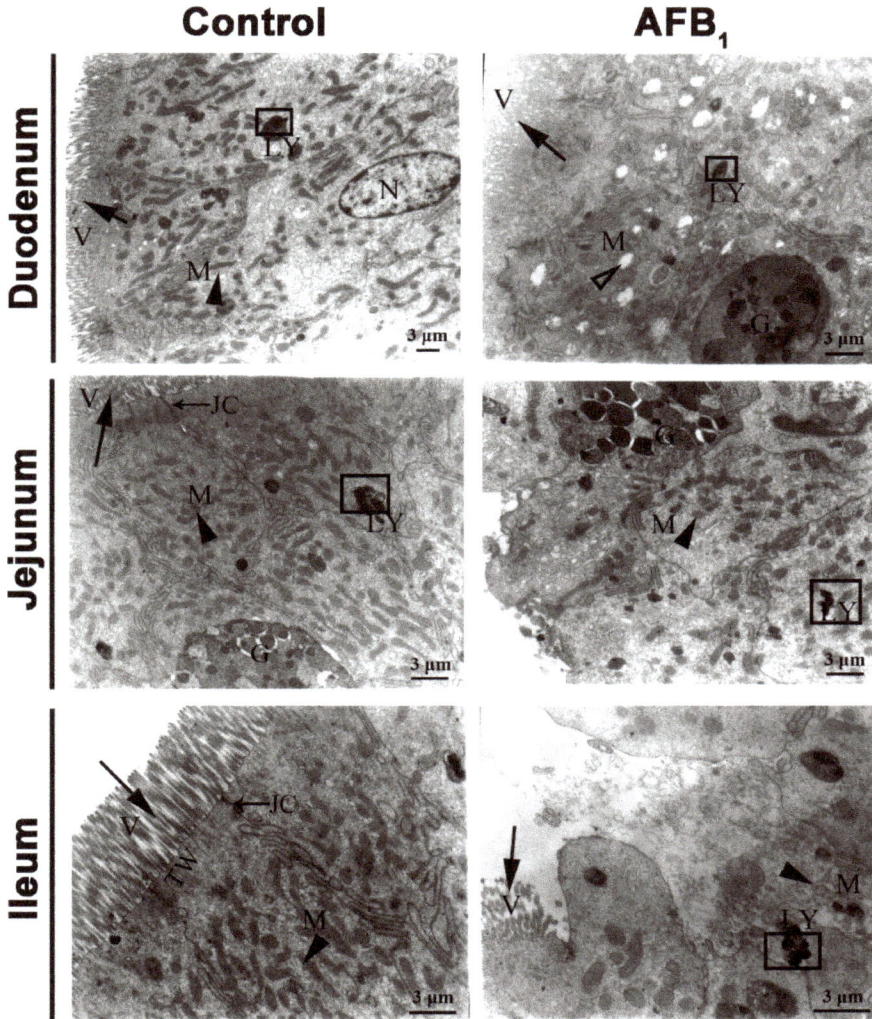

Figure 5. The representative ultrastructure of absorptive cells and goblet cells in the small intestine at 21 days of age. Note: M: mitochondria (▲), V: microvilli (→), G: Goblet cells, LY: lysosomes (□), N: nucleus, JC: Junctional complexes (→), TW: terminal web. Scale bar = 3 μm.

2.4. Number of Goblet Cells Shown by Alcian Blue/PAS

By Alcian Blue/PAS stain, goblet cells locating in mucosal epithelia and crypt were blue or purple in the small intestine of both groups. Compared with the control group, on day 7, the number of goblet cells in jejunum of the AFB_1 group was significantly decreased ($p < 0.05$). On days 14 and 21, the numbers of goblet cells in the AFB_1 group were evidently decreased ($p < 0.05$ or $p < 0.01$) (Figures 6 and 7).

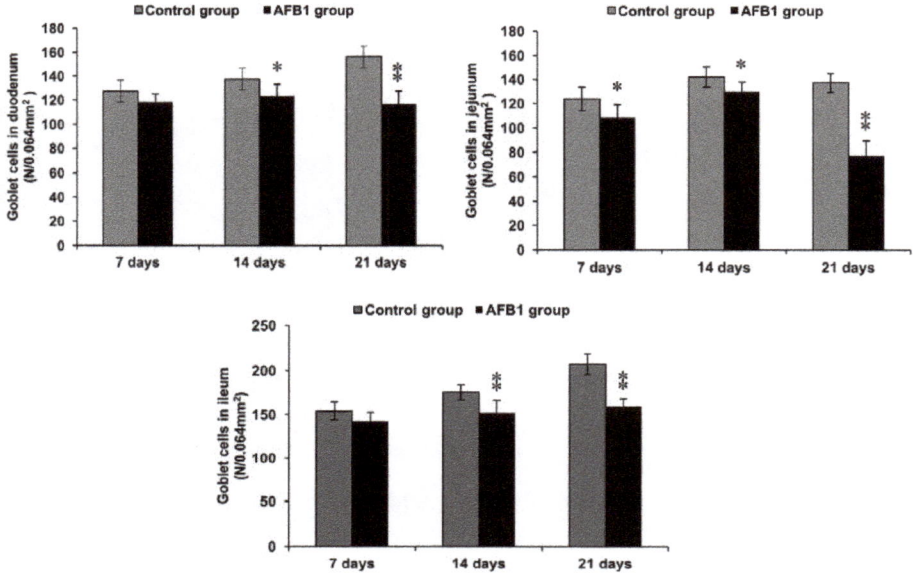

Figure 6. The numbers of goblet cells in the small intestine. Note: 0.064 mm^2 was the area of one field under 400× magnification. * $p < 0.05$, ** $p < 0.01$.

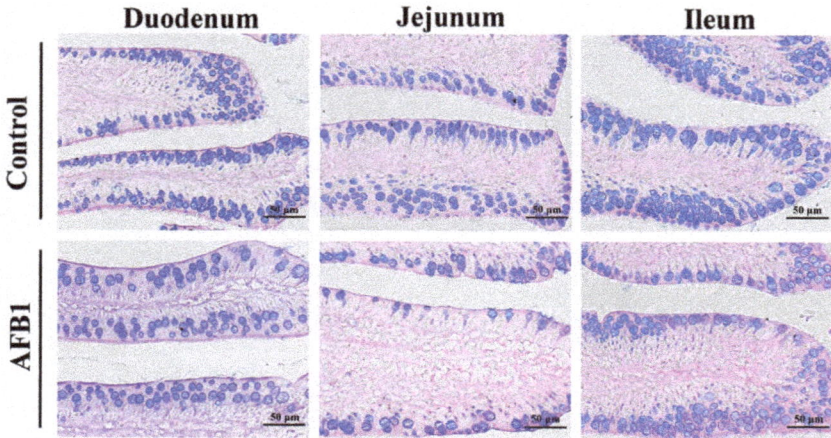

Figure 7. The representative goblet cells in the mucous epithelial cells of villi in the small intestine on day 21 (Alcian Blue/PAS stain, scale bar = 50 μm).

2.5. mRNA Expression of TLR2-2, TLR-4 and TLR-7

The mRNA expression of TLR2-2, TLR-4, and TLR7 in both the duodenum and jejunum in the AFB$_1$ group significantly decreased in comparison to the control group on day 14 and 21 ($p < 0.05$ or $p < 0.01$), except for duodenal TLR2-2 mRNA expression on day 14. The value of ileac TLR2-2 was evidently decreased in the AFB$_1$ group on days 14 and 21 ($p < 0.05$ or $p < 0.01$), and the values of ileac TLR-4 and TLR-7 in the AFB$_1$ group significantly declined during the experiment ($p < 0.05$ or $p < 0.01$) (Figure 8).

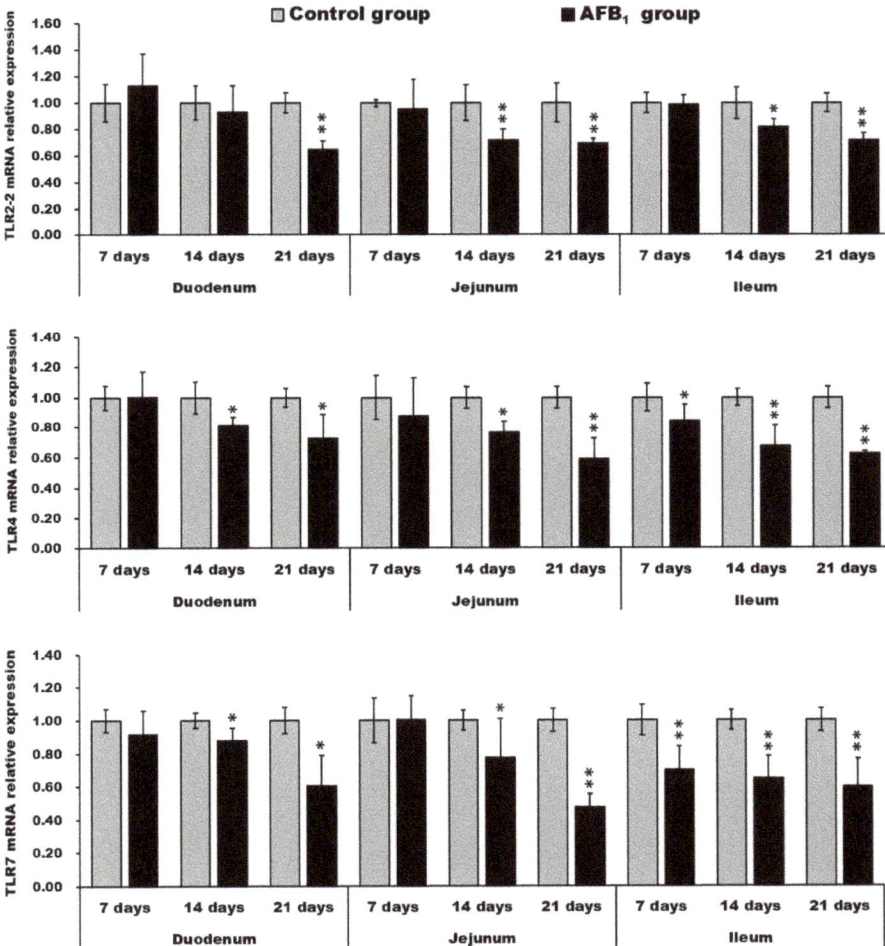

Figure 8. mRNA expression levels (fold of the control) of the TLR2-2, TLR4, and TLR7 in the small intestine. * $p < 0.05$, ** $p < 0.01$.

3. Discussion

Aflatoxin B$_1$, the most common aflatoxin, commonly contaminates various kinds of human food and animal feed elements in tropical and subtropical areas [10]. AFB$_1$ can enter into animals and humans by consumption of AFB$_1$-contaminated feed or food, so the gastrointestinal is the first site to contact AFB_1, especially the small intestine [18]. The mucosal layer of the small intestine, including the lining epithelium, lamina propria with gland, and lamina muscularis, has the specificity to be structured in a way that provides a large surface, thus maximizing the absorption of nutrients. The surface of the mucosa is studded with finger-like projections, the intestinal villi, which are the most characteristic feature of the small intestine [29]. The crypts opening between the bases of the villi penetrate the mucosa as far as the lamina muscularis [29]. The intestinal villus and crypt play a crucial role in nutritional absorption and animal growth [30]. The continuous regeneration of the small intestinal epithelium is ensured by the migration of proliferating crypt cells up the villi [31]. Therefore, the height, width, and area of villus, but especially the area, are positively related with the absorptive efficiency of the small intestine in chickens, as well as epithelium thickness and villus:crypt ratio, while the crypt depth is negatively related. Our study showed decreased villus height and area as well as villus:crypt ratio in the three parts of the small intestine in the AFB_1 group in comparison with the control chickens, suggesting that AFB_1 reduced the small intestine's surface area for absorption in chickens. Our morphological measurements were similar to most previous studies, e.g., one in which Zhang et al. found that 0.3 mg/kg AFB_1 could induce slightly decreased jejunal villus height and shedding of epithelial cells on the tip of the jejunal villus [25]; Aboutalebi reported that 0.7 mg/kg AFB_1-treatment induced more serious damage in the duodenum than 0.35 mg/kg AFB_1-treatment [32]. Thus, AFB_1 may have a dose-dependent effect. However, Feng et al. reported that AFB_1 could increase the villus height and area in the duodenum and jejunum [33], which may result from differences in animal species and doses of AFB_1 used for experiments.

In this study, moreover, AFB_1 caused the shedding of the apical epithelia of villi in the small intestine, which was also observed by other researchers in chickens [18,25]. In murine models, AFB_1 has been found to lead to pathological damage of the intestinal mucosa [34], and to decreased cell proliferation [35]. Furthermore, Akinrinmade et al. observed leucocyte, lymphocyte, and mononuclear cell infiltration in the lamina propria of rats when AFB_1 was administered intraperitoneally [36], which was not observed in our study. These discrepancies may be attributed to different methods of administration and different animal models.

In addition, to explore the relationship between AFB_1 and damage to absorptive cells in the small intestine, we used a transmission electron microscope to examine the ultrastructure of the epithelial cells of the small intestine following AFB_1 exposure. In the duodenum, fewer mitochondrial cristae of absorptive cells and lysis of mitochondrial contents were observed in the AFB_1 group. Also, microvilli on the surface of absorptive cells in the jejunum and ileum of the AFB_1 group were decreased or shedding. Mitochondria play important roles not only in producing ATP, but in controlling apoptosis and contributing to the calcium homeostasis process of cells [37,38]. The involvement of microvilli has been established in various functions such as secretion, mechanotransduction, absorption, and cellular adhesion. Junctional complexes prevent fluid intestinal contents from diffusing into the lamina propria without going through the cells [29]. A terminal web is thought to be responsible for the movement of the microvilli. Damage to the mitochondria and microvilli, along with the disappearance of junctional complexes and the terminal web in some absorptive cells, induced by AFB_1, showed that AFB_1 could cause dysfunction of these structures, resulting in functional disorders of absorptive cells in the small intestine.

To further explore how AFB_1 impaired the epithelial cells of small intestine, we investigated the number of goblet cells by Alcian Blue/PAS staining. Goblet cells are presumed to protect the mucous membrane in the intestine through the synthesis and secretion of several mediators, such as the mucin MUC2 and the small peptide trefoil factor 3 [39,40]. In this research, AFB_1 could decrease the numbers of goblet cells, which may contribute to the damage to small intestine epithelia. Furthermore, the mucins production in goblet cells could be up-regulated by TNF-α [41]. Studies have showed that AFB_1 inhibited the expression of cytokines in the small intestine, including TNF-α [14,42], by which we speculated that the contents of mucins secreted by goblet cells were depressed in the AFB_1 group. Moreover, goblet cells delivered luminal antigen to $CD103^+$ dendric cells in the small intestine [43].

Thus, the decreased goblet cells caused by AFB_1 may be associated with repressed immunity in the small intestine.

Previous in vivo research has shown that AFB_1 impaired the adaptive immunity of the small intestine in chickens. Jiang et al. found that AFB_1 decreased the T cell subset, cytokine expression, IgA^+ cell numbers, and the expression of immunoglobulin in the small intestine of broilers [14,15]. It is still unknown, however, whether AFB_1 impaired the innate immunity of the small intestine of chickens in vivo. In this study, we determined the innate immunity of the small intestine of chickens through the expression levels of three toll-like receptors. By qRT-PCR, we found that the expression levels of TLR2-2, TLR4, and TLR7 mRNA were evidently suppressed by AFB_1 exposure, similarly to zearalenone-induced decrease of TLR-4 in IPEC-1 cells [26] and pig splenocyte [27], and to T2-toxin-induced decrease of TLR-7 in porcine alveolar macrophages [28]. However, mixed aflatoxins B and G could up-regulate TLR2 and TLR4 transcripts in human peripheral blood mononuclear cells [21]. These opposite results may be the consequence of the use of different cell types. Toll-like receptors, expressed on the membranes of immune and non-immune cells, assisted the immune system with the recognition of molecules shared by pathogens, and played vital roles in the innate immune system [44]. TLR2 mediated the host response to Gram-positive bacteria [45], and the functional properties of type 2 TLR2 (TLR2-2) were alike in chickens, humans, and mice [46]. TLR4 could identify lipopolysaccharides (LPS), various viral proteins, polysaccharides, and different kinds of endogenous proteins [47]. TLR7, recognizing single-stranded RNA of viruses such as HCV, played a significant role in the regulation of antiviral immunity [48]. Based on the results of this research, we speculated that AFB_1 may impair the innate immunity of the small intestine in chickens by depressing TLR2-2, TLR4, and TLR7 mRNA levels. Moreover, the activation of NF-κB in various cell types was triggered by the downstream signaling pathway of TLR2 and TLR4 [49,50]. Following NF-κB activation, various cytokines were released, like IL-6 and TNF-α [51]. Our previous data demonstrated that 0.6 mg/kg AFB_1 in the broilers' diet could reduce the expression level of cytokine (like IL-2, IL-4, IL-6, IL-10, IL-17, IFN-γ, and TNF-α) mRNA in the small intestine, implying that the immune function of the intestinal mucosa might be affected [14]. Therefore, the suppressed expression of TLR2 and TLR4 induced by AFB_1 may contribute to the decreased levels of various cytokines [14,42].

4. Conclusions

In conclusion, feed contaminated with 0.6 mg/kg AFB_1 could induce shedding of intestinal epithelial cells; decrease villus height and area, along with villus:crypt ratio; impair the microvilli and mitochondria of absorptive cells; decrease the goblet cell number; and depress the expression of TLR2-2, TLR4, and TLR7 in the chicken small intestine. These findings indicate that AFB_1 may decrease the absorptive capacity and partially impair the innate immunity of the small intestine.

5. Materials and Methods

5.1. Animals and Groups

Ninety healthy male neonatal Cobb chickens, bought from the Chia Tai Group (Wenjiang, Sichuan, China), were randomized into control and AFB_1 groups. There were three replicates/group and 15 animals/replicate. Housed in cages with electrically heated units for 21 days, chickens were provided with water as well as the aforementioned diet *ad libitum*. The animal protocols and all procedures of the experiment in this research were carried out according to the laws and guidelines of Animal Care and Use Committee of Sichuan Agricultural University (Approval No. 2012-024). As the chickens were fed with AFB_1 after hatching, the day of age is the same as the day of the experiment.

5.2. Diets

According to the National Research Council (NRC, 1994) [52] and Chinese Feeding Standard of Chicken (NY/T33-2004), the basal diet was made the control diet. The AFB_1 (Sigma-Aldrich, St. Louis,

MO, USA, A6636) contaminated diet was formulated basically the same as reported earlier [53]. In short, after 27 mg AFB_1 farinose solid was completely dissolved into 30 mL methanol, the 30-mL mixture was mingled into 45 kg corn-soybean basal diet to formulate the AFB_1 diet. For the control diet, equivalent methanol was also added into corn-soybean basal diet. Next, the methanol of both food supplies was evaporated at 98 °F (37 °C). Based on analyses by HPLC (Waters, Milford, MA, USA) with fluorescence detection (Waters, Model 2475, Milford, MA, USA), the AFB_1 concentration was under 0.001 mg/kg in the control group, and 0.601 mg/kg in the AFB_1 group, respectively.

5.3. Histopathological Observation and Microscopic Analyses

The duodenum, jejunum, and ileum from six broilers in each group were collected and fixed in 4% paraformaldehyde on days 7, 14, and 21, and then were dehydrated and embedded in paraffin wax. The sample blocks were sectioned (5 μm) with a microtome (Leica, Wetzlar, Germany, RM2135). The tissue sections were stained with hematoxylin and eosin (H·E), and observed and photographed with a digital camera (Nikon DS-Ri1, Tokyo, Japan).

Five sections of each tissue in a chicken were taken, and five pictures ($400\times$) of each section were taken randomly. The epithelial thickness and villus height, width, and area, as well as crypt depth, were determined by image analysis software (Image-Pro Plus 5.1, Media Cybernetics, Inc., Rockville, MD, USA, 2006). The villus/crypt ratio was calculated by the following formula:

$$\text{Villus/crypt ratio} = \frac{\text{villus height}}{\text{crypt depth}} \tag{1}$$

5.4. Transmission Electron Microscope Observation

On day 21, three chickens from each group were humanely killed. At necropsy, the duodenum, jejunum, and ileum were carved into small pieces and immediately put into 2.5% glutaraldehyde for fixation, and in 2% veronal acetate-buffered OsO_4 for post-fixation. After dehydrating in acetone gradient, the sample tissues were embedded in Epon 812. The sample blocks were sectioned (65–75 nm) in a microtome with a glass knife and put in uncoated copper grids. The tissue sections were stained with uranyl acetate and lead citrate. The ultrastructural architectures of the duodenum, jejunum, and ileum were observed by transmission electron microscope (Hitachi, H-600 transmission, Tokyo, Japan).

5.5. Alcian Blue/Periodic Acid-Schiff (PAS) Stain

De-waxed sections were stained in 1% Alcian blue for 5 min, oxidized in 1% periodic acid, immersed in Schiff's reagent, and mounted and observed by light microscope. With each step, the section was washed in water. The stain showed the goblet cells containing acidic mucins (blue), neutral mucins (magenta), or mixtures of acidic and neutral mucins (purple). Five sections of each tissue in one bird were performed, and five pictures ($400\times$) of each section were taken randomly. The number of goblet cells was calculated on the tip of the villus and the principle for choosing goblet cells was to select the one with more secretion and intact section. All goblet cells in the pictures were counted for further analysis.

5.6. qRT-PCR

The small intestines from six chickens in each group on days 7, 14, and 21 were obtained and stored in liquid nitrogen. Then all samples were transferred and stored at −80 °C. Total RNA was extracted using TriPure isolation reagent (Roche Diagnostics GmbH, Mannheim, Germany). The mRNA was reverse-transcribed into cDNA byTranscription First Strand cDNA Synthesis (Roche Diagnostics GmbH). The cDNA was amplified with primers TLR2-2, 4, 7, and β-actin (specified in Table 1) using methods similar to those described by Jiang et al. [14]. Expression of TLR2-2, 4 and 7 transcripts is shown relative to that of β-actin using the $2^{-\Delta\Delta Ct}$ method of Livak and Schmittgen [54].

Table 1. Primers of TLRs and house-keeping genes.

Gene	Primer	Sequences (5'-3')	Accession Number
TLR2-2	F	CTGGGAAGTGGATTGTGGAC	AB046533.2
	R	CCAGCTCATACTTGCACCAC	
TLR4	F	AGCTACGAGGTTCTGCTCCA	AY064697
	R	TGTCCTGTGCATCTGAAAGC	
TLR7	F	TTATGCCACTCCTCTCTACCG	NM_001011688.2
	R	GCAGCCACCTCTGAAAGATT	
β-actin	F	TGCTGTGTTCCCATCTATCG	L08165
	R	TTGGTGACAATACCGTGTTCA	

5.7. Statistical Analysis

The results were expressed as the mean ± standard deviation, and the significant difference between the two groups was analyzed by variance analysis, which was performed by the independent sample test of SPSS 17.0 software for Windows. Differences were considered to be statistically significant at $p < 0.05$.

Acknowledgments: This work was supported by the Huimin Project of Chengdu Science and Technology (2016-HM01-00337-SF).

Author Contributions: Jing Fang and Xi Peng conceived and designed the experiments; Fengyuan Wang, Kejie Chen, Caixia Gao, and Hetao Song performed the experiments; Fengyuan Wang, Kejie Chen, Zhicai Zuo, and Song Zhao analyzed the data; Ping Ouyang, Yi Zhou, Gang Shu, Bo Jing contributed reagents/materials/analysis tools; Fengyuan Wang and Kejie Chen wrote the paper; Jing Fang, Zhuangzhi Yang, Jianzhen Li and Hengmin Cui assisted with writing the manuscript.

Conflicts of Interest: The authors declare no conflict of interest.

References

1. Murphy, P.A.; Hendrich, S.; Landgren, C.; Bryant, C.M. Food mycotoxins: An update. *J. Food Sci.* **2006**, *71*, 51–65. [CrossRef]
2. Hernandez-Mendoza, A.; González-Córdova, A.F.; Vallejo-Cordoba, B.; Garcia, H.S. Effect of oral supplementation of Lactobacillus reuteri in reduction of intestinal absorption of aflatoxin B$_1$ in rats. *J. Basic Microbiol.* **2011**, *51*, 263–268. [CrossRef] [PubMed]
3. Vineis, P.; Xun, W. The emerging epidemic of environmental cancers in developing countries. *Ann. Oncol.* **2009**, *20*, 205–212. [CrossRef] [PubMed]
4. Teniola, O.D.; Addo, P.A.; Brost, I.M.; Färber, P.; Jany, K.D.; Alberts, J.F.; van Zyl, W.H.; Steyn, P.S.; Holzapfel, W.H. Degradation of aflatoxin B$_1$ by cell-free extracts of Rhodococcus erythropolis and Mycobacterium fluoranthenivorans sp. nov. DSM44556(T). *Int. J. Food Microbiol.* **2005**, *105*, 111–117. [CrossRef] [PubMed]
5. Hedayati, M.T.; Pasqualotto, A.C.; Warn, P.A.; Bowyer, P.; Denning, D.W. Aspergillus flavus: Human pathogen, allergen and mycotoxin producer. *Microbiology* **2007**, *153*, 1677–1692. [CrossRef] [PubMed]
6. Bhat, R.V.; Vasanthi, S.; Rao, B.S.; Rao, R.N.; Rao, V.S.; Nagaraja, K.V.; Bai, R.G.; Prasad, C.A.K.; Vanchinathan, S.; Roy, R.; et al. Aflatoxin B$_1$ contamination in maize samples collected from different geographical regions of India—A multicentre study. *Food Addit. Contam.* **1997**, *14*, 151–156. [CrossRef] [PubMed]
7. Bababunmi, E.A.; Uwaifo, A.O.; Bassir, O. Hepatocarcinogens in Nigerian foodstuffs. *World Rev. Nutr. Diet.* **1978**, *28*, 188–209. [PubMed]
8. Shivachandra, S.B.; Sah, R.L.; Singh, S.D.; Kataria, J.M.; Manimaran, K. Immunosuppression in broiler chicks fed aflatoxin and inoculated with fowl adenovirus serotype-4 (FAV-4) associated with hydropericardium syndrome. *Vet. Res. Commun.* **2003**, *27*, 39–51. [CrossRef] [PubMed]

9.   Peng, X.; Chen, K.; Chen, J.; Fang, J.; Cui, H.; Zuo, Z.; Deng, J.; Chen, Z.; Geng, Y.; Lai, W. Aflatoxin B$_1$ affects apoptosis and expression of Bax, Bcl-2, and Caspase-3 in thymus and bursa of fabricius in broiler chickens. *Environ. Toxicol.* **2015**, *30*, 1113–1120. [CrossRef] [PubMed]

10.   Yunus, A.W.; Razzazi-Fazeli, E.; Bohm, J. Aflatoxin B$_1$ in affecting broiler's performance, immunity, and gastrointestinal tract: A review of history and contemporary issues. *Toxins* **2011**, *3*, 566–590. [CrossRef] [PubMed]

11.   De Kivit, S.; Tobin, M.C.; Forsyth, C.B.; Keshavarzian, A.; Landay, A.L. Regulation of intestinal immune responses through TLR activation: Implications for pro- and prebiotics. *Front. Immunol.* **2014**, *5*, 60. [CrossRef] [PubMed]

12.   Linden, S.K.; Sutton, P.; Karlsson, N.G.; Korolik, V.; McGuckin, M.A. Mucins in the mucosal barrier to infection. *Mucosal Immunol.* **2008**, *1*, 183–197. [CrossRef] [PubMed]

13.   Salzman, N.H.; Hung, K.; Haribhai, D.; Chu, H.; Karlsson-Sjöberg, J.; Amir, E.; Teggatz, P.; Barman, M.; Hayward, M.; Eastwood, D.; et al. Enteric defensins are essential regulators of intestinal microbial ecology. *Nat. Immunol.* **2010**, *11*, 76–83. [CrossRef] [PubMed]

14.   Jiang, M.; Peng, X.; Fang, J.; Cui, H.; Yu, Z.; Chen, Z. Effects of aflatoxin B$_1$ on T-cell subsets and mRNA expression of cytokines in the intestine of broilers. *Int. J. Mol. Sci.* **2015**, *16*, 6945–6959. [CrossRef] [PubMed]

15.   Jiang, M.; Fang, J.; Peng, X.; Cui, H.; Yu, Z. Effect of aflatoxin B$_1$ on IgA$^+$ cell number and immunoglobulin mRNA expression in the intestine of broilers. *Immunopharmacol. Immunotoxicol.* **2015**, *37*, 450–457. [CrossRef] [PubMed]

16.   Kana, J.R.; Teguia, A.; Choumboue, J.T. The evaluation of activated dietary charcoal from Canarium schweinfurthii Engl. seed and maize cob as toxin binder in broiler chickens. *Adv. Anim. Biosci.* **2010**, *1*, 467–468. [CrossRef]

17.   Yunus, A.W.; Ghareeb, K.; Abd-El-Fattah, A.A.; Twaruzek, M.; Böhm, J. Gross intestinal adaptations in relation to broiler performance during chronic aflatoxin exposure. *Poult. Sci.* **2011**, *90*, 1683–1689. [CrossRef] [PubMed]

18.   Grozeva, N.; Valchev, I.; Hristov, T.; Lazarov, L.; Nikolov, Y. Histopathological changes in small intestines of broiler chickens with experimental aflatoxicosis. *Agric. Sci. Technol.* **2015**, *7*, 319–323.

19.   Ledoux, D.R.; Rottinghaus, G.E.; Bermudez, A.J.; Alonso-Debolt, M. Efficacy of a hydrated sodium calcium aluminosilicate to ameliorate the toxic effects of aflatoxin in broiler chicks. *Poult. Sci.* **1999**, *78*, 204–210. [CrossRef] [PubMed]

20.   Takeuchi, O.; Akira, S. Pattern recognition receptors and inflammation. *Cell* **2010**, *140*, 805–820. [CrossRef] [PubMed]

21.   Malvandi, A.M.; Mehrzad, J.; Saleh-Moghaddam, M. Biologically relevant doses of mixed aflatoxins B and G up-regulate MyD88, TLR2, TLR4 and CD14 transcripts in human PBMCs. *Immunopharmacol. Immunotoxicol.* **2013**, *35*, 528–532. [CrossRef] [PubMed]

22.   Sugiyama, K.; Muroi, M.; Kinoshita, M.; Hamada, O.; Minai, Y.; Sugita-Konishi, Y.; Kamata, Y.; Tanamoto, K. NF-κB activation via MyD88-dependent Toll-like receptor signaling is inhibited by trichothecene mycotoxin deoxynivalenol. *J. Toxicol. Sci.* **2016**, *41*, 273–279. [CrossRef] [PubMed]

23.   Yu, Z.; Chen, J.; Peng, X.; Fang, J.; Chen, K.; Yang, H. Effect of aflatoxin B$_1$ pathological changes of immune organs in broilers. *Acta Vet. Zootech. Sin.* **2015**, *46*, 1447–1454. [CrossRef]

24.   Chen, J.; Chen, K.; Yuan, S.; Peng, X.; Fang, J.; Wang, F.; Cui, H.; Chen, Z.; Yuan, J.; Geng, Y. Effects of aflatoxin B$_1$ on oxidative stress markers and apoptosis of spleens in broilers. *Toxicol. Ind. Health* **2016**, *32*, 278–284. [CrossRef] [PubMed]

25.   Zhang, S.; Peng, X.; Fang, J.; Cui, H.; Zuo, Z.; Chen, Z. Effects of aflatoxin B$_1$ exposure and sodium selenite supplementation on the histology, cell proliferation, and cell cycle of jejunum in broilers. *Biol. Trace Elem. Res.* **2014**, *160*, 32–40. [CrossRef] [PubMed]

26.   Taranu, I.; Marin, D.E.; Pistol, G.C.; Motiu, M.; Pelinescu, D. Induction of pro-inflammatory gene expression by Escherichia coli and mycotoxin zearalenone contamination and protection by a lactobacillus mixture in porcine IPEC-1 cells. *Toxicon* **2015**, *97*, 53. [CrossRef] [PubMed]

27.   Pistol, G.C.; Braicu, C.; Motiu, M.; Gras, M.A.; Marin, D.E.; Stancu, M.; Calin, L.; Israel-Roming, F.; Berindan-Neagoe, I.; Taranu, I. Zearalenone mycotoxin affects immune mediators, MAPK signalling molecules, nuclear receptors and genome-wide gene expression in pig spleen. *PLoS ONE* **2015**, *10*, e0127503. [CrossRef] [PubMed]

28. Seeboth, J.; Solinhac, R.; Oswald, I.P.; Guzylack-Piriou, L. The fungal T-2 toxin alters the activation of primary macrophages induced by TLR-agonists resulting in a decrease of the inflammatory response in the pig. *Vet. Res.* **2012**, *43*, 35. [CrossRef] [PubMed]

29. Jo, A.E.; Brian, L.F. *Dellmann's Textbook of Veterinary Histology*; Blackwell Publishing Professional: Ames, IA, USA, 2006, ISBN 0781741483.

30. Hernández, F.; García, V.; Madrid, J.; Orengo, J.; Catalá, P.; Megías, M.D. Effect of formic acid on performance, digestibility, intestinal histomorphology and plasma metabolite levels of broiler chickens. *Br. Poult. Sci.* **2006**, *47*, 50–56. [CrossRef] [PubMed]

31. Geyra, A.; Uni, Z.; Sklan, D. Enterocyte dynamics and mucosal development in the posthatch chick. *Poult. Sci.* **2001**, *80*, 776–782. [CrossRef] [PubMed]

32. Aboutalebi, N. Toxic effects of aflatoxin B_1 on duodenum tissue. *J. Am. Sci.* **2013**, *9*, 115–117.

33. Feng, G.D.; He, J.; Ao, X.; Chen, D.W. Effects of maize naturally contaminated with aflatoxin B_1 on growth performance, intestinal morphology, and digestive physiology in ducks. *Poult. Sci.* **2017**, *96*, 1948–1955. [CrossRef] [PubMed]

34. Gaikwad, S.S.; Pillai, M.M. Effect of aflatoxin B_1 in gastrointestine of mice. *J. Ecophysiol. Occup. Health* **2004**, *4*, 153–159.

35. Fleming, S.E.; Youngman, L.D.; Ames, B.N. Intestinal cell proliferation is influenced by intakes of protein and energy, aflatoxin, and whole-body radiation. *Nutr. Cancer* **1994**, *22*, 11–30. [CrossRef] [PubMed]

36. Akinrinmade, F.J.; Akinrinde, A.S.; Amid, A. Changes in serum cytokine levels, hepatic and intestinal morphology in aflatoxin B_1-induced injury: Modulatory roles of melatonin and flavonoid-rich fractions from Chromolena odorata. *Mycotoxin Res.* **2016**, *32*, 53–60. [CrossRef] [PubMed]

37. Jiang, X.; Wang, X. Cytochrome C-mediated apoptosis. *Annu. Rev. Biochem.* **2004**, *73*, 87–106. [CrossRef] [PubMed]

38. Santulli, G.; Xie, W.; Reiken, S.R.; Marks, A.R. Mitochondrial calcium overload is a key determinant in heart failure. *Proc. Natl. Acad. Sci. USA* **2015**, *112*, 11389–11394. [CrossRef] [PubMed]

39. Moncada, D.M.; Kammanadiminti, S.J.; Chadee, K. Mucin and toll-like receptors in host defense against intestinal parasites. *Trends Parasitol.* **2003**, *19*, 305–311. [CrossRef]

40. Taupin, D.; Podolsky, D.K. Trefoil factors: Initiators of mucosal healing. *Nat. Rev. Mol. Cell Biol.* **2003**, *4*, 721–732. [CrossRef] [PubMed]

41. Andrianifahanana, M.; Moniaux, N.; Batra, S.K. Regulation of mucin expression: Mechanistic aspects and implications for cancer and inflammatory diseases. *Biochim. Biophys. Acta* **2006**, *1765*, 189–222. [CrossRef] [PubMed]

42. He, Y.; Fang, J.; Peng, X.; Cui, H.; Zuo, Z.; Deng, J.; Chen, Z.; Lai, W.; Shu, G.; Tang, L. Effects of sodium selenite on aflatoxin B_1-induced decrease of ileac T cell and the mRNA contents of IL-2, IL-6, and TNF-α in broilers. *Biol. Trace Elem. Res.* **2014**, *159*, 167–173. [CrossRef] [PubMed]

43. McDole, J.R.; Wheeler, L.W.; McDonald, K.G.; Wang, B.; Konjufca, V.; Knoop, K.A.; Newberry, R.D.; Miller, M.J. Goblet cells deliver luminal antigen to CD103$^+$ dendritic cells in the small intestine. *Nature* **2012**, *483*, 345–349. [CrossRef] [PubMed]

44. Delneste, Y.; Beauvillain, C.; Jeannin, P. Innate immunity: Structure and function of TLRs. *Med. Sci.* **2007**, *23*, 67–73. [CrossRef]

45. Borrello, S.; Nicolò, C.; Delogu, G.; Pandolfi, F.; Ria, F. TLR2: A crossroads between infections and autoimmunity? *Int. J. Immunopathol. Pharmacol.* **2011**, *24*, 549–556. [CrossRef] [PubMed]

46. Fukui, A.; Inoue, N.; Matsumoto, M.; Nomura, M.; Yamada, K.; Matsuda, Y.; Toyoshima, K.; Seya, T. Molecular cloning and functional characterization of chicken toll-like receptors. A single chicken toll covers multiple molecular patterns. *J. Biol. Chem.* **2001**, *276*, 47143–47149. [CrossRef] [PubMed]

47. Brubaker, S.W.; Bonham, K.S.; Zanoni, I.; Kagan, J.C. Innate immune pattern recognition: A cell biological perspective. *Annu. Rev. Immunol.* **2015**, *33*, 257–290. [CrossRef] [PubMed]

48. Zhang, Y.; El-Far, M.; Dupuy, F.P.; Abdel-Hakeem, M.S.; He, Z.; Procopio, F.A.; Shi, Y.; Haddad, E.K.; Ancuta, P.; Sekaly, R.P.; et al. HCV RNA Activates APCs via TLR7/TLR8 while virus selectively stimulates macrophages without inducing antiviral responses. *Sci. Rep.* **2016**, *6*, 29447. [CrossRef] [PubMed]

49. Medzhitov, R.; Janeway, C., Jr. Innate immunity. *N. Engl. J. Med.* **2000**, *343*, 338–344. [CrossRef] [PubMed]

50. Anderson, K.V. Toll signaling pathways in the innate immune response. *Curr. Opin. Immunol.* **2000**, *12*, 13–19. [CrossRef]

51. Thoma-Uszynski, S.; Stenger, S.; Takeuchi, O.; Ochoa, M.T.; Engele, M.; Sieling, P.A.; Barnes, P.F.; Rollinghoff, M.; Bolcskei, P.L.; Wagner, M.; et al. Induction of direct antimicrobial activity through mammalian toll-like receptors. *Science* **2001**, *291*, 1544–1547. [CrossRef] [PubMed]
52. National Research Council. *Nutrient Requirement of Poultry*, 9th ed.; National Academy Press: Washington, DC, USA, 1994, ISBN 978-0-309-04892-7.
53. Kaoud, H.A. Innovative methods for the amelioration of aflatoxin (AFB$_1$) effect in broiler chicks. *Spec. J. Biol. Sci.* **2015**, *1*, 19–24.
54. Livak, K.J.; Schmittgen, T.D. Analysis of relative gene expression data using real-time quantitative PCR and the 2(-Delta Delta C(T)) method. *Methods* **2012**, *25*, 402–408. [CrossRef] [PubMed]

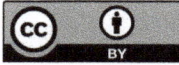

Article

The Impact of T-2 Toxin on Vasoactive Intestinal Polypeptide-Like Immunoreactive (VIP-LI) Nerve Structures in the Wall of the Porcine Stomach and Duodenum

Krystyna Makowska [1], **Kazimierz Obremski** [2] **and Slawomir Gonkowski** [1,*]

[1] Department of Clinical Physiology, Faculty of Veterinary Medicine, University of Warmia and Mazury, Oczapowskiego Str. 13, 10-718 Olsztyn, Poland; krystyna.makowska@uwm.edu.pl

[2] Department of Veterinary Prevention and Feed Hygiene, Faculty of Veterinary Medicine, University of Warmia and Mazury in Olsztyn, Oczapowskiego Str. 13, 10-718 Olsztyn, Poland; kazimierz.obremski@uwm.edu.pl

* Correspondence: slawomir.gonkowski@uwm.edu.pl; Tel.: +48-89-523-4376

Received: 28 February 2018; Accepted: 25 March 2018; Published: 26 March 2018

Abstract: T-2 toxin is a secondary metabolite of some Fusarium species. It is well-known that this substance can harmfully impact living organisms. Among others, thanks to the ability of crossing the blood–brain barrier, T-2 toxin can affect the central nervous system. Mycotoxins mostly get into the organism through the digestive tract; therefore, first of all they have to break the intestinal barrier, wherein the important component is the enteric nervous system (ENS). However, knowledge about the impact of T-2 toxin on the ENS is rather scant. As a result of the influence of various physiological and pathological agents, ENS can undergo adaptive and reparative processes which manifest as changes in the immunoreactivity of perikaryons for neuronal active substances. So, the aim of the present investigation was to study how low doses of T-2 toxin affect vasoactive intestinal polypeptide-like immunoreactive (VIP-LI) nervous structures in the ENS of the porcine stomach and duodenum. Obtained results have shown that T-2 toxin causes an percentage increase of VIP-LI nerve cells and nerve fibers in every enteric plexus in both fragments of gastrointestinal tract studied. This shows that even low doses of T-2 toxin can have an influence on living organisms.

Keywords: T-2 toxin; enteric nervous system; pig; vasoactive intestinal polypeptide

Key contribution: The administration of low doses of T-2 toxin causes the increase in the number of nervous structures immunoreactive to vasoactive intestinal polypeptide (VIP) located in the porcine stomach and duodenum.

---

1. Introduction

Mycotoxins are secondary fungal metabolites that may have a multidirectional negative impact on living organisms. Depending on the type of toxic substance, they may show carcinogenic, mutagenic, allergenic, estrogenic, and/or neurotoxic activities [1–4]. Moreover, due to their widespread presence in the environment, mycotoxins cause not only acute, but also chronic poisoning. Another dangerous consequence of long or intense exposure to these secondary fungal metabolites is the possibility of kidney and/or liver damage resulting in their failure [3,5,6].

Among a broad range of mycotoxins, one of the more dangerous is T-2 toxin, which is synthetized by fungi of the genus Fusarium, namely *Fusarium sporotrichioides, langsethiae, acuminatum*, and *poae*, and occurs ubiquitously in various food products of vegetable origin, including wheat, sorghum, rye, corn, oats, and rice [2,4,7].

T-2 toxin mostly exhibits cytotoxic and immunosuppressive activities [4,8]. Till now, it has been established that this mycotoxin contributes to such gastrointestinal disorders as alimentary toxic aleukia (ATA) and inflammatory bowel disease [7,9]. Moreover, T-2 toxin can cause thymus and spleen impairments [7,8]. However, one of the most dangerous effects of this toxin is the neurologic toxicity caused by its ability to cross the blood–brain barrier, which results in changes within the central nervous system [4,10]. Because of the above-mentioned negative effects, a high resistance to temperature, and its widespread occurrence in food, T-2 toxin constitutes a serious threat to the health and life of both humans and animals [3,6].

Due to the fact that mycotoxins mostly enter into the organism through the digestive tract, first of all they have to break the intestinal barrier, wherein the important component is the enteric nervous system (ENS). The ENS is situated within the digestive tract, from the esophagus to the rectum, in all mammal species and regulates most stomach and intestine activities. The structure of the ENS varies depending on both the animal species as well as the part of the gastrointestinal (GI) tract. Within the stomach of large mammals, including pigs, the ENS is formed of two intramural ganglionated plexuses: the myenteric plexus (MP), which is situated betwixt the longitudinal and circular muscle layers, and the submucous plexus (SP), which is located between the muscularis mucosa and circular muscle layer [7]. Contrary to the stomach, the ENS in the intestine of big mammals species forms three intramural plexuses: MP, which is situated the same as in the stomach, and two submucous plexuses: the outer submucous plexus (OSP), which is located close to the internal side of the circular muscle layer, and the inner submucous plexus (ISP), which lies between the muscularis mucosa and lamina propria [11,12].

On account of the huge amount of enteric neurons, as well as their significant differentiation and autonomy, the ENS is called the "second" or "intestinal" brain [13]. Because the enteric neurons take part in very different regulatory processes connected with all aspects of intestinal physiology, they may contain a vast number of neuronal active substances [14,15]. Till now, several dozen of such substances have been described. Among them, vasoactive intestinal polypeptide (VIP) deserves special attention. This peptide is known to be a non-noradrenergic, non-cholinergic transmitter (NANC) and the most important inhibitory factor within the GI tract [12,16,17]. First of all, VIP causes the relaxation of gastrointestinal muscles and sphincters [18,19]. Moreover, this substance suppresses secretory activity of the stomach and intestine and dilates blood vessels within the wall of the GI tract and mesentery [20,21]. Some previous studies have revealed the neuroprotective and/or adaptive activity of VIP-positive enteric neurons during pathological processes and after toxic substances administration [22–25], but these functions of VIP have not been fully elucidated.

On the other hand, although the knowledge about the negative effects of T-2 toxin is not negligible, many aspects connected with the impact of this substance on living organisms still remain unexplored. One of them is the impact of this toxin on the ENS [4,7], which is known to undergo structural, functional, or chemical changes as a result of some physiological and pathological stimuli [26–29].

So, the present study has been conducted to describe the impact of low doses of T-2 toxin on the distribution of VIP within the enteric perikaryons in the porcine GI tract. Because of the major sensitivity of the ENS to the occurrence of harmful factors in the digestive tract [12,14,26,27,29] and the well-known functions of VIP in intestinal regulatory processes [14,30,31], changes observed during investigations can signify the first subclinical signs of the damage effected by T-2 toxin. The obtained results on the one side can result in a better understanding of the mechanisms connected with the impact of this mycotoxin on living organisms, and on the other side can contribute to an explanation of the roles of VIP during intoxications.

Moreover, the choosing the domestic pig as the laboratory mammal in the investigation allows us to estimate the changes which can occur under the impact of low doses of T-2 toxin in the human enteric nervous system. This assumption is in agreement with previous studies where the neurochemical, histological, and physiological similarities between the human and porcine ENS have been described [12,29,32]. For this reason, the domestic pig seems to be a better animal model for investigations on pathological changes in the human ENS than rodents, which are commonly used for this purpose.

2. Results

During the present investigation, no clinical symptoms were observed after T2 toxin administration. Moreover, there were no differences in the food intake between control and experimental groups.

In this experiment, VIP-positive neurons and nerve fibers were observed in the ENS of the stomach and the duodenum in both control as well as experimental groups of animals. The number of these structures fluctuated depending on the part of the ENS and the fragment of digestive tract studied (Tables 1 and 2, Figures 1–4).

Table 1. Vasoactive intestinal polypeptide (VIP)-positive nerve cells and fibers in the stomach of the pig. CML: circular muscle layer; MP: myenteric plexus; CB: cell bodies; NF: nerve fibers; SP: submucous plexus; S/ML: submucosal/mucosal layer.

STOMACH		Group C	Group T2
CML [1]		4.26 ± 0.21	5.17 ± 0.11 *
MP	CB [2]	37.56 ± 0.84	42.85 ± 0.74 *
	NF [3]	+	+
SP	CB [2]	36.78 ± 0.4	43.83 ± 1.18 *
	NF [3]	−	+
S/ML [1]		2.84 ± 0.07	4.15 ± 0.15 *

[1] Mean number of VIP-positive nerves per microscopic field (mean ± standard error of the mean (SEM)); [2] The percent of VIP-positive nerve cells (mean ± SEM) in regard to perikarya immunoreactive to protein gene-product 9.5 (PGP 9.5) (pan neuronal marker); [3] the consistence of intraganglionic VIP-positive fibers shown in mean units on the scale from (-), presenting the absence of VIP-positive nerves, to (++++), indicating a very dense meshwork of fibers studied. Statistically significant differences ($p \leq 0.05$) are marked with *.

Table 2. VIP-positive nerve cells and fibers in the duodenum of the pig. CML: circular muscle layer; MP: myenteric plexus; CB: cell bodies; NF: nerve fibers; OSP: outer submucous plexus; ISP: inner submucous plexus; S/ML: submucosal/mucosal layer.

DUDODENUM		Group C	Group T2
CML [1]		17.08 ± 0.08	21.22 ± 0.24 *
MP	CB [2]	31.45 ± 0.77	39.24 ± 1.02 *
	NF [3]	+	++
OSP	CB [2]	32.43 ± 1.83	40.59 ± 0.67 *
	NF [3]	++	++
ISP	CB [2]	28.50 ± 1.17	35.42 ± 1.52 *
	NF [3]	+	++
S/ML [1]		32.35 ± 0.32	39.97 ± 1.23 *

[1] Mean number of VIP-positive nerves per microscopic field (mean ± SEM); [2] The percent of VIP-positive nerve cells (mean ± SEM) in regard to perikarya immunoreactive for PGP 9.5 (pan neuronal marker); [3] the consistence of intraganglionic VIP-positive fibers shown in mean units on the scale from (-), presenting the absence of VIP-positive nerves, to (++++), indicating a very dense meshwork of fibers studied. Statistically significant differences ($p \leq 0.05$) are marked with *.

The percentage of vasoactive intestinal polypeptide-like immunoreactive (VIP-LI) neurons with regard to the number of protein gene-products 9.5 (PGP 9.5) LI cells in both the fundus of the stomach as well as the duodenum of control pigs was substantial. However, in the stomach of C group animals this number was higher and amounted to $37.56 \pm 0.84\%$ in the muscular plexus and $36.78 \pm 0.4\%$ in the submucous plexus (Figure 1, Table 1). In the same GI tract fragment, unlike nerve cells, the number of VIP-positive nerves was very slight. There has been observed only a single intraganglionic VIP-LI nerve in the MP, whereas such nerves were absent in most of the SP in the stomach of pigs under physiological conditions. Similarly, in case of the fibers situated in the stomachic wall, the number of these neuronal structures was also low and reached only 4.26 ± 0.21 per observation field in the circular muscle layer and 2.84 ± 0.07 in the submucous/mucous layer (Figure 2, Table 1).

In the duodenum from C group, the number of VIP-LI nerve cells was slightly lower than in the case of the stomach. The percentage of these nerve cells amounted to $31.45 \pm 0.77\%$, $32.43 \pm 1.83\%$, and $28.50 \pm 1.17\%$ in the MP, OSP, and ISP, respectively (Figure 3, Table 2). Although the number of VIP-positive neurons was comparable in the both GI tract parts studied, the amount of VIP-positive nerve fibers was completely different. The number of intraganglionic nerves was higher than in the stomach, and contrary to the gastric SP, in the submucous plexuses of the duodenum were observed single (in the ISP) and rare (in the OSP) VIP-LI nerve fibers. However, the main difference concerned nerve fibers located in the wall of the studied organs. In contrast to a few VIP-positive nerves in the gastric wall, in the duodenum their number was high and amounted to 17.08 ± 0.08 per observation field in the circular muscle and 32.35 ± 0.32 in the submucous/mucous layers (Figure 4, Table 2).

Treatment with T-2 toxin caused changes in the percentage of VIP-LI enteric perikaryons and the density of nerve fibers positive for the studied substance. These alterations consisted mainly in an increase in the number of VIP-positive nerve structures. However, the intensity of these deviations clearly depended on both the GI tract fragment and part of the ENS studied. The biggest changes concerned the MP and OSP in the duodenum, where the percentage of VIP-positive perikaryons increased about eight percentage points (pp). Considerably lower alterations were observed in the duodenal inner submucous plexus (about a seven pp increase) (Figure 3, Table 2). Similar changes have been noted in the gastric MP (increase of five pp) and SP (increase of six pp) (Figure 1, Table 1). In the experimental group, the concentration of intraganglionic VIP-positive nerves was also greater than in the C group; however, these alterations were not so significant and were noted in the stomachic SP and the duodenal MP and ISP. Furthermore, marked changes in the density of VIP-LI nerves in the muscle and mucous layers were noted in the T2 group. The clearest increase in the number of nerves per observation field was noted in the duodenal submucous/mucous layer: from 32.35 ± 0.32 to 39.97 ± 1.23, whereas in the stomach, these values accelerated from 2.84 ± 0.07 to 4.15 ± 0.15. Alterations in the amount of VIP-LI nerve fibers in the muscle layer were less observable and reached about 5.17 ± 0.11 in the duodenum and about 21.22 ± 0.24 within the stomach (Tables 1 and 2, Figures 2 and 4).

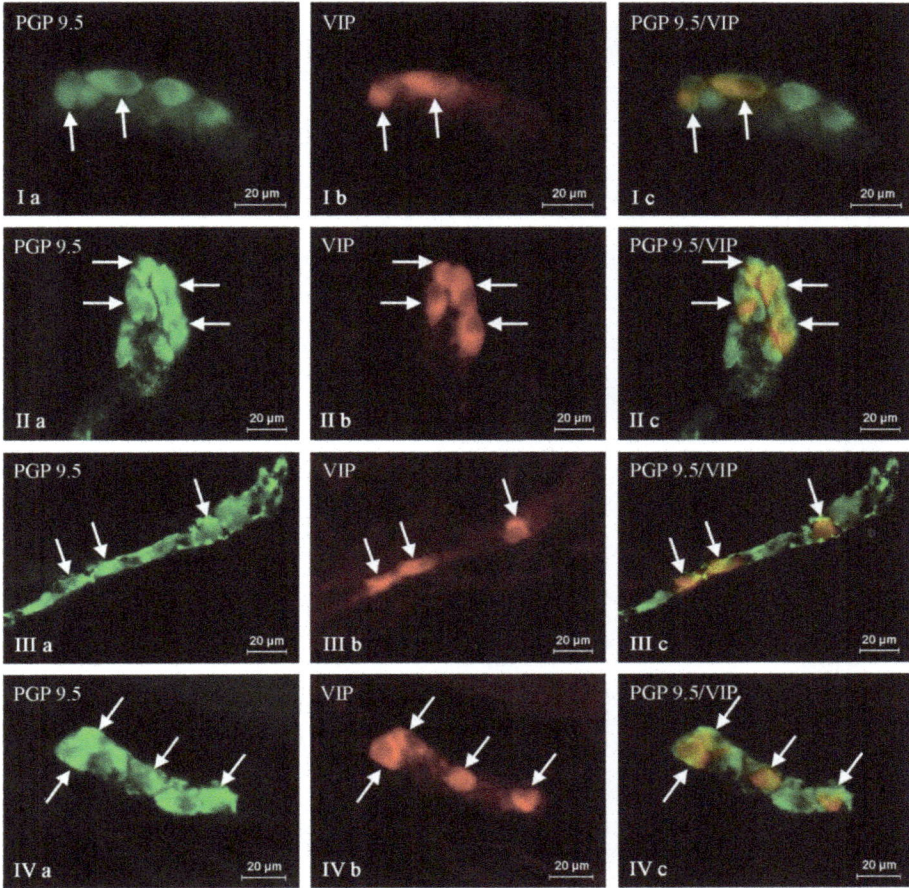

Figure 1. Nerve cell bodies containing the protein gene-product 9.5 (PGP 9.5) pan-neuronal marker (**a**) and vasoactive intestinal polypeptide (VIP) (**b**) within the porcine gastric wall in control animals (I, III) and after T-2 toxin giving (II, IV). I, II: submucous plexus; III, IV: myenteric plexus. Arrows indicate VIP-positive neurons. Photos Ic, IIc, IIIc, and IVc came from the merger of green (PGP 9.5) and red (VIP) fluorescent channels. The pictures were captured with an Olympus XM10 camera.

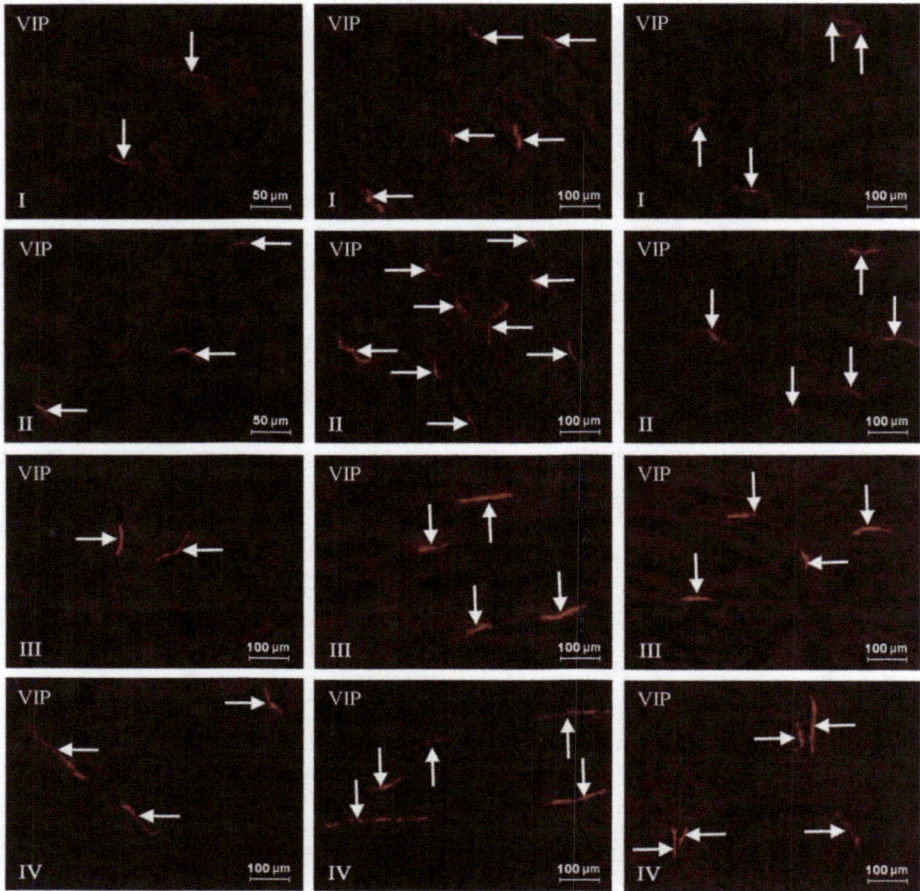

Figure 2. Vasoactive intestinal polypeptide (VIP)-positive nerve fibers in the porcine stomach in control animals (I, III) and after T-2 toxin giving (II, IV). I, II: mucosal layer; III, IV: muscle layer. VIP-positive nerve fibers are indicated by arrows. The pictures were captured with an Olympus XM10 camera.

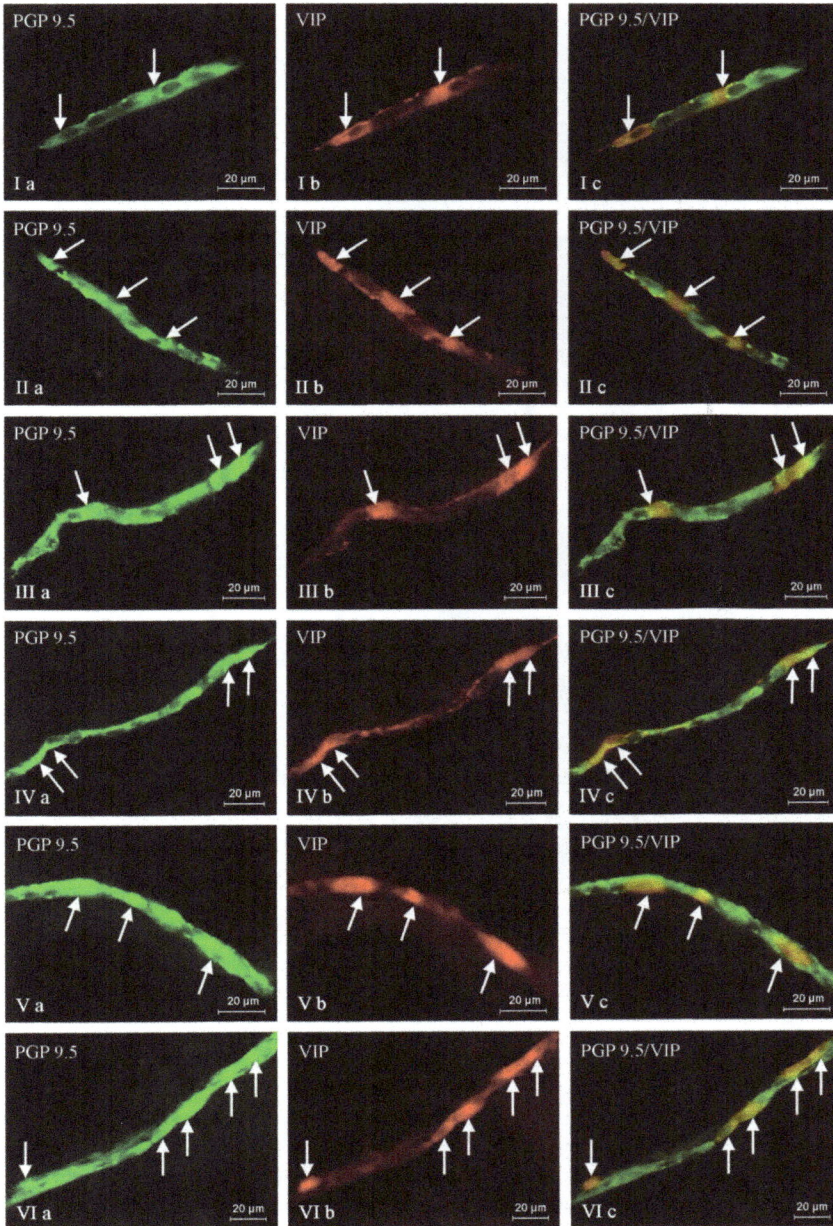

Figure 3. Nerve cell bodies containing the protein gene-product 9.5 (PGP 9.5) pan-neuronal marker (**a**) and vasoactive intestinal polypeptide (VIP) (**b**) within the porcine duodenal wall in control animals (I, III) and after T-2 toxin giving (II, IV). I, II: submucous plexus; III, IV: myenteric plexus. Arrows indicate VIP-positive neurons. Photos Ic, IIc, IIIc, and IVc came from the merger of green (PGP 9.5) and red (VIP) fluorescent channels. The pictures were captured with an Olympus XM10 camera.

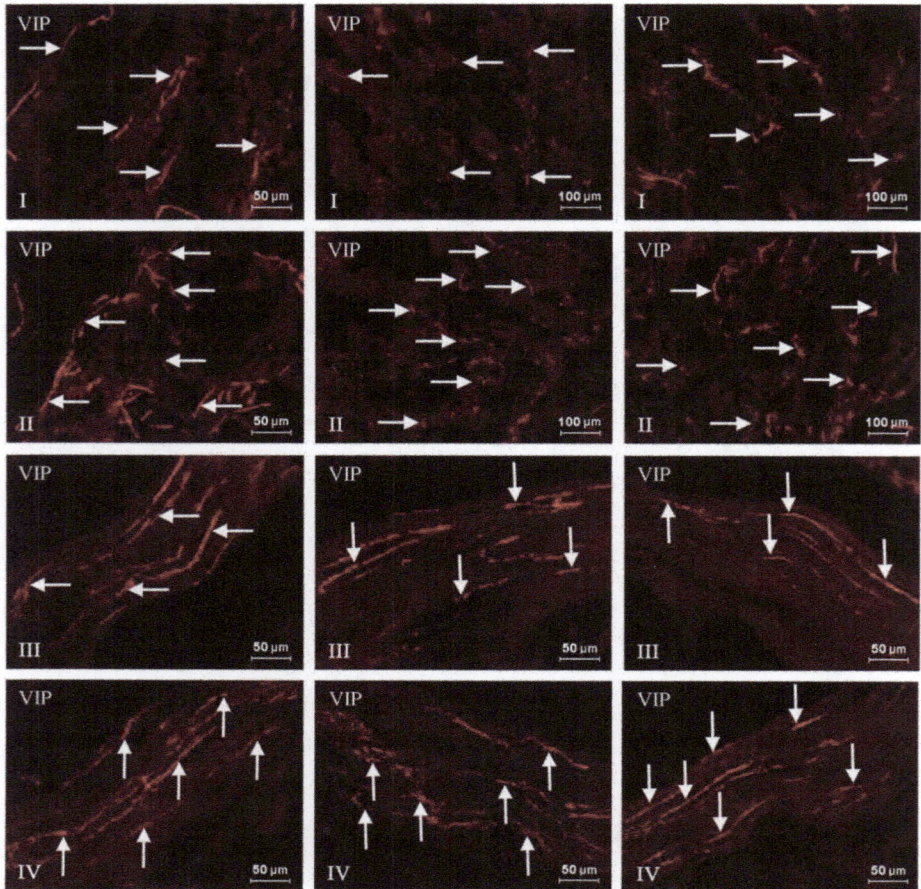

Figure 4. Vasoactive intestinal polypeptide (VIP)-positive nerve fibers in the porcine duodenum in control animals (I, III) and after T-2 toxin giving (II, IV). I, II: mucosal layer; III, IV: muscle layer. VIP-positive nerve fibers are indicated by arrows. The pictures were captured with an Olympus XM10 camera.

3. Discussion

The present observations have confirmed that VIP is present in the enteric neurons and nerve fibers of the porcine stomach and duodenum. It is compatible with previous investigations describing this substance as an important neurotransmitter in the ENS of a wide range of mammals species, including humans [22,24,31,33,34]. It is known that enteric neurons capable of VIP synthesis first of all have inhibitory effects and their stimulation causes the relaxation of the intestinal smooth muscles and a decrease in the secretory activity of the digestive tract. Inhibitory effects on gastrointestinal activities are not the only functions of VIP, because this substance also takes part in the regulation of immune processes [35,36] and intestinal blood flow [12,37] as well as may influence intestinal commensal and pathogenic bacteria populations [38]. Moreover, some studies have described the presence of VIP in enteric sensory neurons [39]. In spite of the relatively numerous studies concerning VIP in the GI tract, some aspects connected with the functions of this peptide remain unexplained. One of them is the physiological factors that influence the number of VIP-positive enteric neurons. The percentage of neurons immunoreactive to VIP observed in control animals during the present study differ from the values described in previous studies [22,24,31,33,34], which suggests that the synthesis of this peptide by enteric neuronal cells depends on unidentified stimuli that would probably include (apart from individual variations) type of diet, farming conditions, and/or environmental factors. Moreover, differences in the number of VIP-LI enteric nerve cells between the stomach and duodenum observed during the present experiment strongly imply that the precise roles of VIP in the digestive tract vary depending on the part of the GI tract studied.

During the present study, the impact of low doses of T-2 toxin on the number of neurons immunoreactive to VIP was noted in all parts of the ENS within the stomach and duodenum. Due to the fact that knowledge about the impact of T-2 toxin on the ENS is extremely scant, and VIP may have multidirectional functions in enteric neurons, the exact elucidation of the observed fluctuations is rather difficult. Moreover, observed changes may arise from various processes, including disorders in the transcription and/or translation stage of VIP synthesis as well as from disturbance of the peptide inside neuronal cells.

These changes are probably connected with the neurotoxic effects of this mycotoxin, which are the result of reactions of epoxides included in the molecules of the described substance with DNA and proteins of neuronal cells [40]. Furthermore, T-2 toxin is a commonly known inhibitor of cellular protein synthesis and a factor causing changes in the metabolism of membrane phospholipids [41,42]. Admittedly, the knowledge concerning T-2 toxin-induced changes in the ENS is extremely scant. Namely, our previous observations have shown that even low dosages of this mycotoxin may influence the number of enteric neurons immunoreactive to cocaine- and amphetamine-regulated transcripts in various parts of the GI tract [7] as well as affect the neurochemical characterization of calcitonin gene-related peptide-positive structures of the ENS within the descending colon [4]. Nevertheless, the mechanisms underlying the above-mentioned fluctuations in chemical coding of the enteric neurons remain unknown. On the other hand, it can be expected that processes connected with the neurotoxicity of T-2 toxin in the ENS are similar to those observed in the other parts of the nervous system. According to previous investigations, it is known that T-2 toxin causes alterations in the levels of brain biogenic monoamines [43] and induces apoptosis in brain neuronal cells [44]. The reason of the exacerbation of apoptotic reactions in the nervous tissue is probably connected with dysfunction of mitochondria caused by a T-2 toxin-induced decrease in the levels of mitochondrial NADH-dehydrogenase and cytochrome oxidase enzymes occurring in mitochondria-related genes [45]. The thesis about connections of observed changes with neurotoxic effects of T-2 toxin is strongly supported by the fact that VIP is known to be an important neuroprotective factor. Some previous works have described that this peptide has multidirectional neurotrophic activities. Among others, VIP stimulates mitosis within the astrocytes [46], supports neuronal differentiation of embryonic stem cells [47], and increases neuronal survival under various pathological factors [48]. Furthermore, it is known that VIP has neuroprotective functions during excitotoxicity, i.e., pathological processes consisting in neuronal cell damage by excessive stimulation by some neurotransmitters [49], and therefore inhibits the lesion of neurons in the brain cortex [50]. The neuroprotective effects of VIP are probably connected with direct actions on microglial cells, which are the main source of inflammatory factors damaging neurons in the central nervous system [51,52]. The above-mentioned VIP properties have caused this substance as well as its analogs to be tested as drugs to treat neurodegenerative diseases [48]. Contrary to the central nervous system, knowledge about the neuroprotective roles of VIP within the enteric nervous system is more limited. Nevertheless, the previous investigations have shown that this substance increases the survival of cultured enteric nerve cells undergoing some pathological factors, including axotomy or bacterial lipopolysaccharide [23,53]. In view of the foregoing, it is very likely that dissimilarities in VIP-LI observed during the present investigation are an effect of neurotoxic activity of T-2 and are the result of neuroprotective and/or adaptive processes within the ENS, which aim to maintain homeostasis in the GI tract under the influence of the toxin.

The other mechanisms connected with observed changes may result from pro-inflammatory and damaging properties of T-2. T-2 toxin may cause multidirectional disorders, among which is alimentary toxic aleukia (ATA). During these processes, inflammatory changes and GI tract injuries occur, which result in intestinal epithelial barrier disruption and manifest by vomiting, nausea, and diarrhea [2,54]. It should be pointed out that inflammatory changes in the intestine have been also observed after relatively low doses of T-2 toxin administration [55]. These changes may influence indirectly the ENS. This is all the more likely as the interdependences between intestinal epithelial cells and the ENS are commonly known [56]. Moreover, VIP is one of the factors that is are involved in gastrointestinal inflammatory processes, and enteric neurons respond to these processes with the growth of VIP expression [22–24,36,37].

Changes in VIP expression observed during this investigation can be also caused by the stimulation of the gastrointestinal immune system, because this substance is considered to be a major immunoregulatory neuropeptide. Previous investigations have described VIP as an anti-inflammatory factor, which first of all, through the VPAC1 type of receptor, inhibits macrophage activity [57]. These effects on the one side lead to a decrease in the synthesis of pro-inflammatory cytokines, including TNFα, IL-6, and IL-12, and on the other side result in a simultaneous increase in the levels of IL-10, which is the main anti-inflammatory factor [57,58]. Moreover, it is known that VIP may affect the phagocytosis, migration, and adherence of macrophages, but the exact mechanisms connected with these activities have not been fully elucidated. Some studies have described that VIP stimulates the above-mentioned processes, whereas other investigations have reported inhibitory effects [59]. The described polypeptide also inhibits the synthesis and activity of the inducible isoform of nitric oxide synthase (iNOS) within immunological cells [57].

The second type of immune cells that may be subject to the influence of VIP are lymphocytes. Previous studies have reported that this polypeptide influences Th1/Th2 cells' balance by the inhibition of Th1 cells, the support of Th2 cells [57], and the reduction of T cells migration through intestinal Peyer's patches [59]. Moreover, as in the case of macrophages, VIP changes the levels of cytokines synthesized in Th1 and Th2 cells. For example, VIP suppresses the production of IL-2 but increases IL-5 synthesis [59]. The above-mentioned immunoregulatory functions of VIP have made this polypeptide a potential therapeutic agent during various inflammatory and autoimmune diseases, including lupus, autoimmune thyroiditis, and arthritis [57]. The hypothesis that fluctuations in the VIP-like immunoreactivity observed during the present investigation are the result of the cooperation of the ENS with the gastrointestinal immune system and may be the answer of the enteric nervous structures to the inflammatory processes induced by T-2 toxin is probable in the light of previous studies. These studies have shown the described mycotoxin to have an influence on the number of types of lymphocytes and the expression of cytokines within the porcine ileal Peyer's patches [60]. Since during the present study low doses of T-2 toxin have been used, and symptoms of inflammation in the experimental animals were not observed, it cannot be excluded that the observed fluctuations were the first sign of a subclinical inflammatory process.

4. Conclusions

The obtained results have shown that even low doses of T-2 toxin are not neutral for mammal organisms and may change the chemical coding of the neurons and nerve fibers in the stomach and duodenum. Moreover, they confirm the important roles of VIP within the ENS under physiological conditions and after administration of T-2 toxin. The fluctuations of VIP-like immunoreactivity observed during the study are probably connected with neuroprotective functions of this substance and/or its participation in immune processes. Nevertheless, due to the multidirectional negative activities of T-2 toxin and the various functions of VIP within the digestive tract, the exact elucidation of mechanisms taking part in observed changes remains for further studies.

5. Materials and Methods

The experiment was performed on 10 immature female pigs of the Large White Polish breed (8 weeks old, 20 kg body weight (b.w.)). Both the division of animals into groups as well as doses of T-2 toxin were performed as described previously by Makowska et al. [4]. In short, after a five-day adaptation period, animals were randomly divided into two equal groups (five animals in each). Animals of both groups received capsules per os, once a day for 42 days. In the control group (C group), the administered capsules were empty, while in the experimental group (T2 group), capsules contained T-2 toxin (12 µg/kg b.w. per day).

All animals were fed with feed appropriate for age and species "WIGOR 3" (WIPASZ S.A, Olsztyn, Poland) of known composition, which is available on the producer's website. Furthermore, to eliminate additional mycotoxins contamination of the feed, the presence of Aflatoxin B1, T-2 toxin, ochratoxin A (OTA), ZEN, alpha-zearalenol (α-ZEL), and deoxynivalenol (DON) were evaluated using common separation techniques with immunoaffinity columns (Afla-TestR P Aflatoxin testing system, G1010, VICAM, Watertown, MA, USA; T-2-TestTM HPLC Mycotoxin Testing System G1028, VICAM, Watertown, MA, USA; Ochra-TestTM WB Mycotoxin Testing System, G1033, VICAM, Watertown, MA, USA; Zearala-Test™ Zearalenone Testing System, G1012, VICAM, Watertown, MA, USA; DON-Test™ DON Testing System, VICAM, Watertown, MA, USA) and high performance liquid chromatography (HPLC) (Hewlett Packard, type 1050 and 1100) with fluorescent and/or UV detection methods. All of the above-mentioned mycotoxins were absent in the studied feed.

Throughout the duration of the investigation, gilts stayed under standard experimental conditions and all procedures were conducted in agreement with the directions of the Local Ethical Committee for Animal Experiments in Olsztyn (Poland) (decision from 28 November 2012, No. 73/2012/DTN).

After 42 days, animals from both groups were premedicated with Stressnil (Janssen, Beerse, Belgium, 75 µL/kg b.w.) then, after 15 min, euthanized with high doses of sodium thiopental (Thiopental, Sandoz, Kundl-Rakúsko, Austria). Directly after euthanasia, the fragments (with a length of about 2 cm) of the stomach fundus (20 cm before the pylorus) and duodenum (5 cm after the pylorus) were collected from all pigs and fixed for one hour in a solution of 4% buffered paraformaldehyde (pH 7.4). Afterward, the taken fragments of the stomach and duodenum were put in phosphate buffer (0.1 M, pH 7.4, at 4 °C). This procedure lasted for three days with a daily exchange of the buffer. Later on, the tissues were inserted into 18% phosphate-buffered sucrose and storage for 3 weeks at 4 °C. Then, after freezing at −22 °C, the tissue fragments of both stomach and duodenum were cut perpendicular to the lumen of the digestive tract into 14-µm-thick sections with freezing microtome (Microm, HM 525, Walldorf, Germany).

Such prepared tissue fragments were subjected to a routine double-labelling immunofluorescence method as previously described by Gonkowski 2013 [29].

In brief, the immunofluorescence labelling was carried out as follows. Frozen fragments of the stomach and duodenum were dried (45 min, room temperature (rt)) and incubated with blocking solution (10% goat serum, 0.1% bovine serum albumin (BSA), 0.01% NaN3, Triton X-100, and thimerosal in PBS) for 1 h at rt. Next, fragments of the GI tract were incubated with a mixture of two antibodies: mouse monoclonal antibody directed towards protein gene-product 9.5 (PGP 9.5, Biogenesis, UK, catalogue No. 7863-2004, working dilution 1:2000, used here as a pan-neuronal marker) and rabbit polyclonal anti-VIP antibody (Cappel, Aurora, OH, USA, catalogue No. 11428, working dilution 1:5000). For the incubation process, slices covered with antibodies mixture were left overnight at rt in a humid chamber. The next day, for visualization of the primary antibodies connected with suitable antigens, an incubation with the mixture of species-specific secondary antisera conjugated to selected fluorochromes (Alexa fluor 488 donkey anti-mouse IgG and Alexa fluor 546 donkey anti-rabbit IgG, both antibodies from Invitrogen, Carlsbad, CA, USA, working dilution 1:1000) has been performed. This incubation process lasted 1 h at rt. After every stage of the immunofluorescence method, samples were rinsed with PBS (3 × 15 min, pH 7.4).

During the present investigation, routine specificity tests of antibodies were performed. Pre-absorption of the antibodies with appropriate antigens and omission and replacement tests were performed to eliminate non-specific labelling.

To evaluate the percentage of VIP-like immunoreactive perikaryons in relation to all enteric neurons, no less than 500 cells labelled with PGP-9.5 (treated as 100%) in the particular type of enteric plexus from each part of the digestive tract and each animal were examined for the presence of VIP. Only nerve cells with clearly visible nuclei were considered in the present study. The received results were pooled and presented as mean $\pm$ SEM. To obviate double counting of the same perikaryons, the investigated sections of the GI tract were located no less than 150 μm apart.

To define the density of intraganglionic nerves positive for VIP, an arbitrary scale was used. In this scale, (-) indicated the absence of nerve fibers, (+) single fibers, (++) rare fibers, (+++) a dense network of fibers, and (++++) a very dense meshwork of VIP-LI fibers. The evaluation of VIP-LI nerve fibers in the muscular and mucosal layers in the stomach and duodenum was carried out on the basis of the counting of all VIP-positive nerves per area studied (0.1 mm^2). Such evaluation was carried out in four sections per animal (in five fields per section) and the obtained results were presented as a mean $\pm$ SEM.

All indications during the present study were performed using an Olympus BX51 microscope with epi-fluorescence and appropriate filter sets connected with an Olympus XM10 camera.

Statistical analysis was performed with Student's t-test (Statistica 12, StatSoft, Inc., Cracow, Poland). The differences were considered statistically significant at $p < 0.05$.

Acknowledgments: This study was a part of a research project, No. NN 308 237936, financed by the National Science Centre in Poland and the KNOW (Leading National Research Centre) Scientific Consortium "Healthy Animal—Safe Food", decision of Ministry of Science and Higher Education No. 05-1/KNOW2/2015.

Author Contributions: K.M. and S.G. conceived and designed the experiments; K.M. performed the experiments; K.M. and S.G. analyzed the data; K.O. contributed reagents/materials/analysis tools; K.M. and S.G. wrote the paper.

Conflicts of Interest: There are no conflict of interest to declare.

References

1. Lewis, L.; Onsongo, M.; Njapau, H.; Schurz-Rogers, H.; Luber, G.; Kieszak, S.; Nyamongo, J.; Backer, L.; Dahiye, A.M.; Misore, A.; et al. Kenya Aflatoxicosis Investigation Group. Aflatoxin contamination of commercial maize products during an outbreak of acute aflatoxicosis in eastern and central Kenya. *Environ. Health Perspect.* **2005**, *113*, 1763–1767. [CrossRef] [PubMed]
2. De Ruyck, K.; De Boevre, M.; Huybrechts, I.; De Saeger, S. Dietary mycotoxins, co-exposure, and carcinogenesis in humans: Short review. *Mutat. Res. Rev. Mutat. Res.* **2015**, *766*, 32–41. [CrossRef] [PubMed]
3. Moretti, A.; Logrieco, A.F.; Susca, A. Mycotoxins: An underhand food problem. *Methods Mol. Biol.* **2017**, *1542*, 3–12. [PubMed]
4. Makowska, K.; Obremski, K.; Zielonka, L.; Gonkowski, S. The Influence of Low Doses of Zearalenone and T-2 Toxin on Calcitonin Gene Related Peptide-Like Immunoreactive (CGRP-LI) Neurons in the ENS of the Porcine Descending Colon. *Toxins* **2017**, *9*, 98. [CrossRef] [PubMed]
5. Ruiz, M.J.; Macáková, P.; Juan-García, A.; Font, G. Cytotoxic effects of mycotoxin combinations in mammalian kidney cells. *Food Chem. Toxicol.* **2011**, *49*, 2718–2724. [CrossRef] [PubMed]
6. Adhikari, M.; Negi, B.; Kaushik, N.; Adhikari, A.; Al-Khedhairy, A.A.; Kaushik, N.K.; Choi, E.H. T-2 mycotoxin: Toxicological effects and decontamination strategies. *Oncotarget* **2017**, *8*, 33933–33952. [CrossRef] [PubMed]
7. Makowska, K.; Gonkowski, S.; Zielonka, L.; Dabrowski, M.; Calka, J. T2 Toxin-Induced Changes in Cocaine- and Amphetamine-Regulated Transcript (CART)-Like Immunoreactivity in the Enteric Nervous System Within Selected Fragments of the Porcine Digestive Tract. *Neurotox. Res.* **2017**, *31*, 136–147. [CrossRef] [PubMed]

8.   Weidner, M.; Huwel, S.; Ebert, F.; Schwerdtle, T.; Galla, H.J.; Humpf, H.U. Influence of T-2 and HT-2 toxin on the blood-brain barrier in vitro: New experimental hints for neurotoxic effects. *PLoS ONE* **2013**, *8*, e60484. [CrossRef] [PubMed]

9.   Lutsky, I.; Mor, N. Alimentary toxic aleukia (septic angina, endemic panmyelotoxicosis, alimentary hemorrhagic aleukia): T-2 toxin-induced intoxication of cats. *Am. J. Pathol.* **1981**, *104*, 189–191. [PubMed]

10. Martin, L.J.; Doebler, J.A.; Anthony, A. Scanning cytophotometric analysis of brain neuronal nuclear chromatin changes in acute T-2 toxin-treated rats. *Toxicol. Appl. Pharmacol.* **1986**, *85*, 207–214. [CrossRef]

11. Gonkowski, S.; Kamińska, B.; Landowski, P.; Całka, J. Immunohistochemical distribution of cocaine- and amphetamine-regulated transcript peptide—Like immunoreactive (CART-LI) nerve fibers and various degree of co-localization with other neuronal factors in the circular muscle layer of human descending colon. *Histol. Histopathol.* **2013**, *28*, 851–858. [CrossRef] [PubMed]

12. Makowska, K.; Gonkowski, S. The Influence of Inflammation and Nerve Damage on the Neurochemical Characterization of Calcitonin Gene-Related Peptide-Like Immunoreactive (CGRP-LI) Neurons in the Enteric Nervous System of the Porcine Descending Colon. *Int. J. Mol. Sci.* **2018**, *19*, 548. [CrossRef]

13. Furness, J.B.; Callaghan, B.P.; Rivera, L.R.; Cho, H.J. The enteric nervous system and gastrointestinal innervation: Integrated local and central control. *Adv. Exp. Med. Biol.* **2014**, *817*, 39–71. [CrossRef] [PubMed]

14. Makowska, K.; Gonkowski, S. Cocaine-And Amphetamine-Regulated Transcript (Cart) Peptide in Mammals Gastrointestinal System—A Review. *Ann. Anim. Sci.* **2017**, *17*, 3–21. [CrossRef]

15. Furness, J.B. Types of neurons in the enteric nervous system. *J. Autonom. Nerv. Syst.* **2000**, *81*, 87–96. [CrossRef]

16. Kasparek, M.S.; Fatima, J.; Iqbal, C.W.; Duenes, J.A.; Sarr, M.G. Role of VIP and Substance P in NANC innervation in the longitudinal smooth muscle of the rat jejunum -influence of extrinsic denervation. *J. Surg. Res.* **2007**, *141*, 22–30. [CrossRef] [PubMed]

17. Rytel, L.; Palus, K.; Calka, J. Co-expression of PACAP with VIP, SP and CGRP in the porcine nodose ganglion sensory neurons. *Anat. Histol. Embryol.* **2015**, *44*, 86–91. [CrossRef] [PubMed]

18. Nakashima, M.; Morrison, K.J.; Vanhoutte, P.M. Hyperpolarization and relaxation of canine vascular smooth muscle to vasoactive intestinal polypeptide. *J. Cardiovasc. Pharmacol.* **1997**, *30*, 273–277. [CrossRef] [PubMed]

19. Van Geldre, L.A.; Lefebvre, R.A. Interaction of NO and VIP in gastrointestinal smooth muscle relaxation. *Curr. Pharm. Des.* **2004**, *10*, 2483–2497. [CrossRef] [PubMed]

20. Nassar, C.F.; Abdallah, L.E.; Barada, K.A.; Atweh, S.F.; Saadé, N.F. Effects of intravenous vasoactive intestinal peptide injection on jejunal alanine absorption and gastric acid secretion in rats. *Regul. Pept.* **1995**, *55*, 261–267. [CrossRef]

21. Burleigh, D.E.; Banks, M.R. Stimulation of intestinal secretion by vasoactive intestinal peptide and cholera toin. *Auton. Neurosci. Basic Clin.* **2007**, *133*, 64–75. [CrossRef] [PubMed]

22. Kaleczyc, J.; Klimczuk, M.; Franke-Radowiecka, A.; Sienkiewicz, W.; Majewski, M.; Łakomy, M. The distribution and chemical coding of intramural neurons supplying the porcine stomach—The study on normal pigs and on animals suffering from swine dysentery. *Anat. Histol. Embryol.* **2007**, *36*, 186–193. [CrossRef] [PubMed]

23. Arciszewski, M.B.; Sand, E.; Ekblad, E. Vasoactive intestinal peptide rescues cultured rat myenteric neurons from lipopolysaccharide induced cell death. *Regul. Pept.* **2008**, *146*, 218–223. [CrossRef] [PubMed]

24. Pidsudko, Z.; Kaleczyc, J.; Wasowicz, K.; Sienkiewicz, W.; Majewski, M.; Zajac, W.; Lakomy, M. Distribution and chemical coding of intramural neurons in the porcine ileum during proliferative enteropathy. *J. Comp. Pathol.* **2008**, *138*, 23–31. [CrossRef] [PubMed]

25. Gonkowski, S.; Obremski, K.; Calka, J. The Influence of Low Doses of Zearalenone on Distribution of Selected Active Substances in Nerve Fibers within the Circular Muscle Layer of Porcine Ileum. *J. Mol. Neurosci.* **2015**, *56*, 878–886. [CrossRef] [PubMed]

26. Vasina, V.; Barbara, G.; Talamonti, L.; Stanghellini, V.; Corinaldesi, R.; Tonini, M.; de Ponti, F.; de Giorgio, R. Enteric neuroplasticity evoked by inflammation. *Auton. Neurosci.* **2006**, *126–127*, 264–272. [CrossRef] [PubMed]

27. Gonkowski, S.; Burlinski, P.; Calka, J. Proliferative enteropathy (PE)-induced changes in galanin-like immunoreactivity in the enteric nervous system of the porcine distal colon. *Acta Vet.* **2009**, *59*, 321–330.

28. Gonkowski, S.; Burliński, P.; Skobowiat, C.; Majewski, M.; Całka, J. Inflammation- And Axotomy-Induced Changes In Galanin-Like Immunoreactive (Gal-Li) Nerve Structures In The Porcine Descending Colon. *Acta Vet. Hung.* **2010**, *58*, 91–103. [CrossRef] [PubMed]

29. Gonkowski, S. Substance P as a neuronal factor in the enteric nervous system of the porcine descending colon in physiological conditions and during selected pathogenic processes. *Biofactors* **2013**, *39*, 542–551. [CrossRef] [PubMed]

30. Timmermans, J.P.; Adriaensen, D.; Cornelissen, W.; Scheuermann, D.W. Structural organization and neuropeptide distribution in the mammalian enteric nervous system, with special attention to those components involved in mucosal reflexes. *Comp. Biochem. Physiol. A Physiol.* **1997**, *118*, 331–340. [CrossRef]

31. Gonkowski, S.; Wojtkiewicz, J.; Bossowska, A.; Kaleczyc, J.; Sienkiewicz, W.; Majewski, M. Proliferative enteropathy (PE)-induced changes in the number of vasoactive intestinal polypeptide-immunoreactive (VIP-IR) neural elements in the porcine descending colon. *Pol. J. Vet. Sci.* **2004**, *7*, 53–55.

32. Verma, N.; Rettenmeier, A.W.; Schmitz-Spanke, S. Recent advances in the use of Sus scrofa (pig) as a model system for proteomic studies. *Proteomics* **2011**, *11*, 776–793. [CrossRef] [PubMed]

33. Johnson, R.J.; Schemann, M.; Santer, R.M.; Cowen, T. The effects of age on the overall population and on sub-populations of myenteric neurons in the rat small intestine. *J. Anat.* **1998**, *192*, 479–488. [CrossRef] [PubMed]

34. Kleinschmidt, S.; Nolte, I.; Hewicker-Trautwein, M. Structural and functional changes of neuronal and glial components of the feline enteric nervous system in cats with chronic inflammatory and non-inflammatory diseases of the gastrointestinal tract. *Res. Vet. Sci.* **2011**, *91*, 129–135. [CrossRef] [PubMed]

35. Brenneman, D.E.; Philips, T.M.; Hauser, J.; Hill, J.M.; Spong, C.Y.; Gozes, I. Complex array of cytokines released by vasoactive intestinal peptide. *Neuropeptides* **2003**, *37*, 111–119. [CrossRef]

36. Vota, D.; Aguero, M.; Grasso, E.; Hauk, V.; Gallino, L.; Soczewski, E.; Pérez Leirós, C.; Ramhorst, R. Progesterone and VIP cross-talk enhances phagocytosis and anti-inflammatory profile in trophoblast-derived cells. *Mol. Cell Endocrinol.* **2017**, *443*, 146–154. [CrossRef] [PubMed]

37. Obremski, K.; Gonkowski, S.; Wojtacha, P. Zearalenone-induced changes in the lymphoid tissue and mucosal nerve fibers in the porcine ileum. *Pol. J. Vet. Sci.* **2015**, *18*, 357–365. [CrossRef] [PubMed]

38. Bednarska, O.; Walter, S.A.; Casado-Bedmar, M.; Ström, M.; Salvo-Romero, E.; Vicario, M.; Mayer, E.A.; Keita, Å.V. Vasoactive Intestinal Polypeptide and Mast Cells Regulate Increased Passage of Colonic Bacteria in Patients With Irritable Bowel Syndrome. *Gastroenterology* **2017**, *153*, 948–960. [CrossRef] [PubMed]

39. Kirchgessner, A.L.; Dodd, J.; Gershon, M.D. Markers shared between dorsal root and enteric ganglia. *J. Comp. Neurol.* **1988**, *276*, 607–621. [CrossRef] [PubMed]

40. Li, Y.; Wang, Z.; Beier, R.C.; Shen, J.; De Smet, D.; De Saeger, S.; Zhang, S. T-2 toxin, a trichothecene mycotoxin: Review of toxicity, metabolism, and analytical methods. *J. Agric. Food Chem.* **2011**, *59*, 3441–3453. [CrossRef] [PubMed]

41. Chang, I.M.; Mar, W.C. Effect of T-2 toxin on lipid peroxidation in rats: Elevation of conjugated diene formation. *Toxicol. Lett.* **1988**, *40*, 275–280. [PubMed]

42. Shifrin, V.I.; Anderson, P. Trichothecene mycotoxins trigger a ribotoxic stress response that activates c-jun N-terminal kinase and p38 mitogen-activated protein kinase and induces apoptosis. *J. Biol. Chem.* **1999**, *274*, 13985–13992. [CrossRef] [PubMed]

43. Wang, J.; Fitzpatrick, D.W.; Wilson, J.R. Effects of the trichothecene mycotoxin T-2 toxin on neurotransmitters and metabolites in discrete areas of the rat brain. *Food Chem. Toxicol.* **1998**, *36*, 947–953. [CrossRef]

44. Sehata, S.; Kiyosawa, N.; Makino, T.; Atsumi, F.; Ito, K.; Yamoto, T.; Teranishi, M.; Baba, Y.; Uetauka, K.; Nakayama, H.; et al. Morphological and microarray analysis of T-2 toxin-induced rat fetal brain lesion. *Food Chem. Toxicol.* **2004**, *42*, 1727–1736. [CrossRef] [PubMed]

45. Doi, K.; Uetsuka, K. Mechanisms of mycotoxin-induced neurotoxicity through oxidative stress-associated pathways. *Int. J. Mol. Sci.* **2011**, *12*, 5213–5237. [CrossRef] [PubMed]

46. Brenneman, D.E.; Nicol, T.; Warren, D.; Bowers, L.M. Vasoactive intestinal peptide: A neurotrophic releasing agent and an astroglial mitogen. *J. Neurosci. Res.* **1990**, *25*, 386–394. [CrossRef] [PubMed]

47. Cazillis, M.; Gonzalez, B.J.; Billardon, C.; Lombet, A.; Fraichard, A.; Samarut, J.; Gressens, P.; Vaudry, H.; Rostène, W. VIP and PACAP induce selective neuronal differentiation of mouse embryonic stem cells. *Eur. J. Neurosci.* **2004**, *19*, 798–808. [CrossRef] [PubMed]

48. Passemard, S.; Sokolowska, P.; Schwendimann, L.; Gressens, P. VIP-induced neuroprotection of the developing brain. *Curr. Pharm. Des.* **2011**, *17*, 1036–1039. [CrossRef] [PubMed]

49. Rangon, C.M.; Dicou, E.; Goursaud, S.; Mounien, L.; Jégou, S.; Janet, T.; Muller, J.M.; Lelièvre, V.; Gressens, P. Mechanisms of VIP-induced neuroprotection against neonatal excitotoxicity. *Ann. N. Y. Acad. Sci.* **2006**, *1070*, 512–517. [CrossRef] [PubMed]

50. Gressens, P.; Marret, S.; Hill, J.M.; Brenneman, D.E.; Gozes, I.; Fridkin, M.; Evrard, P. Vasoactive intestinal peptide prevents excitotoxic cell death in the murine developing brain. *J. Clin. Investig.* **1997**, *100*, 390–397. [CrossRef] [PubMed]

51. Carniglia, L.; Ramírez, D.; Durand, D.; Saba, J.; Turati, J.; Caruso, C.; Scimonelli, T.N.; Lasaga, M. Neuropeptides and Microglial Activation in Inflammation, Pain, and Neurodegenerative Diseases. *Mediat. Inflamm.* **2017**, *2017*, 5048616. [CrossRef] [PubMed]

52. Chandrasekharan, B.; Nezami, B.G.; Srinivasan, S. Emerging neuropeptide targets in inflammation: NPY and VIP. *Am. J. Physiol. Gastrointest. Liver Physiol.* **2013**, *304*, G949–G957. [CrossRef] [PubMed]

53. Sandgren, K.; Lin, Z.; Ekblad, E. Differential effects of VIP and PACAP on survival of cultured adult rat myenteric neurons. *Regul. Pept.* **2003**, *111*, 211–217. [CrossRef]

54. Goossens, J.; Pasmans, F.; Verbrugghe, E.; Vandenbroucke, V.; De Baere, S.; Meyer, E.; Haesebrouck, F.; De Backer, P.; Croubels, S. Porcine intestinal epithelial barrier disruption by the Fusarium mycotoxins deoxynivalenol and T-2 toxin promotes transepithelial passage of doxycycline and paromomycin. *BMC Vet. Res.* **2012**, *8*, 245. [CrossRef] [PubMed]

55. Obremski, K.; Zielonka, L.; Gajecka, M.; Jakimiuk, E.; Bakuła, T.; Baranowski, M.; Gajecki, M. Histological estimation of the small intestine wall after administration of feed containing deoxynivalenol, T-2 toxin and zearalenone in the pig. *Pol. J. Vet. Sci.* **2008**, *11*, 339–345. [PubMed]

56. Moriez, R.; Abdo, H.; Chaumette, T.; Faure, M.; Lardeux, B.; Neunlist, M. Neuroplasticity and neuroprotection in enteric neurons: Role of epithelial cells. *Biochem. Biophys. Res. Commun.* **2009**, *382*, 577–582. [CrossRef] [PubMed]

57. Ganea, D.; Hooper, K.M.; Kong, W. The neuropeptide vasoactive intestinal peptide: Direct effects on immune cells and involvement in inflammatory and autoimmune diseases. *Acta Physiol* **2015**, *213*, 442–452. [CrossRef] [PubMed]

58. Delgado, M.; Munoz-Elias, E.J.; Gomariz, R.P.; Ganea, D. Vasoactive intestinal peptide and pituitary adenylate cyclase-activating polypeptide enhance IL-10 production by murine macrophages: In vitro and in vivo studies. *J. Immunol.* **1999**, *162*, 1707–1716. [PubMed]

59. Delgado, M.; Pozo, D.; Ganea, D. The significance of vasoactive intestinal peptide in immunomodulation. *Pharmacol. Rev.* **2004**, *56*, 249–290. [CrossRef] [PubMed]

60. Obremski, K.; Podlasz, P.; Zmigrodzka, M.; Winnicka, A.; Woźny, M.; Brzuzan, P.; Jakimiuk, E.; Wojtacha, P.; Gajecka, M.; Zielonka, Ł.; et al. The effect of T-2 toxin on percentages of CD4+, CD8+, CD4+ CD8+ and CD21+ lymphocytes, and mRNA expression levels of selected cytokines in porcine ileal Peyer's patches. *Pol. J. Vet. Sci.* **2013**, *16*, 341–349. [CrossRef] [PubMed]

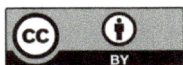

toxins

MDPI

Article

Response of Intestinal Bacterial Flora to the Long-Term Feeding of Aflatoxin B1 (AFB1) in Mice

Xiai Yang, Liangliang Liu, Jing Chen and Aiping Xiao *

Institute of Bast Fiber Crops, Chinese Academy of Agricultural Sciences, Changsha 410205, China;
yangxiai@caas.cn (X.Y.); liuliangliang@caas.cn (L.L.); 17673116054@163.com (J.C.); xap5@sina.com (A.X.)
* Correspondence: xap5@sina.com

Academic Editors: Isabelle P. Oswald, Philippe Pinton and Imourana Alassane-Kpembi
Received: 9 August 2017; Accepted: 30 September 2017; Published: 12 October 2017

Abstract: In order to investigate the influence of aflatoxin B1 (AFB1) on intestinal bacterial flora, 24 Kunming mice (KM mice) were randomly placed into four groups, which were labeled as control, low-dose, medium-dose, and high-dose groups. They were fed intragastrically with 0.4 mL of 0 mg/L, 2.5 mg/L, 4 mg/L, or 10 mg/L of AFB1 solutions, twice a day for 2 months. The hypervariable region V3 + V4 on 16S rDNA of intestinal bacterial flora was sequenced by the use of a high-flux sequencing system on a Miseq Illumina platform; then, the obtained sequences were analyzed. The results showed that, when compared with the control group, both genera and phyla of intestinal bacteria in the three treatment groups decreased. About one third of the total genera and one half of the total phyla remained in the high-dose group. The dominant flora were *Lactobacillus* and *Bacteroides* in all groups. There were significant differences in the relative abundance of intestinal bacterial flora among groups. Most bacteria decreased as a whole from the control to the high-dose groups, but several beneficial and pathogenic bacterial species increased significantly with increasing dose of AFB1. Thus, the conclusion was that intragastric feeding with 2.5~10 mg/mL AFB1 for 2 months could decrease the majority of intestinal bacterial flora and induce the proliferation of some intestinal bacteria flora.

Keywords: mice; aflatoxin B1; intestinal bacterial flora; response

1. Introduction

Intestinal microflora play important roles in affecting the health of hosts through many aspects, including nutrition decomposition and transformation, immunity intrusion, biological antagonism and anti-aging [1,2]. Some degree of internal and external stimulation or interference of the body may trigger a change in the numbers or the components of intestinal microflora, cause physiochemical reactions, and lead to diseases [3,4]. Intestinal microflora were proved to be able to bind, transform, degrade, and transfer mycotoxins [5–7]. Some intestinal bacterial strains isolated from intestines and other environments were able to transform and degrade some mycotoxins in vitro [8–10]. Considering the functional influences, scientists attempted to find methods which could balance or optimize intestinal microflora communities to achieve normal or active levels in intestinal tracts and keep the body healthy. For instance, one could feed hosts with curing drugs, nutritional elements, probiotics or symbiotic foods, etc. To a large extent, the normality of intestinal microflora could symbolize the health level of the body [11–13].

Aflatoxins are highly hazardous contaminants in common food and feed, mainly originating from secondary metabolites in *Aspergillus flavus* and *Aspergillus parasiticus* [14,15]. Aflatoxin B1 (AFB1) is the predominant type in aflatoxins and was demonstrated to be highly toxic, mutagenic, teratogenic, and carcinogenic to many animals [16,17]. As a potent carcinogen, AFB1 reacts mainly with liver DNA and serum albumin in a dose-dependent manner [18]. Toxicity from AFB1 can lead to a reduction in production, hepatotoxicity, nephrotoxicity, disturbance in the gastrointestinal tract and reproduction, immune suppression, and disease susceptibility. Contamination of feed with aflatoxins, especially AFB1, is one of the major concerns in poultry industry [19,20]. Because of its high toxicity, strict regulations are placed on foods and feeds containing AFB1, on a world-wide basis [21].

Like most mycotoxins, AFB1 not only damages body organs directly but also disturbs the normal activities of intestinal microflora in animals [22,23]. While previous studies have mainly focused on its toxicology and binding and while some have also attempted to transform and remove AFB1 to decrease the toxicity in some poultry species [24,25], the influential mechanism underlying the effect of AFB1 on intestinal microflora has not been found so far. Based on this investigation, a continuous feeding procedure was performed with KM mice in this study by using AFB1 solutions with various concentrations, which was designed comprehensively according to the dose of chronic aflatoxicosis in mice [26–29]. The research results might lay a foundation for discovering whether the disturbance of intestinal microflora under the toxicity of AFB1 is related to liver cancer or for finding feasible ways to reduce the toxicity through modulating intestinal bacterial flora.

2. Results

2.1. Operational Taxonomic Units (OTUs) and Rarefaction Curves

The OTUs of each group and the overlapped OTUs among groups were drawn as a Venn picture [30]. The similarity of overlapped OTUs between or among groups was $\geq$97%. There were 167 OTUs contained in all groups, whereas the specific OTUs in the control, low, medium, and high dose groups were 31, 16, 3, and 7, respectively. Although the high-dose group had slightly higher OTUs than the medium-dose group, the OTUs in each group showed a decrease tendency as a whole (Figure 1).

When the measured Operational Taxonomic Units (OTUs) [31] reached about 250, the rarefaction curves for the control and low-dose groups plateaued. However, when the measured OTUs were about 200 and 150, the rarefaction curves plateaued for the high- and medium-dose groups, respectively (Figure 2). All rarefaction curves of the four groups plateaued, which meant that the majority of sequences were involved in the analysis process for each group. Both OTUs and sequence numbers of the medium-dose group (less than 20,000 reads) were lower than those of the remaining groups (about 20,000 reads) based on Figure 2. The changing trend of the rarefaction curves was consistent with OTUs among groups.

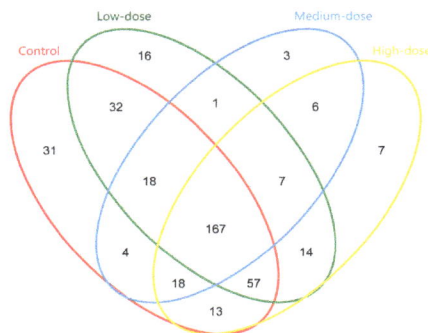

Figure 1. Venn map of OTU distribution in each group and between and among groups (97% similarity of OTUs). Different colors represent different samples. If, for instance, figure 100 was simultaneously marked in two different circles, this meant that the two samples had the same sequences categorized in the same OTUs, and the OTUs were 100.

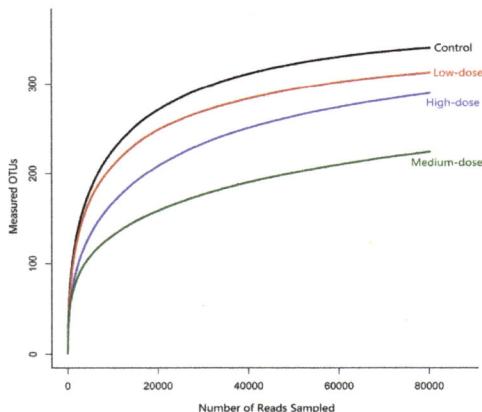

Figure 2. Rarefaction curves (97% similarity of OTUs). Horizontal ordinate: Sequences sampled randomly; Vertical ordinate: Measured OTUs. Rarefaction curves could estimate the depth of sequencing; the plateau indicates that the measured OTUs could reasonably represent the sampled sequences.

2.2. Genera and Phyla Performances

The genus and phylum types and the relative abundances of intestinal bacteria were clustered as a Heatmap [32], where darker colors indicate a higher abundance of the bacterial flora. According to the Heatmap, the control and the low-dose groups had higher abundances and also more types of genera and phyla than the medium- and high-dose groups (Figure 3). The high-dose group had the fewest types of genera. Although there were more genera for both the control and low-dose groups, the genera types differed greatly between the two groups. The two genera with high abundance in the four groups were *Lactobacillus* and *Bacteroides*. The four genera with the second highest abundance in the four groups were *Candiatus*, *Desulfovibrio*, *Bacteroides* and *Acinetobacter* (Figure 3A). Except for the control group, which had an extra phylum *Tenericutes*, there were 4 phyla with high relative abundances in each group. These 4 phyla were *Firmicutes*, *Bacteroidetes*, *Proteobacteria* and *Actinobacteria*. There was no evident difference for each phylum among all the groups, and *Firmicutes* had the highest abundance in each group (Figure 3B).

The genus and phylum types and relative abundances of intestinal bacteria were drawn as column pictures [33]. These pictures contain similar information as in the Heatmap, showing that *Lactobacillus* and *Bacteroides* had high abundances in the four groups, while the other 4 genera mentioned in Figure 3 were also present as the second highest. There were visually fewer genera in the high-dose group compared with the rest of groups, and especially with respect to the control group. There was an interesting phenomenon that the abundance of *Lactobacillus* decreased, but the abundance of *Bacteroides* increased evidently in the medium-dose group, while the two genera increased, reaching a large proportion in the high-dose group that was nearly the same as in the control group (Figure 4A). With respect to the phyla, more than six phyla were present in the control and the low-dose groups, whereas only 4 phyla were present in the medium- and high-dose groups (Figure 4B).

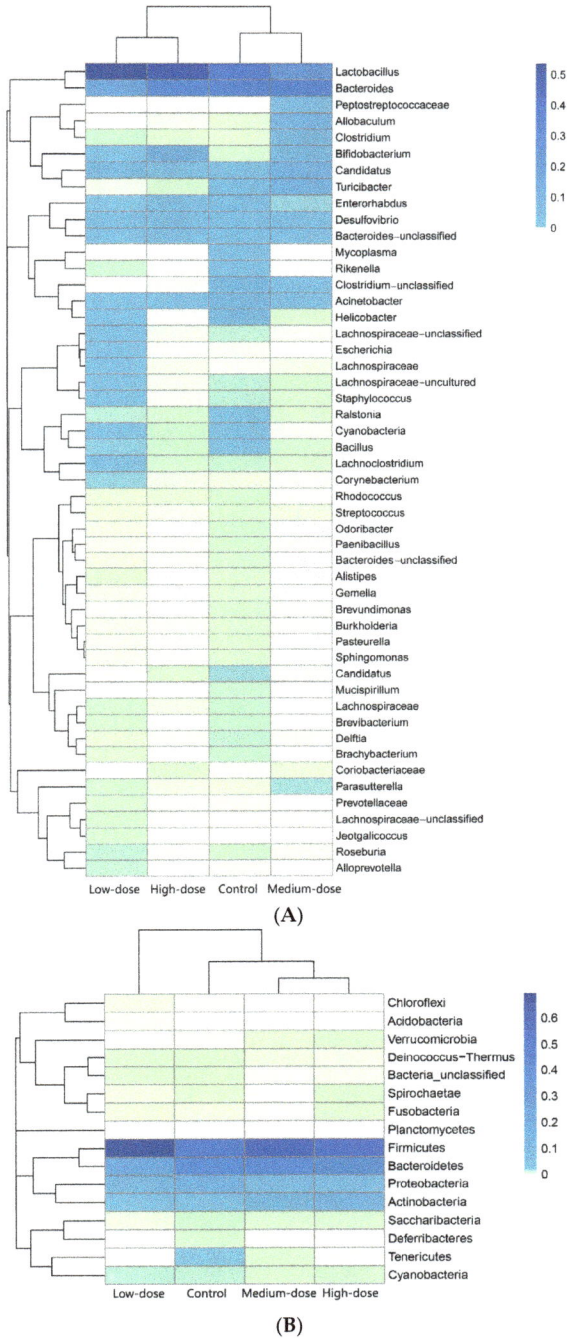

Figure 3. Heatmap of genus and phylum types and relative abundance of intestinal bacteria flora. (**A**) Heatmap of genus types; (**B**) Heatmap of phylum types. Different colors represent the relative abundances of different intestinal bacteria; the darker color indicates higher abundance.

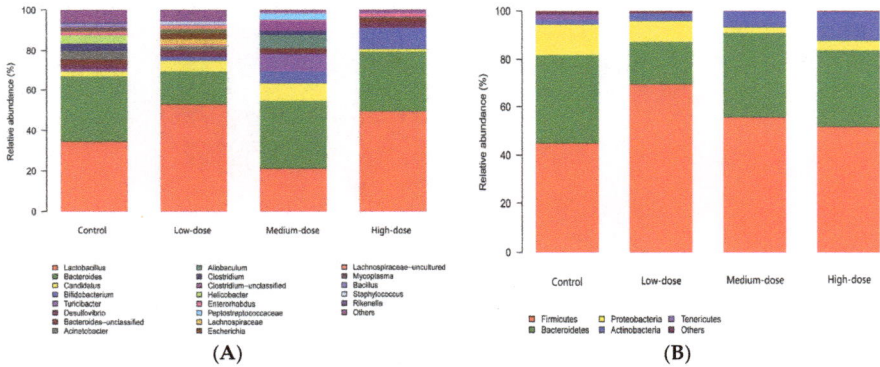

(A)

(B)

Figure 4. Column pictures of genus and phylum types and relative abundance of intestinal bacteria. Others: Intestinal bacterial flora with relative abundance <1% were included as others. (**A**) Column pictures of genera; (**B**) Column pictures of phyla. Different colors represent different intestinal bacteria; the percentage on the vertical ordinate indicates the relative abundance of intestinal bacteria.

2.3. Phylogenetic Tree

The phylogenetic tree was built based on the Hierarchical clustering method [34]. The intestinal bacteria of the control and the low-dose groups were clustered together (Figure 5), indicating that most bacteria in the two groups had a relatively close genetic relationship. The intestinal bacteria of the medium- and high-dose groups were clustered together, showing a close genetic relationship.

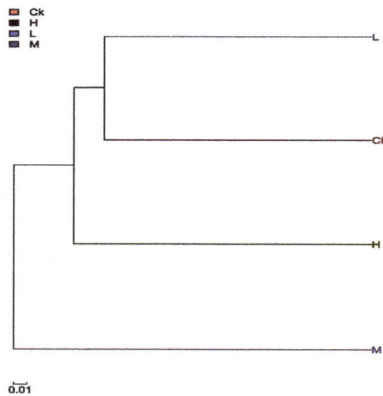

Figure 5. Phylogenetic clustering tree based on the Hierarchical clustering method. Branch size represents the genetic distance between samples; different colors represent different samples.

2.4. Differences in Relative Abundance of Bacterial Flora

The significance of the difference in the relative abundance of bacterial flora between groups is shown in Figure 6. Compared with the control, *Lactobacillus* increased significantly in the low-dose and the high-dose groups but decreased significantly in the medium-dose group. *Bacteroides* showed a significant decrease in the low-dose group and a slight decrease in the high-dose group, while no evident change occurred in the medium-dose group. *Bifidobacterium* showed a significant increase in the high-dose group. *Candidatus, Turicibacter, Allobaculum, Clostridium*, and *Peptostreptococcaceae* had a significant increase in the medium-dose group and then decreased dramatically in the high-dose group. *Escherichia* and *Lachnospiraceae* increased significantly in the low-dose group and then decreased dramatically in the medium-dose and the high-dose groups (Figure 6A). The majority of the intestinal bacterial flora at the genus level decreased as a whole, and the results in Figure 6 confirm the results in Figures 3 and 4. At the phylum level, *Firmicutes* showed a significant increase in all treatment groups, *Bacteroidetes* showed a significant decrease in the low-dose group, while no evident change occurred in the other two treatment groups, and *Actinobacteria* showed an increase in all treatment groups, especially in the high-dose group. The remaining phyla showed a decreasing tendency from the control to the high-dose groups (Figure 6B). The statistical data of the relative abundance of intestinal microflora are shown in Table 1.

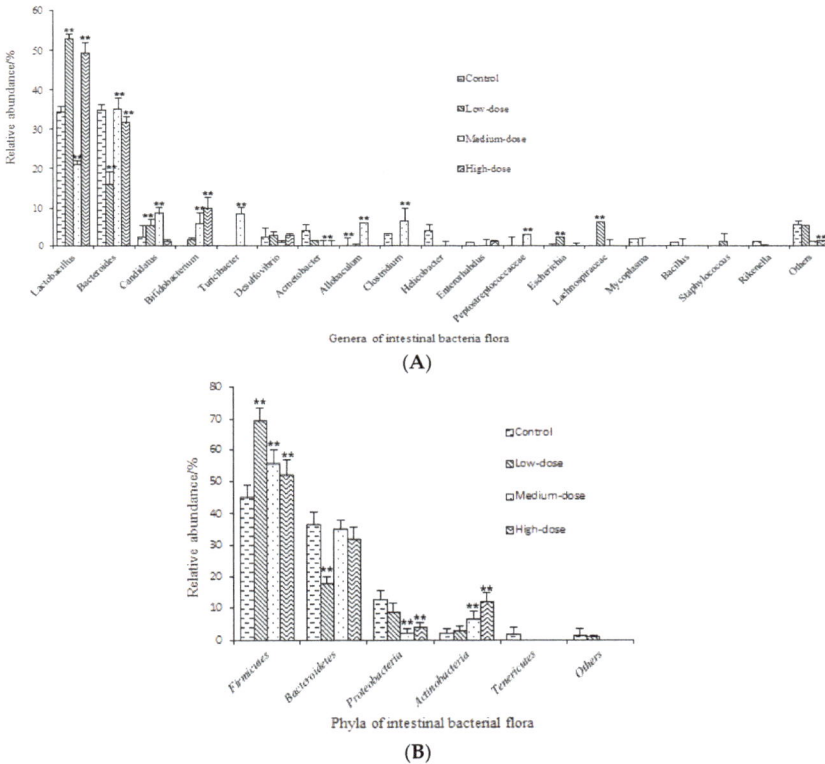

Figure 6. Difference in relative abundance of intestinal microflora between the control and the treatment groups. (**A**) Difference in relative abundance of intestinal microflora at the genus level; (**B**) Difference in relative abundance of intestinal microflora at the phylum level. ** means a significant difference ($p < 0.01$). Data were analyzed using one-way ANOVA. Difference between the control and the treatment groups was assessed by Duncan's test.

Table 1. Relative abundance of intestinal microflora in mice treated with different doses of AFB1.

Taxon	Control	Low-Dose	Medium-Dose	High-Dose
Lactobacillus	34.45 ± 0.69	52.99 ± 1.91 **	21.16 ± 2.01 **	49.40 ± 2.20
Bacteroides	32.32 ± 1.86	16.27 ± 1.64 **	33.36 ± 2.21	29.91 ± 1.80
Candidatus	2.52 ± 0.10	5.65 ± 0.13 **	8.80 ± 0.14 **	1.32 ± 0.05

Table 1. *Cont.*

Taxon	Control	Low-Dose	Medium-Dose	High-Dose
Bifidobacterium	0.11 ± 0.04	1.71 ± 0.15	5.98 ± 0.42 **	10.19 ± 0.75 **
Turicibacter	0.96 ± 0.06	0.05 ± 0.01	8.70 ± 0.33 **	0.11 ± 0.03
Desulfovibrio	2.57 ± 0.11	2.97 ± 0.12	1.07 ± 0.05	2.89 ± 0.14
Bacteroides-unclassified	2.63 ± 0.10	0.57 ± 0.05	1.83 ± 0.06	1.98 ± 0.10 **
Acinetobacter	4.20 ± 0.01	1.56 ± 0.01	0.55 ± 0.01 **	0.66 ± 0.01 **
Allobaculum	0.07 ± 0.00	0.08 ± 0.00	6.20 ± 0.20 **	0.03 ± 0.00
Clostridiium	3.52 ± 0.08	0.01 ± 0.00	4.83 ± 0.05 **	0.02 ± 0.00 **
Helicobacter	4.23 ± 0.15	0.66 ± 0.01	0.08 ± 0.00	0.01 ± 0.00 **
Enterorhabdus	1.15 ± 0.10	0.54 ± 0.02	0.43 ± 0.02	1.43 ± 0.04
Peptostreptococcaceae-unclassified	0.00 ± 0.00	0.00 ± 0.00	3.22 ± 0.50 **	0.00 ± 0.00
Lachnospiraceae-unclassified	0.26 ± 0.01	2.52 ± 0.07	0.03 ± 0.00	0.04 ± 0.01
Escherichia	0.03 ± 0.01	2.62 ± 0.05 **	1.25 ± 0.02	0.02 ± 0.00
Lachnospiraceae	0.03 ± 0.00	2.36 ± 0.12 **	0.05 ± 0.01	0.04 ± 0.00
Lachnospiraceae-uncultured	0.30 ± 0.01	1.64 ± 0.02	0.14 ± 0.01	0.04 ± 0.00
Mycoplasma	2.03 ± 0.07	0.00 ± 0.00	0.00 ± 0.00	0.00 ± 0.00
Bacillus	1.04 ± 0.07	0.48 ± 0.02	0.12 ± 0.01	0.17 ± 0.00
Staphylococcus	0.29 ± 0.00	1.38 ± 0.12	0.09 ± 0.00	0.03 ± 0.00
Rikenella	1.31 ± 0.05	0.18 ± 0.01	0.02 ± 0.00	0.05 ± 0.00 **
Others	05.90 ± 0.17	5.63 ± 0.15	1.32 ± 0.05 **	1.6 ± 0.08 **

Each value is the mean ± standard deviation ($n = 3$). Data were analyzed using one-way ANOVA. Differences between control and treatment groups were assessed by Duncan's test. ** means values are significantly different ($p < 0.01$).

3. Discussion

Although knowledge of microflora in animal intestinal tracts is very limited, the view about their mediation and maintenance roles in host health is highly agreeable. Many important immune and metabolic disorders, including diabetes, obesity, behavioral disorders, and chronic inflammation, are known to be partially caused by the imbalance of interactions between host and intestinal microflora [35–37]. It is crucial to keep intestinal microflora in balance for host health.

It is well accepted that the two dominant normal intestinal microflora in mammalians belong to the phyla *Firmicutes* and *Bacteroidetes*, which are strict anaerobic bacteria [38]. *Bacteroides, Lactobacillus, Streptococcus, Clostridium, Enterococcus, Bifidobacterium, Candidatus*, etc. are the main genera with a larger quantity of microflora which inhabit the intestines [39–41]. However, major mycotoxins including deoxynivalenol, zearalenone, ochratoxin A, fumonisin B1 and aflatoxin B1 are proven to be able to disturb the stability of mammalian intestinal microflora [42]. Feeding with a certain dose of deoxynivalenol for 4 weeks by oral gavage increased *Bacteroides* and *Prevotella* but decreased *Escherichia coli* in rat intestines [43]. Zearalenone, given by oral gavage, reduced the total cultivable aerobic bacteria in pig intestines [44]. Ochratoxin A enhanced the *Lactobacilliaceae* family, increased the facultative anaerobes and decreased the microbial α-diversity in rat intestines [45]. Fumonisin B1 changed the similarity between microbial CE-SSCP profiles in pigs after a fumonisin-based feeding [46].

In our study, both genus and phylum showed a decreasing tendency from the control to the high-dose group as a whole, which was consistent with the finding that there was a reduction in microbial diversity in the colon from the healthy rats exposed chronically to AFB1 for 4 weeks [47]. There were about 8 genera with higher relative abundances in the high-dose group, which contained the least genera among all the groups (Figure 3A). Compared with the control group, the high-dose group had about one third of the total genera and nearly half of the total microflora (Figure 4A). There were about 4 phyla in both the medium-dose and the high-dose groups (Figure 4B). Compared with the control group, the high-dose group had about one half of the total phyla. The statistical analysis showed the same decreasing tendency for most bacterial flora except for several special ones (Table 1, Figure 6). However, a chronic exposure to AFB1 could not change the proportion of *Firmicutes* and *Bacteroidetes* [47].

The two dominant flora in mice were *Lactobacillus* and *Bacteroides*. However, their relative abundances were different among the groups. This observation might be explained that AFB1 with different doses disturbed the two dominant bacteria and led to different results. These two dominant bacteria showed similar total proportions in the control, the low-dose, and the high-dose groups but displayed the lowest proportion in the medium-dose group (Figure 4). Different abundance with a similar total proportion under different AFB1 doses meant that these two types of bacteria finally recovered to the normal proportion, even though they were fed with AFB1 at a high dose for 2 months. They showed strong viabilities, indicating that the two bacteria were tolerant and adaptable to a certain dose of AFB1. Wang et al. also found that different bacterial flora had different tolerances to AFB1, three *Clostridiales* species had the largest increase while 2 *Lactobacillales* species had the largest decrease with increasing AFB1 dose in their study [47]. Using a cultural method, Galarza-Seeber et al. discovered that the facultative anaerobe (coliforms) population was 10-fold higher than the control in cecum of broilers exposed to AFB1, whereas there was only a numerical non-significant rise observed for other microbial populations [48].

There were five genera with high relative abundances in the medium-dose group but not in other 3 groups, especially not in the high-dose group. They were *Peptostreptococcaceae*, *Allobaculum*, *Clostridium*, *Turicibacter*, and *Cadidatus* (Figures 3A and 6A). Among these genera, *Clostridium* contains several significant human pathogens, including the causative agent of botulism and an important cause of diarrhea [49,50]. A high-fat diet can lead to the expansion of the cluster XI of genus *Clostridium*, which could produce secondary bile acid, causing a phenotypic change in hepatic stellate cells to secrete proinflammatory cytokines, and eventually resulting in hepatocellular carcinoma in mice [51]. *Turicibacter* spp. has been strongly associated with immune function and bowel disease [52]. The proportion of *Turicibacter* was significantly more abundant in Inflammatory Colorectal Polyps (ICRPs)-affected in miniature dachshunds [53]. The high abundances of these bacteria may have resulted from the animals been maintained under unhealthy conditions. However, all these genera were not found in the high-dose group. The mechanism needs to be further explored to understand whether a high dose of AFB1 killed these genera or other factors led to the phenomenon.

Since there are only two research papers published that are relevant to the influence of AFB1 on gut microflora [47,48], more studies are required.

4. Conclusions

In conclusion, the intestinal bacterial flora in mice could be strongly disturbed by intragastric feeding with AFB1 solutions ranging from 2.5 mg/L to 10.0 mg/L for 2 months. *Lactobacillus* and *Bacteroides* were the two dominant bacterial flora, which could be induced to the same level as the control group under a high dose of AFB1 in this study. Nearly two thirds of the total genera and two more phyla finally disappeared. There might be several tolerant, adaptable, and inducible bacterial flora in mouse intestines under a certain dose of AFB1, but this possibility needs be investigated further.

5. Materials and Methods

5.1. Diet Information

With no antibiotics, hormones, and preservatives, the food ingredients were 27.0% corn starch, 19.0% wheat bran, 16% rice starch, 16.0% soybean dreg, 13.0% fish powder, 3.0% bone powder, 2.3% yeast powder, 0.5% salt, 0.1% compound vitamin and 0.1% trace elements; sterile water was added to ensure a 10% water content. After being mixed evenly, the mixture was sterilized at 121 °C for 20 min in a high pressure steam sterilizer.

5.2. AFB1 Solutions Preparation

The AFB1 stock solution was prepared by dissolving 0.01g AFBI powder (99.9% of purity, Solarbio Company, Beijing, China) in 500 mL of 2% sterile aqueous ethanol. The solution was stirred with a magnet stirring bar at 150 rpm under 50 °C for 30 min and then diluted with sterile water to reach the concentrations of 2.5 mg/L, 4 mg/L, and 10 mg/L.

5.3. Animal Trial

All animal experiments were approved by the Animal Care and Use Committee of Institute of Bast Fiber Crops, Chinese Academy of Agricultural Sciences (Changsha, Hunan). A total of 24 KM mice (SPF grade, Silaida Co., Ltd.. Hunan, China) with no specific pathogens were used in this study. Their average weight was about 20 ± 2 g. Equal numbers of males and females were adaptively fed in a quiet environment at 24 °C temperature and 65% humidity. The mice were then randomly divided into 4 groups, which were labeled as the control, low-dose, medium-dose, and high-dose groups. Each group was consisted of an equal number of males and females. The control group was fed intragastrically with sterile water, while the low-dose, the medium-dose, and the high-dose groups were fed intragastrically with 2.5 mg/L, 4 mg/L, and 10 mg/L of AFB1 solutions, respectively. The feeding dosage was 0.4 mL per mouse each time and 2 times a day for 2 months. Other conventional food was administered normally.

5.4. Sample Collection

The animals were killed by cervical dislocation and dissected aseptically on a laminar flow bench after the feeding treatment was over. Small intestinal contents (from jejunum to rectum) were collected from 2 randomly chosen mice (one male and one female) in each group, then stirred evenly with a sterile glass rod under a sterile environment, and considered as one replicate. Three replicates were used to analyze intestinal bacteria.

5.5. Intestinal Bacterial Flora Information

The total DNA was extracted from the obtained intestinal contents according to the instruction of the FastDNA® Spin Kit for Feces (MP Company, CA, USA) and then tested by electrophoresis on a 1% agarose gel. After being recycled and purified with AxyPrepDNA (Axygen Company, CA, USA), the bands were amplified with primers 338F: ACTCCTACGGGAGGCAGCA and 806R: GGACTACHVGGGTWTCTAAT, which were specifically designed for testing the hypervariable region V3 + V4 zones of intestinal bacteria DNA. The PCR reaction mixture contained 4 μL of 5 × Fast Pfu buffer, 2 μL of 2.5 mM dNTPs, 0.8 μL of 5 μM Forward Primer, 0.8 μL of 5 μM Reverse Primer, 0.4 μL FastPfu Polymerase, 0.2 μL BSA, and 10 ng Template DNA. Dd H_2O was added to reach the final volume to 20 μL. The reaction conditions as follows: an initial denaturing cycle at 95 °C for 3 min, with 28 cycles, denaturation at 95 °C for 30 s, annealing at 55 °C for 30 s, and extension at 72 °C for 45 s, with a final extension step at 72 °C for 10 min. Electrophoresis on 2% agarose gels was used to test the PCR products, the gene library was built, and the sequences were analyzed by Frasergene company (Wuhan, Hubei, China) with the Miseq Illumina System.

5.6. Statistical Analysis

SPSS software 22.0 (IBM Corp, Armonk, NY, USA) was used to analyze the significance of differences in the relative abundances of intestinal bacterial flora between groups.

Acknowledgments: The acknowledgments are given to Ministry of Agriculture of the People's Republic of China for funding this work (the Project No. GJFP2016010).

Author Contributions: Aiping Xiao and Xiai Yang conceived and designed the experiments; Xiai Yang and Jing Chen performed the experiments; Xiai Yang and Liangliang Liu analyzed the data and wrote the paper.

Conflicts of Interest: The authors declare no conflicts of interest.

References

1. Lu, L.; Walker, W.A. Pathologic and physiologic interactions of bacteria with the gastro intestinal epithelium. *Am. J. Clin. Nutr.* **2001**, *73*, 1124S–1130S. [PubMed]
2. Blaut, M.; Clavel, T. Metabolic diversity of the intestinal microbiota: Implications for health and disease. *J. Nutr.* **2007**, *137*, 751S–755S. [PubMed]
3. Cani, P.D.; Neyrinck, A.M.; Fava, F.; Knauf, C.; Burcelin, R.G.; Tuohy, K.M.; Gibson, G.R.; Delzenne, N.M. Selective increases of *bifidobacteria* in gut microflora improve high-fat-diet-induced diabetes in mice through a mechanism associated with endotoxaemia. *Diabetologia* **2007**, *50*, 2374–2383. [CrossRef] [PubMed]
4. Croswell, A.; Amir, E.; Teggatz, P.; Barman, M.; Salzman, N.H. Prolonged impact of antibiotics on intestinal microbial ecology and susceptibility to enteric salmonella infection. *Infect. Immun.* **2009**, *77*, 2741–2753. [CrossRef] [PubMed]
5. Eriksen, G.S.; Pettersson, H.; Johnsen, K.; Lindberg, J.E. Transformation of trichothecenes in ileal digesta and faeces from pigs. *Arch. Anim. Nutr.* **2002**, *56*, 263–274. [CrossRef]
6. Wang, J.C.; Tang, L.L.; Glenn, T.C.; Wang, J.S. Ameliorating effects of *Bacillus subtilis* ANSB060 on growth performance, antioxidant functions, and aflatoxin residues in ducks fed diets contaminated with aflatoxins. *Toxicol. Sci.* **2016**, *150*, 54–63. [CrossRef] [PubMed]
7. Young, J.C.; Zhou, T.; Yu, H.; Zhu, H.; Gong, J. Degradation of trichothecene mycotoxins by chicken intestinal microbes. *Food Chem. Toxicol.* **2007**, *45*, 136–143. [CrossRef] [PubMed]
8. Kollarczik, B.; Gareis, M.; Hanelt, M. In vitro transformation of the Fusarium mycotoxins deoxynivalenol and zearalenone by the normal gut microflora of pigs. *Nat. Toxins* **1994**, *2*, 105–110. [CrossRef] [PubMed]
9. Niderkorn, V.; Boudra, H.; Morgavi, D.P. Binding of Fusarium mycotoxins by fermentative bacteria in vitro. *J. Appl. Microbiol.* **2006**, *101*, 849–856. [CrossRef] [PubMed]
10. Hathout, A.S.; Aly, S.E. Biological detoxification of mycotoxins: A review. *Ann. Microbiol.* **2014**, *64*, 905–919. [CrossRef]
11. Vitali, B.; Ndagijimana, M.; Cruciani, F.; Carnevali, P.; Candela, M.; Guerzoni, M.E.; Brigidi, P. Impact of a synbiotic food on the gut microbial ecology and metabolic profiles. *BMC Microbiol.* **2010**, *10*, 1471–2180. [CrossRef] [PubMed]
12. Qi, H.W.; Xiang, Z.T.; Han, G.Q.; Chen, D.W. Effects of different dietary protein sources on cecal microflora in rats. *Afr. J. Biotechnol.* **2011**, *10*, 3704–3708.
13. Chassard, C.; Scott, K.P.; Marquet, P.; Martin, J.C.; Del'homme, C.; Dapoigny, M.; Flint, H.J.; Bernalier-Donadille, A. Assessment of metabolic diversity within the intestinal microbiota from healthy humans using combined molecular and cultural approaches. *FEMS Microbiol. Ecol.* **2008**, *66*, 496–504. [CrossRef] [PubMed]
14. Wogan, G.N. Aflatoxins as risk factors for hepatocellular carcinoma in humans. *Cancer Res.* **1992**, *52*, 2114s–2118s. [PubMed]
15. Windham, G.L.; Hawkins, L.K.; Williams, W.P. Aflatoxin accumulation and kernel infection of maize hybrids inoculated with *Aspergillus flavus* and *Aspergillus parasiticus*. *World Mycotoxin J.* **2010**, *3*, 89–93. [CrossRef]
16. Bennett, J.W.; Klich, M. Mycotoxins. *Clin. Microbiol. Rev.* **2003**, *16*, 497–516. [CrossRef] [PubMed]
17. Cuccioloni, M.; Mozzicafreddo, M.; Barocci, S.; Ciuti, F.; Re, L.; Eleuteri, A.M.; Angeletti, M. Aflatoxin B1 misregulates the activity of serine proteases: Possible implications in the toxicity of some mycotoxins. *Toxicol. In Vitro* **2009**, *23*, 393–399. [CrossRef] [PubMed]
18. Sabbioni, G. Chemical and physical properties of the major serum albumin adduct of aflatoxin B1 and their implications for the quantification in biological samples. *Chem. Biol. Interact.* **1990**, *75*, 1–15. [CrossRef]
19. Rawal, S.; Kim, J.E.; Coulombe, R.J. Aflatoxin B1 in poultry: Toxicology, metabolism and prevention. *Res. Vet. Sci.* **2010**, *89*, 325–331. [CrossRef] [PubMed]
20. Mughal, M.J.; Peng, X.; Kamboh, A.A.; Zhou, Y.; Fang, J. Aflatoxin B1 induced systemic toxicity in poultry and rescue effects of Selenium and Zinc. *Biol. Trace Elem. Res.* **2017**, *178*, 292–300. [CrossRef] [PubMed]
21. Liu, B.H.; Hsu, Y.T.; Lu, C.C.; Yu, F.Y. Detecting aflatoxin B1 in foods and feeds by using sensitive rapid enzyme-linked immunosorbent assay and gold nanoparticle immunochromatographic strip. *Food Control.* **2013**, *30*, 184–189. [CrossRef]

22. He, J.; Zhang, K.Y.; Chen, D.W.; Ding, X.M.; Feng, G.D.; Ao, X. Effects of maize naturally contaminated with aflatoxin B1 on growth performance, blood profiles and hepatic histopathology in ducks. *Livest. Sci.* **2013**, *152*, 192–199. [CrossRef]

23. Wache, Y.J.; Valat, C.; Postollec, G.; Bougeard, S.; Burel, C.; Oswald, I.P.; Fravalo, P. Impact of deoxynivalenol on the intestinal microflora of pigs. *Int. J. Mol. Sci.* **2009**, *10*, 1–17. [CrossRef] [PubMed]

24. El-Nezami, H.; Mykkänen, H.; Kankaanpää, P.; Salminen, S.; Ahokas, J. Ability of *Lactobacillus* and *Propionibacterium* strains to remove aflatoxin B, from the chicken duodenum. *J. Food Prot.* **2000**, *63*, 549–552. [CrossRef] [PubMed]

25. Gratz, S.; Täubel, M.; Juvonen, R.O.; Viluksela, M.; Turner, P.C.; Mykkänen, H.; El-Nezami, H. *Lactobacillus rhamnosus* Strain GG Modulates Intestinal Absorption, Fecal Excretion, and Toxicity of Aflatoxin B1 in Rats. *Appl. Environ. Microbiol.* **2006**, *72*, 7398–7400. [CrossRef] [PubMed]

26. Egbunike, G.N.; Emerole, G.O.; Aire, T.A.; Ikegwuonu, F.I. Sperm production rates, sperm physiology and fertility in rats chronically treated with sublethal doses of aflatoxin B1. *Andrologia* **1980**, *12*, 467–475. [CrossRef] [PubMed]

27. Wild, C.P.; Garner, R.C.; Montesano, R.; Tursi, F. Aflatoxin B1 binding to plasma albumin and liver DNA upon chronic administration to rats. *Carcinogenesis* **1986**, *7*, 853–858. [CrossRef] [PubMed]

28. Hinton, D.M.; Myers, M.J.; Raybourne, R.A.; Franckecarroll, S.; Sotomayor, R.E.; Shaddock, J.; Warbritton, A.; Chou, M.W. Immunotoxicity of aflatoxin B1 in rats: Effects on lymphocytes and the inflammatory response in a chronic intermittent dosing study. *Toxicol. Sci.* **2003**, *73*, 362–377. [CrossRef] [PubMed]

29. Wogan, G.N.; Newberne, P.M. Dose-response characteristics of aflatoxin B1 carcinogenesis in rats. *Cancer Res.* **1968**, *27*, 2370–2376.

30. Fouts, D.E.; Szpakowski, S.; Purushe, J.; Torralba, M.; Waterman, R.C. Next generation sequencing to define prokaryotic and fungal diversity in the bovine rumen. *PLoS ONE* **2012**, *7*, e48289. [CrossRef] [PubMed]

31. Amato, K.R.; Yeoman, C.J.; Kent, A.; Righini, N.; Carbonero, F.; Estrada, A.; Gaskins, H.R.; Stumpf, R.M.; Yildirim, S.; Torralba, M.; et al. Habitat degradation impacts black howler monkey (*Alouatta pigra*) gastrointestinal microbiomes. *ISME. J.* **2013**, *7*, 1344–1353. [CrossRef] [PubMed]

32. Jami, E.; Israel, A.; Kotser, A.; Mizrahi, I. Exploring the bovine rumen bacterial community from birth to adulthood. *ISME J.* **2013**, *7*, 1069–1079. [CrossRef] [PubMed]

33. Oberauner, L.; Zachow, C.; Lackner, S.; Högenauer, C.; Smolle, K.H.; Berg, G. The ignored diversity: Complex bacterial communities in intensive care units revealed by 16S pyrosequencing. *Sci. Rep.* **2013**, *3*, 1413–1422. [CrossRef] [PubMed]

34. Noval, M.R.; Burton, O.T.; Wise, P.; Zhang, Y.Q.; Hobson, S.A.; Lloret, M.G.; Chehoud, C.; Kuczynski, J.; DeSantis, T.; Warrington, J.; et al. A microbita signature associated with experimental food allergy promotes allergic senitization and anaphylaxis. *J. Allergy Clin. Immunol.* **2013**, *131*, 201–212. [CrossRef] [PubMed]

35. Musso, G.; Gambino, R.; Cassader, M. Interactions between gut microbiota and host metabolism predisposing to obesity and diabetes. *Annu. Rev. Med.* **2011**, *62*, 361–380. [CrossRef] [PubMed]

36. Tremaroli, V.; Bäckhed, F. Functional interactions between the gut microbiota and host metabolism. *Nature* **2012**, *489*, 242–249. [CrossRef] [PubMed]

37. Lee, W.J.; Hase, K. Gut microbiota-generated metabolites in animal health and disease. *Nat. Chem. Biol.* **2014**, *10*, 416–424. [CrossRef] [PubMed]

38. Lozupone, C.A.; Stombaugh, J.I.; Gordon, J.I.; Jansson, J.K.; Knight, R. Diversity, stability and resilience of the human gut microbiota. *Nature* **2012**, *489*, 220–230. [CrossRef] [PubMed]

39. Salzman, N.H.; De, J.H.; Paterson, Y.; Harmsen, H.J.; Welling, G.W. Analysis of 16S libraries of mouse gastrointestinal microflora reveals a large new group of mouse intestinal bacteria. *Microbiology* **2002**, *148*, 3651–3660. [CrossRef] [PubMed]

40. Dick, L.K.; Bernhard, A.E.; Brodeur, T.J.; Domingo, J.W.S.; Simpson, J.M.; Walters, S.P.; Field, K.G. Host distributions of uncultivated fecal *Bacteroidales* bacteria reveal genetic markers for fecal source identification. *Appl. Environ. Microbiol.* **2005**, *71*, 3184–3191. [CrossRef] [PubMed]

41. Shenghua, G.; Dandan, C.; Jinna, Z.; Xiaoman, L.; Kun, W.; Liping, D.; Yong, N.; Xiaolei, W. Bacterial community mapping of the mouse gastrointestinal tract. *PLoS ONE* **2013**, *8*, e74957.

42. Robert, H.; Payros, D.; Pinton, P.; Theodorou, V.; Mercier-Bonin, M.; Oswald, I.P. Impact of mycotoxins on the intestine: Are mucus and microbiota new targets? *J. Toxicol. Environ. Health B Crit. Rev.* **2017**, *20*, 249–275. [CrossRef] [PubMed]

43. Saint-Cyr, M.J.; Perrin-Guyomard, A.; Houée, P.; Rolland, J.G.; Laurentie, M. Evaluation of an oral subchronic exposure of deoxynivalenol on the composition of human gut microbiota in a model of human microbiotaassociated rats. *PLoS ONE* **2013**, *8*, e80578. [CrossRef] [PubMed]

44. Piotrowska, M.; Śliżewska, K.; Nowak, A.; Zielonka, L.; Zakowska, Z.; Gajęcka, M.; Gajęcki, M. The effect of experimental fusarium mycotoxicosis on microbiota diversity in porcine ascending colon contents. *Toxins* **2014**, *6*, 2064–2081. [CrossRef] [PubMed]

45. Guo, M.; Huang, K.; Chen, S.; Qi, X.; He, X.; Cheng, W.H.; Luo, Y.; Xia, K.; Xu, W. Combination of metagenomics and culture-based methods to study the interaction between ochratoxin A and gut microbiota. *Toxicol. Sci.* **2014**, *141*, 314–323. [CrossRef] [PubMed]

46. Burel, C.; Tanguy, M.; Guerre, P.; Boilletot, E.; Cariolet, R.; Queguiner, M.; Postollec, G.; Pinton, P.; Salvat, G.; Oswald, I.P.; et al. Effect of low dose of fumonisins on pig health: Immune status, intestinal microbiota and sensitivity to *Salmonella*. *Toxins* **2013**, *5*, 841–864. [CrossRef] [PubMed]

47. Wang, J.; Tang, L.; Glenn, T.C.; Wang, J.S. Aflatoxin B1 induced compositional changes in gut microbial communities of male F344 rats. *Toxicol. Sci.* **2016**, *150*, 54–63. [CrossRef] [PubMed]

48. Galarza-Seeber, R.; Latorre, J.D.; Bielke, L.R.; Kuttappan, V.A.; Wolfenden, A.D.; Hernandez-Velasco, X.; Merino-Guzman, R.; Vicente, J.L.; Donoghue, A.; Cross, D.; et al. Leaky gut and mycotoxins: Aflatoxin B1 does not increase gut permeability in broiler chickens. *Front. Vet. Sci.* **2016**, *3*, 10. [CrossRef] [PubMed]

49. Bartlett, J.G. Narrative review: The new epidemic of Clostridium difficile-associated enteric disease. *Ann. Intern. Med.* **2006**, *145*, 758–764. [CrossRef] [PubMed]

50. Pépin, J.; Routhier, S.; Gagnon, S.; Brazeau, I. Management and outcomes of a first recurrence of *Clostridium difficile*-associated disease in Quebec, Canada. *Clin. Infect. Dis.* **2006**, *42*, 758–764. [CrossRef] [PubMed]

51. Yoshimoto, S.; Loo, T.M.; Atarashi, K.; Kanda, H.; Sato, S.; Oyadomari, S.; Iwakura, Y.; Oshima, K.; Moria, H.; Hattori, M.; et al. Obesity-induced gut microbial metabolite promotes liver cancer through senescence secretome. *Nature* **2013**, *499*, 97–101. [CrossRef] [PubMed]

52. Allen, J.M.; Miller, M.E.B.; Pence, B.D.; Whitlock, K.; Nehra, V. Voluntary and forced exercise differentially alters the gut microbiome in C57BL/6J mice. *J. Appl. Physiol.* **2015**, *118*, 1059–1066. [CrossRef] [PubMed]

53. Igarashi, H.; Ohno, K.; Horigome, A.; Fujiwara-Igarashi, A.; Kanemoto, H.; Fukushima, K.; Odamaki, T.; Tsujimoto, H. Fecal dysbiosis in miniature dachshunds with inflammatory colorectal polyps. *Res. Vet. Sci.* **2016**, *105*, 41–46. [CrossRef] [PubMed]

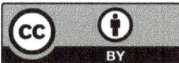

toxins

MDPI

Article

Colon Microbiome of Pigs Fed Diet Contaminated with Commercial Purified Deoxynivalenol and Zearalenone

Kondreddy Eswar Reddy [1,†], Jin Young Jeong [1,†], Jaeyong Song [1], Yookyung Lee [1], Hyun-Jeong Lee [1], Dong-Wook Kim [1,2], Hyun Jung Jung [1], Ki Hyun Kim [1], Minji Kim [1], Young Kyoon Oh [1], Sung Dae Lee [1,*] and Minseok Kim [1,3,*]

[1]   Animal Nutrition & Physiology Team, National Institute of Animal Science, Rural Development Administration, #1500 Kongjwipatjwi-ro, Iseo-myeon, Wanju 55365, Korea; dreswar4u@gmail.com (K.E.R.); jeong73@korea.kr (J.Y.J.); jysong76@korea.kr (J.S.); yoo3930@korea.kr (Y.L.); hyunj68@korea.kr (H.-J.L.); poultry98@korea.kr (D.-W.K.); hyjjung@korea.kr (H.J.J.); kihyun@korea.kr (K.H.K.); mjkimen@naver.com (M.K.); oh665@korea.kr (Y.K.O.)
[2]   Department of Poultry Science, Korea National College of Agriculture and Fisheries, #1515 Kongjwipatjwi-ro, Deokjin-gu, Jeonju-si 54874, Korea
[3]   Department of Animal Science, College of Agriculture and Life Sciences, Chonnam National University, Gwangju 61186, Korea
*   Correspondence: leesd@korea.kr (S.D.L.); mkim2276@gmail.com (M.K.); Tel.: +82-632-387-454 (S.D.L.); +82-632-387-459 (M.K.)
†   These authors contributed equally to this work.

Received: 9 June 2018; Accepted: 27 August 2018; Published: 29 August 2018

Abstract: Deoxynivalenol (DON) and zearalenone (ZEN) can seriously affect animal health, with potentially severe economic losses. Previous studies have demonstrated that gut microbiota plays a significant role in detoxification. We analyzed the colon contents from three groups of pigs (fed either a standard diet, or a diet with 8 mg/kg DON or ZEN). Bacterial 16S rRNA gene amplicons were obtained from the colon contents, and sequenced using next-generation sequencing on the MiSeq platform. Overall, 2,444,635 gene sequences were generated, with $\geq$2000 sequences examined. Firmicutes and Bacteroidetes were the dominant phyla in all three groups. The sequences of *Lactobacillus*, *Megasphaera*, and *Faecalibacterium* genera, and the unclassified Clostridiaceae family, represented more than 1.2% of the total, with significantly different abundances among the groups. *Lactobacillus* was especially more abundant in the DON (7.6%) and ZEN (2.7%) groups than in the control (0.2%). A total of 48,346 operational taxonomic units (OTUs) were identified in the three groups. Two OTUs, classified as *Lactobacillus*, were the most dominant in the DON and ZEN groups. The abundances of the remaining OTUs were also significantly different among the groups. Thus, the mycotoxin-contaminated feed significantly affected the colon microbiota, especially *Lactobacillus*, which was the most abundant. Therefore, we speculate that *Lactobacillus* plays a major role in detoxification of these mycotoxins.

Keywords: deoxynivalenol; zearalenone; pig; colon microbiota; *Lactobacillus*; detoxification

Key contribution: Collectively, our results indicate that *Lactobacillus* was the most abundant in the DON and ZEN dietary groups and less abundant in the control, suggesting that members of this genus may play a key role in the detoxification of dietary DON and ZEN in pigs.

1. Introduction

Deoxynivalenol (DON) and zearalenone (ZEN) are *Fusarium* mycotoxins that cause significant economic losses of crops globally, and frequently contaminate food and animal feed, such as maize, wheat, barley, rice, rye, oats, sorghum, and triticale. DON and ZEN cause damage to the gastrointestinal and immune systems in both humans and farm animals, resulting in vomiting, diarrhea, hemorrhage, leukopenia, and shock [1–3]. Among animal species, pigs show a comparatively high sensitivity to DON and ZEN, likely because of a high percentage of cereals in the porcine diet, posing a greater risk of exposure to these two mycotoxins. Furthermore, the front portion of the pig small intestine lacks microorganisms that are able to degrade mycotoxins before they are absorbed by the small intestine [4,5].

DON has been known to cause toxic effects in both animals and humans. Following DON exposure, the initial adverse effect in pigs is a reduced feed intake. DON adversely affects the growth performance, immune response, and reproductive performance in growing pigs [6,7]. A DON-contaminated diet influences the gastrointestinal tract, causing epithelial wounds in the stomach and intestine and, foremost, an intestinal inflammatory response in pigs [8,9]. According to Pierron et al. [10], in vitro and in vivo studies confirmed that DON severely inhibited intestinal nutrient absorption, changed the intestinal cell functions, and caused severe intestinal barrier damage.

ZEN and its metabolites clinically cause hyperestrogenism and reproductive disorders. ZEN metabolites compete with endogenous estrogens for estrogen receptor binding sites, and ultimately affect RNA and protein synthesis, leading to the deregulation of estrogenic activities [11]. Compared to chickens and ruminants, pigs are more sensitive to ZEN exposure, even at low levels [12]. According to Dänicke et al. [13], ZEN is regularly found in piglets under normal conditions, and these animals are initially exposed to ZEN in the uterus through placental transfer from the exposed sow, or through release of stored ZEN via suckling. ZEN also shows numerous genotoxic and cytotoxic effects in vitro and ex vivo, and is potentially carcinogenic [14]. Further, ZEN is recognized to be immunotoxic; nonetheless, its function in the inflammatory response is not yet completely understood [15].

The animal gastrointestinal tract is colonized by a rich variety of microorganisms, and quantitative and qualitative permanence of these organisms is an important factor in the maintenance of animal health [16]. The gut microbiota exerts obvious effects on basic host physiology and metabolism [17]. According to Richards et al. [16], the animal intestinal microbiota exhibits nutritional and protective functions, stimulates the immunity, produces fermentation products, and prevents colonization by pathogens. Bauer and his team [18] have demonstrated that the gut microbiota is influenced by various factors, such as the animal health, individual characteristics of the animal, and the feed type and quality. Microorganisms may also prevent harmful effects on animal health; in fact, it has been suggested that intestinal microbiota may play a protective role against mycotoxins as potential risk factors for inflammatory bowel disease [19]. As shown by Bauer and Williams [18], pathogenic microorganisms produce toxic metabolites and fecal enzymes that may increase the levels of carcinogenic substances, or convert procarcinogenic compounds into carcinogenic ones.

However, studies of the effects of the DON and ZEN mycotoxins on the pig gastrointestinal microbiota are lacking; in particular, the effect of ZEN on the pig gut microbiota remains unclear. Recently, Li et al. [20] have studied the intestinal microbial diversity in pigs fed a basal diet, naturally DON-contaminated wheat, and a feed contaminated with *Clostridium* sp. WJ06. In another study, DON and ZEN, separately and together, induced negative effects on the microbial diversity in the ascending colon of pigs [21].

Recently, 16S rRNA gene (*rrs*) sequencing using the Illumina MiSeq platform was used to compare the intestinal bacterial biota in DON-contaminated wheat-fed pigs and the rumen microbiota of steers fed various diets, demonstrating that DON and different diets greatly affected the microbiota of pigs and cattle, respectively [20,22]. However, direct effects of purified DON and ZEN on the colon microbiota composition have not yet been reported in pigs. Therefore, the main aim of this study was to comparatively investigate the abundance of unculturable microorganisms in control and mycotoxin-treated groups of pigs to gain insights into the community structure of the pig colon microbiota. We hypothesized that the community structure of the colon microbiome of pigs would be influenced by toxic effects of DON and ZEN.

2. Results

2.1. Sequencing and Bacterial Abundance

Quality control of clean *rrs* sequences, obtained from the colon contents of the control, DON, and ZEN dietary groups, resulted in a total of 2,444,635 sequences, with read lengths averaging 500 nucleotides. Of these, 740,744 sequences represented control feces, while 884,437 and 819,454 represented DON and ZEN feces (Table 1). The numbers of *rrs* sequences from individual control samples ranged from 158,817 to 192,996; those from DON-treated samples ranged from 166,967 to 196,160, while those from ZEN-treated samples ranged from 140,276 to 195,822.

Table 1. Diversity statistics of the reads in control and dietary deoxynivalenol (DON) and zearalenone (ZEN) treatment samples.

Sample Group	Sampling Type	No. of Sequences	No. of Observed OTUs [1]	Chao1	Phylogenetic Diversity Whole Tree	Shannon	Sample Group
Control (*n* = 4)	Subsampled reads	100,000	16,961 [a]	58,020 [a]	791 [a]	9.805 [a]	0.990 [a]
DON (*n* = 5)	Subsampled reads	100,000	16,003 [a]	52,108 [a,b]	772 [a]	9.692 [a]	0.991 [a]
ZEN (*n* = 5)	Subsampled reads	100,000	14,565 [a]	45,882 [b]	696 [a]	9.353 [a]	0.989 [a]

[1] The number of operational taxonomic units (OTUs) was normalized by subsampling 100,000 sequences from each colon contents. Means among the three groups were compared using analysis of variance, followed by Duncan's test. Values with different superscript letters in the same row are significantly different ($p < 0.05$).

Almost 99.8% of all *rrs* sequences from the colon contents of the three groups were classified into known phyla. As shown in Figure 1 and Supplementary Table S1, the phyla Firmicutes and Bacteroidetes were highly abundant, and were represented by 57.3% and 35.00% of all *rrs* sequences, respectively. The next most abundant phylum was Proteobacteria, which was represented by 3.2% of the total sequences; the remaining phyla were each represented by <2.00% of all *rrs* sequences. The phyla Spirochaetes and Actinobacteria were represented by 1.7% and 1.0% of all *rrs* sequences, respectively. Planctomycetes, Tenericutes, and candidate division TM7 were represented by less than 1.00% of all *rrs* sequences. The genus *Prevotella* comprised 23.7% of the 5,279,245 *rrs* sequences.

At the genus level, *Prevotella* was highly abundant, being represented by 18.8% of the 2,444,635 *rrs* sequences. Other genera, represented by at least 0.5% of the total sequences, were *Lactobacillus* (3.8%), *Dialister* (2.3%), *Bacteroides* (2.3%), *Megasphaera* (2.1%), *Phascolarctobacterium* (1.6%), *Treponema* (1.6%), *Ruminococcus* (1.4%), *Faecalibacterium* (1.2%), CF231 (1.2%), *Oscillospira* (1.1%), *Lachnospira* (1.0%), *Bulleidia* (0.9%), *Coprococcus* (0.8%), *Parabacteroides* (0.8%), *Blautia* (0.8%), *Campylobacter* (0.8%), *Shuttleworthia* (0.7%), p-75-a5 (0.5%), *Dorea* (0.5%), *Roseburia* (0.5%), *Acidaminococcus* (0.5%), *Clostridium* (0.5%), and *Desulfovibrio* (0.5%). Some taxa were not classified at the genus level but showed high abundance at the phylum level, such as Firmicutes and Bacteroidetes. The orders Clostridiales (8.5%) and Bacteroidales (2.8%) were dominant, and at the family level, Ruminococcaceae (14.4%) was highly abundant, followed by S24-7 (5.7%), Lachnospiraceae (3.9%), Veillonellaceae (2.7%), Paraprevotellaceae (2.5%), Clostridiaceae (1.3%), Christensenellaceae (0.5%), and Erysipelotrichaceae (0.5%).

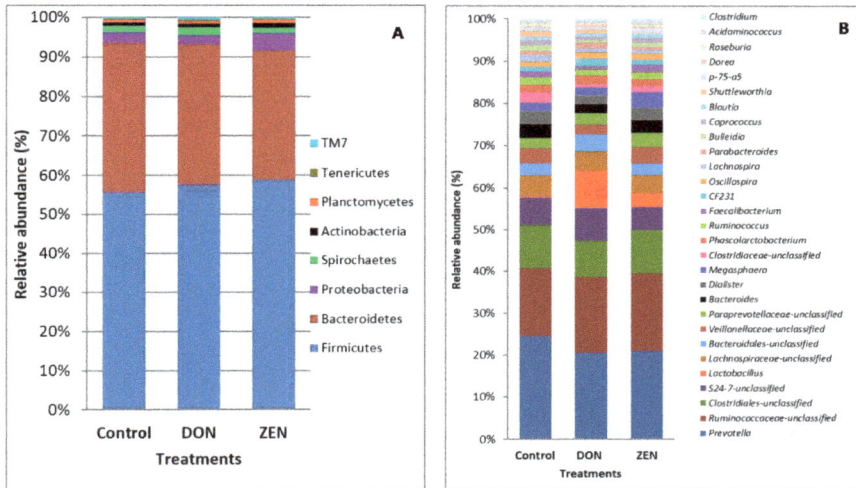

Figure 1. Microbial taxonomic profiles from the colon contents of the three dietary treatment groups at the phylum (**A**) and genus (**B**) levels, classified by the representation of >1% of the total sequences. Taxonomic compositions of the colon microbiota among the control, deoxynivalenol (DON), and zearalenone (ZEN) groups were compared based on the relative abundance (taxon reads/total reads in the colon contents).

A total of 192,724 operational taxonomic units (OTUs) were identified at a 0.03 dissimilarity cutoff level for all samples. All reads were normalized and analyzed using the Shannon diversity index, Chao1 richness estimator, and the Simpson index. OTUs of normalized samples did not vary ($p > 0.05$) among the three dietary treatment groups. The data of the richness estimate showed significant differences ($p < 0.05$) in the numbers of OTUs among the groups (Table 1).

2.2. Taxonomic Composition

Analysis of the taxonomic abundance in samples from the control, DON, and ZEN dietary groups showed differences at the phylum and genus levels (Figure 1A,B and Supplementary Table S1). The microbial data for all three dietary treatment groups were analyzed to determine the mean comparative abundance (taxon reads/total reads in a sample). At the genus level, *Lactobacillus* ($p = 0.002$), *Megasphaera* ($p = 0.01$), and *Faecalibacterium* ($p = 0.045$), as well as the order Clostridiales ($p = 0.05$), showed significant differences in the abundance among the DON, ZEN, and control groups. Analysis of the abundances at the taxonomic levels from the phylum to genus revealed differences among the DON, ZEN, and control groups. These variations were most obvious for Firmicutes, Bacteroidetes, *Prevotella*, *Lactobacillus*, the family Ruminococcaceae, and the order Clostridiales.

As shown in Figure 2A, the phyla Firmicutes and Bacteroidetes were highly abundant, while the remaining phyla were represented by <5% of all sequences. Furthermore, no significant differences were observed at the phylum level among the three dietary treatment groups. *Prevotella* was the most abundant known genus, represented by 18.8% of all sequences. The abundance of *Prevotella* was higher ($p = 0.72$) in the control group (21.7%) than in the DON (17.5%) and ZEN (17.7%) groups (Figure 2B). The abundance of *Lactobacillus*, which was represented by 3.8% of the total sequences, was significantly different ($p = 0.002$) among the groups. Interestingly, *Lactobacillus* was significantly ($p = 0.002$) more abundant in the DON group (7.6%), compared to 2.7% and 0.2% in the ZEN and control groups, respectively. The abundance of *Megasphaera*, which was represented by 2.1% of all sequences, was significantly higher ($p = 0.01$) in the ZEN group (3.0%) than in the control group (1.7%), but no significant difference was observed between the DON (1.6%) and control groups. The abundance of *Faecalibacterium*, which was represented by 1.2% of the total sequences, was also significantly different ($p = 0.045$) among the three dietary treatment groups; compared with that in the control group (1.3%), the abundance was lower (0.7%) in the DON group, and slightly higher (1.5%) in the ZEN group. The abundance of the unclassified family Clostridiaceae was significantly different ($p = 0.05$) among the three dietary treatment groups, being much lower in the DON group (0.6%) and moderately lower in the ZEN group (1.2%) than that in the control group (2.1%).

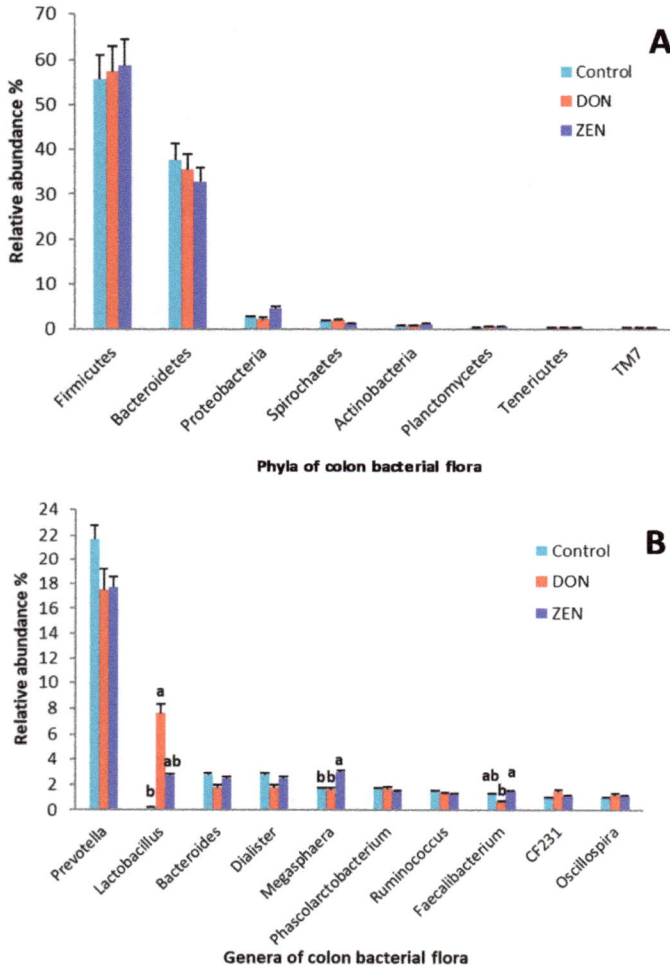

Figure 2. Relative abundances of the colon microbiota between the control and deoxynivalenol (DON) and zearalenone (ZEN) mycotoxin groups. (**A**) Variations in the relative abundance of the colon microbiota at the phylum level. (**B**) Variations in the relative abundance of the colon microbiota at the genus level. Different letters indicate significant differences ($p < 0.05$). Data were analyzed using one-way analysis of variance, followed by Duncan's test.

Approximately 60% of the Firmicutes sequences could not be classified at the genus level. The following five unclassified groups were dominant: Ruminococcaceae (14.4%), Clostridiales (8.5%), Lachnospiraceae (3.8%), Veillonellaceae (2.7%), and Clostridiaceae (1.3%). Similar results have been reported for the feces of cattle fed different diets [23]; however, in the present study, none of the unclassified groups showed significant differences ($p > 0.05$) among the three dietary treatments. Approximately 32% of Bacteroidetes could not be classified at the genus level either, including S24-7, Bacteroidales, and Paraprevotellaceae, nor did these taxa show any differences ($p > 0.05$) among the dietary treatments.

2.3. Analysis of Diversity

The diversity of the pig colon microbiota was compared among the control and two mycotoxin-treated groups. We analyzed the species-level OTUs at a cutoff of 0.03 from all the samples to evaluate the diversity of the colon microbiota from the three dietary groups, and identified a total of 48,346 OTUs from all the samples. Nine of the 48,346 OTUs were represented by $\geq 0.1\%$ of all sequences in at least one dietary group, but three of the nine OTUs could not be classified into known genera (Table 2).

Table 2. Relative abundances of significantly different operational taxonomic units (OTUs), calculated for the control, deoxynivalenol (DON), and zearalenone (ZEN) dietary groups.

OTU ID [1]	Classification	Percentage of Total Sequences [2]					
		Collective Data	Control	DON	ZEN	SEM	*p*-Value
denovo28392	*Lactobacillus*	1.03	0.01 [b]	2.77 [a]	0.29 [a,b]	0.005	0.006
denovo31941	Unclassified Ruminococcaceae	2.32	2.39 [a,b]	1.34 [b]	3.23 [a]	0.005	0.025
denovo47686	*Prevotella*	0.17	0.06 [b]	0.14 [a,b]	0.31 [a]	0.001	0.001
denovo63294	Unclassified Clostridiales	0.21	0.32 [a]	0.10 [b]	0.21 [a,b]	0.001	0.005
denovo92866	*Megasphaera*	1.13	0.63 [b]	1.88 [a]	0.89 [b]	0.002	0.006
denovo218634	*Lactobacillus*	0.90	0.07 [b]	1.57 [a]	1.05 [a,b]	0.004	0.049
denovo231303	Unclassified Clostridiaceae	0.39	0.77 [a]	0.04 [b]	0.34 [a,b]	0.002	0.019
denovo254063	*Bulleidia*	0.18	0.29 [a]	0.04 [b]	0.22 [a,b]	0.001	0.011
denovo274039	*Faecalibacterium*	0.39	0.45 [a,b]	0.21 [b]	0.52 [a]	0.001	0.001

[1] A total of 192,724 de novo OTUs were numbered in consecutive order. [2] Values represent the means. Values with different superscript letters in the same row are significantly different ($p < 0.05$).

OTU denovo31941, classified into Ruminococcaceae, was the most dominant among the nine OTUs in the collective data, and its abundance was the highest ($p = 0.025$) in the ZEN group and the lowest ($p = 0.025$) in the DON group (Table 2). The second most dominant OTU was that representing the genus *Megasphaera* (denovo92866), and it showed the highest abundance ($p = 0.006$) in the DON group and the lowest abundance ($p = 0.006$) in the control group. The next most abundant OTU was that representing the genus *Lactobacillus* (denovo28392), which was the most abundant ($p = 0.006$) in the DON group, moderately abundant ($p = 0.006$) in the ZEN group, and of the lowest abundance ($p = 0.006$) in the control group. Moreover, another OTU, also belonging to *Lactobacillus* (denovo218634), was highly, moderately, and lowly abundant ($p = 0.049$) in the DON, ZEN, and control groups, respectively. The abundances of three additional OTUs, representing Clostridiaceae (denovo231303; $p = 0.019$), *Bulleidia* (denovo254063; $p = 0.011$), and Clostridiales (denovo63294; $p = 0.005$), were much lower in the DON and ZEN groups than in the control group. An OTU of the genus *Prevotella* (denovo47686) was highly abundant in the ZEN group, moderately abundant in the DON group, and of the lowest abundance in the control group ($p = 0.001$). One OTU, classified as *Faecalibacterium*, was highly abundant in the ZEN group, and of relatively low abundance in the DON group compared with that in the control group ($p = 0.001$).

3. Discussion

Until now, few studies have been conducted to investigate the effects of the DON and ZEN mycotoxins on the pig gastrointestinal microbiota; in particular, the effects of ZEN on the gastrointestinal microbiota are largely unknown. Previous studies have examined the effects of naturally mycotoxin-contaminated feeds on the gut microbiota, but no reports are available on the microbial composition of the colonic contents of pigs fed commercially purified DON and ZEN [20,24]. Therefore, we analyzed the colon contents of pigs fed commercially purified DON and ZEN, to compare microbial abundances in the control, DON, and ZEN dietary groups, for the first time.

The animal digestive tract is suitable for microbial mass reproduction. Usually, various bacterial species are preferentially localized in different regions of the gastrointestinal tract, and not all regions are heavily colonized. According to Jia et al. [25], microbial communities in the small and large intestines play an important role in managing the host's health, including the energy intake from food, immune system function, generation of important metabolites, and the response to gastrointestinal diseases. Swanson et al. [26] have reported the function of fecal and intestinal microbiota in the metabolism of trichothecenes, which was studied by anaerobically incubating microbial suspensions from the feces of swine, cattle, horses, dogs, chickens, and rats with diacetoxyscirpenol (DAS). The microbiota from pigs, cattle, and rats fully transformed DAS, primarily to de-epoxy monoacetoxyscirpenol and de-epoxy scirpentriol. This research clearly indicated that the function of intestinal microbiota involves more than just binding DAS. A study by McCormick [27] has reported anaerobic bacterial degradation of trichothecenes in animal systems. The toxic impact of trichothecenes on animals was mitigated by intestinal or rumen bacteria that could detoxify the compounds. Kabak and Dobson [28,29] have also discussed in their reviews the role of microorganisms in detoxification.

In the present study, Firmicutes (57.3%) and Bacteroidetes (35.0%) were the most abundant groups of bacteria in the colon contents from the DON, ZEN, and control groups at the phylum level, but their levels were not significantly different between the control and treatment groups. By contrast, abundances of Firmicutes and Bacteroidetes were significantly different in the ileum, cecum, and colon of growing pigs fed naturally DON-contaminated wheat [20]. Feeding a diet with a 100 µg/kg body weight dose of DON for 4 weeks by oral gavage increased the abundances of *Bacteroides* and *Prevotella* in rat intestines [30]. In another study, compared with the control group, the DON-treated mouse group showed significantly lower species abundances of Bacteroidetes and higher abundances of Proteobacteria [31]. According to Scaldaferri et al. [32], the abundance of Bacteroidetes significantly decreased as a result of intestinal ulceration or inflammation in humans. We speculated that these inconsistencies were due to variations in the type and age of animals, dietary concentrations of DON and ZEN, conditions of toxins (natural contamination or a purified powder), the duration of treatment, weather conditions, and the diet composition.

At the genus level, *Lactobacillus* was significantly more abundant in the DON and ZEN groups, particularly in the DON group, than in the control. Similar to our findings, *Lactobacillus* was the most abundant in the ileum, cecum, and colon of growing pigs fed a diet naturally contaminated with DON [20]. Some studies have already proven the many physiological effects of *Lactobacillus* on the host, including microbial interference, antimicrobial effects, nutritional supplementation, a decrease in the serum cholesterol, antitumor effects, a decrease in the necessary antibiotic treatments, and immunomodulatory effects, among others [20,33,34]. Investigators have previously found that the pig small intestine is commonly dominated by *Lactobacillus*, and generally, the bacterial density increases quickly as the animal grows [35,36]. *Lactobacillus* is an important natural constituent of the intestinal microbiota in healthy animals and humans; in fact, bacteria of this genus have been shown in in vitro and in vivo studies to bind various mycotoxins [37,38]. *Lactobacillus* spp. are also able to rapidly form a complex bacterial community, which protects the host from infections by pathogenic bacteria [39]. *Lactobacillus* can successfully remove trichothecenes, such as DON, fusarenon, and DAS from liquid media [40]. *Lactobacillus* species are potential probiotics, shown to participate in the removal of ZEN in an in vitro study [41]. El-Nezami and his team [42] have investigated the binding affinity interactions of ZEN and its derivative α-zearalenol with two food-grade strains of *Lactobacillus*. *Lactobacillus* spp. can produce lactic acid as a byproduct of carbohydrate fermentation, and have been reported to extracellularly bind ZEN, DON, and aflatoxins [42–44]. Cell wall polysaccharides and peptidoglycans are two key elements accountable for the binding of mutagens to *Lactobacillus* cells [45]. Consequently, the high proportion of *Lactobacillus*, detected in the current study, might have resulted from a competitive advantage related to the capability of *Lactobacillus* to metabolize DON and ZEN. Many investigators have examined the interactions between bacteria and trichothecenes and revealed that those can occur through metabolic degradation and the conversion of trichothecenes into considerably less toxic forms [46–48]. The effects of DON on the intestinal microbial abundance and diversity in mice have also been explored using an Illumina MiSeq high-throughput sequencing method [31]. Robert et al. [49] have demonstrated that the mucus and microbiota are important targets for dietary mycotoxins, especially DON. Using in vitro and ex vivo models, Pinton et al. [50] demonstrated that the inhibitory effect of DON on mucus secretion by human and porcine goblet cells relies on its ability to suppress the expression of the resistin-like molecule beta (RELM-beta). Generally, the presence of the gastrointestinal mucus can lower the capacity of probiotics to bind mycotoxins because the mucus may interfere with the adsorption of a mycotoxin to the bacterial cell wall of the probiotic. However, in the current study, the regular administration of the probiotic *Lactobacillus* during the dietary treatment period may have reduced the effect of the mucus. Consequently, it could be hypothesized that, as the number of colony-forming units increased, the effect of the mucus on the adsorption of DON and ZEN by the *Lactobacillus* cell wall was reduced. Previously, similar results have been reported by Gratz et al. [51] who used the probiotic *Lactobacillus* in aflatoxin B1-fed rats.

In the present study, the abundances of *Faecalibacterium* and the family Clostridiaceae were significantly lower in the DON and ZEN groups than in the control group. However, the relative abundances of these two bacterial taxa differed between the DON and ZEN dietary groups. This difference might have been caused by the use of DON and ZEN at different doses, which led to different effects on these two dominant bacterial taxa. These results suggest that the growth of these bacteria was inhibited by the highly toxic DON, and slightly inhibited by the low-toxic ZEN. Similarly, the abundance of *Clostridium* significantly decreased in the ileum and colon of DON-treated pigs, but increased in the colon of pigs fed DON-contaminated wheat in combination with *Clostridium* sp. WJ06, which is used as a detoxicant [20]. According to a study by Rotter et al. [52], before mycotoxin-contaminated food enters the small intestine of poultry and ruminants, DON comes into contact with high concentrations of microbes, which can change DON to de-epoxy-deoxynivalenol (DOM-1). These results suggest that DON may have induced intestinal lesions by destroying the integrity of the intestinal barrier in pigs, consistent with the data from previous studies on DON-fed pigs [20,53]. In the current study, bacteria of the genus *Megasphaera* were highly abundant in the ZEN and DON treatment groups, with no significant difference between the dietary groups. This genus is an important member of the gut microbiota, and exerts useful effects on the host [54]. Shetty et al. [55] have reported that *Megasphaera* plays a key role in the complex gut environment and performs the complete metabolic functions of the human gut microbiome. We assumed that because of the low concentration of ZEN, *Megasphaera* may have developed resistance to the low-toxic condition and, therefore, was abundant in the ZEN dietary group. Currently, there has been no published research on the microbial effects in ZEN-fed pigs. The absorption rates of DON and ZEN show substantial variance among animals; pigs show the highest absorption rate (82%), followed by chickens (19%), sheep (9.9%), and cows (1%) [56,57]. Frey et al. [58] have demonstrated that differences in absorption are mostly associated with the distribution of microorganisms before or after the small intestine. In particular, in monogastric animals and humans, bacteria are absent in the front portion of the small intestine; thus, compared to ruminants and poultry, pigs and humans are highly sensitive to DON [59,60]. Waché et al. [2] have revealed that DON-contaminated feed could increase the abundance of anaerobic bacteria in pigs, while decreasing the number of anaerobic sulfite-reducing bacteria. Based on the above observations, we speculated that the colon microbial structure and composition were mainly affected by the DON and ZEN doses, animal type, age, and health, as well as by environmental conditions and the duration of treatment.

To date, no OTU information has been available for intestinal or fecal samples from DON- or ZEN-treated pigs. In the present study, nine OTUs were identified whose abundances were significantly different among the three dietary treatment groups. Among these OTUs, two represented *Lactobacillus* and one each represented *Prevotella*, *Megasphaera*, *Bulleidia*, *Faecalibacterium*, unclassified Ruminococcaceae, unclassified Clostridiales, and unclassified Clostridiaceae. Similarly, except for *Megasphaera* and *Bulleidia*, the remaining seven OTU species were found in the colon contents of cattle fed different diets [23]. Species related to these nine main OTUs may have considerably contributed to the colon bacterial ecosystem, irrespective of the dietary treatment group. In particular, two OTUs representing *Lactobacillus* and *Megasphaera* were highly abundant in the DON group, and three OTUs, including *Prevotella*, *Faecalibacterium*, and Ruminococcaceae, were dominant in the ZEN group. Species associated with these OTUs may have played a major role in the metabolism of DON and ZEN. In particular, the *Lactobacillus* species corresponding to the two OTUs were shown to be highly abundant in the DON and ZEN groups, compared with their abundances in the control, and might have bound the DON and ZEN mycotoxins and detoxified them, protecting the pig immune system. For further clarification, isolation and characterization of *Lactobacillus* species will need to be performed to reveal their function in the pig gastrointestinal microbial community.

In summary, our results showed that the abundances of microbiota components were significantly different in the pig colon contents from the control, DON, and ZEN groups; in particular, the DON group showed the highest abundance of *Lactobacillus* among the treatment groups, possibly indicating a major role of *Lactobacillus* in detoxification. Based on the El-Nezami et al. [42] data, we believe that our results are due to the physical phenomenon of the binding of the DON and ZEN toxins to *Lactobacillus* via weak non-covalent bond interactions, such as those related to hydrophobic pockets on the bacterial surface. Consistent with this phenomenon, the *Lactobacillus* abundance was higher in the DON- and ZEN-treated groups than in the control group. There may be numerous tolerant, adaptable, and inducible members of the microbiota in the pig gastrointestinal tract following exposure to particular doses of DON and ZEN, but this possibility needs to be examined further. Additional studies are needed to investigate the chemical nature of mycotoxin-binding sites of *Lactobacillus*, and the types of chemical interactions involved in the binding mechanism. These future studies may also clarify the potential relationships between DON and ZEN, and the gut microbiota, facilitating the development of effective therapeutic methods to control DON- and ZEN-induced diseases.

4. Materials and Methods

4.1. Ethics Statement

The protocols for the animal experimental procedures were reviewed and approved by the Institutional Animal Care and Use Committee of the National Institute of Animal Science, South Korea (No. 2015-147, 29 May 2015).

4.2. Animals

The current study was carried out with 14 castrated 8-week-old male piglets (Landrace × Yorkshire = Large White Landrace; ~19 kg) obtained from a commercial pig farm. All piglets, which originated from different litters, were randomly selected. Each piglet was housed in a separate pen (2.1 m × 1.4 m) with free access to water from drinking nipples, and they were fed individually. The piglets were allowed to acclimate to their new housing conditions for 1 week at 25 ± 1 °C, and were subsequently allocated to three dietary groups, the control ($n = 4$), DON ($n = 5$), and ZEN ($n = 5$) groups, with approximately equal body weights. Piglets in the control group were supplied a standard diet (Table 3) to meet their nutritional requirements [61], and those in the treatment groups were supplied the control diet with added DON or ZEN. Commercially available purified DON and ZEN powders (Biomin Singapore Pte. Ltd., Singapore) were properly mixed into the feed at 8 mg/kg and 0.8 mg/kg, respectively. During the entire 4-week experimental period, the control and DON- and ZEN-contaminated diets, as well as water, were supplied to the pigs ad libitum. Ethical guidelines for animal protection rights were observed.

Table 3. Ingredients and chemical composition of the piglet standard diet (as-fed basis).

Item	Control Diet
Ingredients	**(%)**
Ground corn	58.56
Soybean meal (46% crude protein)	14.00
Extruded soybean meal	12.00
Whey powder (12% crude protein)	7.00
Fish meal	3.45
Soybean oil	1.60
L-Lysine-HCl (78%)	0.43
DL-Methionine (99%)	0.14
L-Threonine (99%)	0.12
Calcium hydrophosphate	1.08
Limestone	0.60
Choline chloride (50%)	0.20
Sodium chloride	0.32
Vitamin–trace mineral premix [1]	0.50
Calculated nutrients	**(%)**
Metabolizable energy (kcal/kg)	3444
Crude fiber	2.29
Crude protein	20.78
Crude fat	3.44
Ash	4.35
Lysine	1.47
Methionine	0.49
Calcium	0.75
Phosphorus	0.45

[1] The following quantities (per kilogram of complete diet) were provided: vitamin A, 11,000 IU; vitamin D3, 1500 IU; vitamin E, 44.1 IU; vitamin K3, 4.0 mg; vitamin B1, 1.4 mg; vitamin B2, 5.22 mg; vitamin B5, 20.0 mg; vitamin B12, 0.01 mg; niacin, 26.0 mg; pantothenic acid, 14 mg; folic acid, 0.8 mg; biotin, 44 mg; Fe, 100.0 mg (as iron sulfate); Cu, 16.50 mg (as copper sulfate); Zn, 90.0 mg (as zinc sulfate); Mn, 35.0 mg (as manganese sulfate); I, 0.30 mg (as calcium iodate).

4.3. Mycotoxin Analysis

The DON and ZEN quantities in the DON- and ZEN-supplemented corn feed were examined by ultra-performance liquid chromatography (UPLC). A homogenized DON-contaminated grain sample (1 g) was extracted with 20 mL of distilled water by shaking for 30 min. A ZEN-contaminated corn sample (1 g) was mixed with 0.5 g of NaCl and 20 mL of acetonitrile (ACN), and then shaken for 1 h. After filtering the extracts through Whatman No. 1 paper, 5 mL of the DON-contaminated filtrate was diluted in 20 mL of phosphate-buffered saline (PBS), and 5 mL of the ZEN-mixed grain filtrate was diluted in 20 mL of a 1% Tween 20 solution. The extracted DON- and ZEN-mixed samples were loaded separately onto immunoaffinity chromatography columns. The DON column was allowed to dry, then washed with 10 mL each of PBS and distilled water, and eluted with 0.5 mL of methanol (MeOH) and 1.5 mL of ACN. In the case of ZEN, the column was washed with 10 mL of distilled water and eluted with 1.5 mL of MeOH. The eluates were dried under N_2 gas, and 10 µL of each sample was injected into a UPLC instrument (Acquity UPLC® H Class; Waters, Milford, MA, USA). The mobile phase used to separate DON and ZEN consisted of water/ACN/MeOH (90:5:5 for DON and 43:35:22 for ZEN). The samples were separated isocratically at a flow rate of 0.3 mL/min. Photodiode array and fluorescence detectors were used to detect DON and ZEN, respectively. Waters Acquity UPLC® BEH C18 columns (2.1 × 100 mm, 1.7 μm particle size) were used for both DON and ZEN toxin analyses. The complete details of the mass spectrometry system running method, the excitation and emission wavelengths, and the limits of detection and quantification, were as described by Reddy et al. [7]. We found that the amounts of DON and ZEN in the mixed corn feed were 7.38 and 0.67 mg/kg, respectively; these values were close to the original concentrations. No DON and ZEN contamination was found in the control feed.

4.4. Sampling and Processing

A total of 14 male piglets were used to examine the colon microbiota composition in the standard diet and DON and ZEN mycotoxin-contaminated feed groups. After 4 weeks of treatment, all pigs were euthanized by an overdose of the anesthetic pentobarbital. After cardiac arrest, the colon contents of all pigs were aseptically collected directly into sample containers, rapidly frozen in liquid nitrogen, and then stored at −80 °C for further analysis.

4.5. DNA Extraction and 16S rRNA Gene Sequencing

Total community DNA was extracted from the 14 samples of colon contents using the repeated bead beating plus column method [62], and stored at −20 °C before sequencing. From each DNA sample, 14 amplicon libraries were generated using the 341F (5′-CCTACGGGNGGCWGCAG-3′) and 805R (5′-GACTACHVGGGTATCTAATCC-3′) primers, which produce approximately 450 bp products. The resultant 14 amplicon libraries were sequenced using a 2 × 300 bp paired-end protocol with the MiSeq platform (Illumina, San Diego, CA, USA) at the Macrogen sequencing facility (Macrogen, Inc., Seoul, Korea). Paired reads were assembled using the FLASH program [63]. The assembled sequences were demultiplexed using the default parameters and quality filtered using a Q20 minimum value with the QIIME software package 1.9.1 [64]. Taxa were identified using the Greengenes reference database [65], while OTUs were determined at 97% sequence similarity using the uclust program [66]. After 100,000 sequences were subsampled from each colon sample to normalize the number of OTUs, alpha diversity indices (number of OTUs, Chao1, PD_whole_tree distance, and Shannon diversity index) were determined.

4.6. Statistical Analysis

Taxa (or OTUs) representing, on average, ≥0.2% of the total sequences were regarded as major taxa (or OTUs), and used for statistical analysis. The mean proportion of each taxon or OTU in the total sequences was compared among the three diet groups using analysis of variance, followed by Duncan's test, in the XLSTAT statistical software version 18.07 (Addinsoft, New York, NY, USA). A significant difference was considered at $p < 0.05$.

4.7. Nucleotide Sequence Accession Number

The 16S rRNA gene sequence data used in the current study are available from the EMBL European Nucleotide Archive under accession number PRJEB27663.

Supplementary Materials: The following is available online at http://www.mdpi.com/2072-6651/10/9/347/s1, Table S1: Relative abundance of taxa in the control and DON and ZEN mycotoxin dietary treatment groups.

Author Contributions: S.D.L., M.K. (Minseok Kim), and K.E.R. designed and performed the experiments; J.Y.J. and J.S. developed methods and contributed reagents/materials; H.-J.L., D.-W.K., Y.L., and H.J.J. performed the experiments; K.H.K. and M.K. (Minji Kim) analyzed and discussed the data; Y.K.O. created the illustrations; K.E.R. wrote the manuscript.

Acknowledgments: This work was carried out with the support of the Cooperative Research Program for Agriculture Science & Technology Development (Project No. PJ01093202) and the 2017 RDA Fellowship Program of the National Institute of Animal Sciences, Rural Development Administration, Republic of Korea.

Conflicts of Interest: The authors declare no conflict of interest.

References

1. Creppy, E.E. Update of survey, regulation and toxic effects of mycotoxins in Europe. *Toxicol. Lett.* **2002**, *127*, 19–28. [CrossRef]
2. Wache, Y.J.; Valat, C.; Postollec, G.; Bougeard, S.; Burel, C.; Oswald, I.P.; Fravalo, P. Impact of deoxynivalenol on the intestinal microflora of pigs. *Int. J. Mol. Sci.* **2009**, *10*, 1–17. [CrossRef] [PubMed]
3. Smith, M.C.; Madec, S.; Coton, E.; Hymery, N. Natural co-occurrence of mycotoxins in foods and feeds and their in vitro combined toxicological effects. *Toxins* **2016**, *8*, 94. [CrossRef] [PubMed]
4. Ghareeb, K.; Awad, W.A.; Böhm, J.Q.; Zebeli, K.G. Impacts of the feed contaminant deoxynivalenol on the intestine of monogastric animals: Poultry and swine. *J. Appl. Toxicol.* **2015**, *35*, 327–340. [CrossRef] [PubMed]
5. Lewczuk, B.B.; Przybylska-Gornowicz, M.; Gajecka, K.; Targonska, N.; Ziolkowska, M.; Gajecki, M. Histological structure of duodenum in gilts receiving low doses of zearalenone and deoxynivalenol in feed. *Exp. Toxicol. Pathol.* **2016**, *68*, 157–166. [CrossRef] [PubMed]
6. Etienne, M.; Wache, Y. Biological and physiological effects of deoxynivalenol (DON) in the pig. In *Mycotoxins in Farm Animals*, 1st ed.; Oswald, I.P., Taranu, I., Eds.; Research Signpost: Kerala, India, 2008; pp. 113–130.
7. Reddy, K.E.; Song, J.; Lee, H.-J.; Kim, M.; Kim, D.-W.; Jung, H.J.; Kim, B.; Lee, Y.; Yu, D.; Kim, D.-W.; et al. Effects of high levels of deoxynivalenol and zearalenone on growth performance, and hematological and immunological parameters in pigs. *Toxins* **2018**, *10*, 114. [CrossRef] [PubMed]
8. Romero, A.A.; Ramos, I.; Castellano, E.; Martinez, V.; Martinez-Larranaga, M.; Anadon, M.R.; Martinez, M.A. Mycotoxins modify the barrier function of Caco-2 cells through differential gene expression of specific claudin isoforms: Protective effect of illite mineral clay. *Toxicology* **2016**, *353*, 21–33. [CrossRef] [PubMed]
9. Yu, M.L.; Chen, Z.; Peng, A.K.; Nussler, Q.; Wu, L.; Liu, W.Y. Mechanism of deoxynivalenol effects on the reproductive system and fetus malformation: Current status and future challenges. *Toxicol. In Vitro* **2017**, *41*, 150–158. [CrossRef] [PubMed]
10. Pierron, A.; Alassane-Kpembi, I.; Oswald, I.P. Impact of two mycotoxins deoxynivalenol and fumonisin on pig intestinal health. *Porc. Health Manag.* **2016**, *2*, 2–8. [CrossRef] [PubMed]
11. Döll, S.; Dänicke, S. The Fusarium toxins deoxynivalenol (DON) and zearalenone (ZON) in animal feeding. *Prev. Vet. Med.* **2011**, *102*, 132–145. [CrossRef] [PubMed]
12. Zhang, Y.; Gao, R.; Liu, M.; Shi, B.; Shan, A.; Cheng, B. Use of modified halloysite nanotubes in the feed reduces the toxic effects of zearalenone on sow reproduction and piglet development. *Theriogenology* **2015**, *83*, 932–941. [CrossRef] [PubMed]
13. Dänicke, S.; Brüssow, K.P.; Goyarts, T.; Valenta, H.; Ueberschär, K.H.; Tiemann, U. On the transfer of the *Fusarium* toxins deoxynivalenol (DON) and zearalenone (ZON) from the sow to the full-term piglet during the last third of gestation. *Food Chem. Toxicol* **2007**, *45*, 1567–1574.
14. Ghedira-Chekir, L.; Maaroufi, K.; Creppy, E.E.; Bacha, H. Cytotoxic and genotoxic effects of zearalenone: Prevention by vitamin E. *J. Toxicol. Toxin Rev.* **1999**, *18*, 355–368. [CrossRef]
15. Reddy, K.E.; Lee, W.; Jeong, J.Y.; Lee, Y.; Lee, H.-J.; Kim, M.; Kim, D.-W.; Yu, D.; Cho, A.; Oh, Y.K.; et al. Effects of deoxynivalenol- and zearalenone-contaminated feed on the gene expression profiles in the kidneys of piglets. *Asian-Australas J. Anim. Sci.* **2018**, *31*, 138–148. [CrossRef] [PubMed]
16. Richards, J.D.; Gong, J.; de Lange, C.F.M. The gastrointestinal microbiota and its role in monogastric nutrition and health with an emphasis on pigs: Current understanding, possible modulations, and new technologies for ecological studies. *Can. J. Anim. Sci.* **2005**, *85*, 421–435. [CrossRef]
17. Sommer, F.; Backhed, F. The gut microbiota-masters of host development and physiology. *Nat. Rev. Microbiol.* **2013**, *11*, 227–238. [CrossRef] [PubMed]
18. Bauer, E.; Williams, B.A.; Smidt, H.; Mosenthin, R.; Verstegen, M.W.A. Influence of dietary components on development of the microbiota in single-stomached species. *Nutr. Res. Rev.* **2006**, *19*, 63–78. [CrossRef] [PubMed]
19. Maresca, M.; Fantini, J. Some food-associated mycotoxins as potential risk factors in humans predisposed to chronic intestinal inflammatory diseases. *Toxicon* **2010**, *56*, 282–294. [CrossRef] [PubMed]
20. Li, F.; Wang, J.; Huang, L.; Chen, H.; Wang, C. Effects of adding *Clostridium* sp. WJ06 on intestinal morphology and microbial diversity of growing pigs fed with natural deoxynivalenol contaminated wheat. *Toxins* **2017**, *9*, 383. [CrossRef] [PubMed]

21. Stich, N.; Model, N.; Samstag, A.; Gruener, C.S.; Wolf, H.M.; Eibl, M.M. Toxic shock syndrome toxin-1-mediated toxicity inhibited by neutralizing antibodies late in the course of continual in vivo and in vitro exposure. *Toxins* **2014**, *6*, 1724–1741. [CrossRef] [PubMed]

22. Myer, P.R.; Smith, T.P.L.; Wells, J.E.; Kuehn, L.A.; Freetly, H.C. Rumen microbiome from steers differing in feed efficiency. *PLoS ONE* **2015**, *10*, e0129174. [CrossRef] [PubMed]

23. Kim, M.; Kuehn, L.A.; Bono, J.L.; Berry, D.D.; Kalchayanand, N.; Freetly, H.C.; Benson, A.K.; Well, J.E. Investigation of bacterial diversity in the feces of cattle fed different diets. *J. Anim. Sci.* **2014**, *92*, 683–694. [CrossRef] [PubMed]

24. Piotrowska, M.; Śliżewska, K.; Nowak, A.; Zielonka, L.; Zakowska, Z.; Gajęcka, M.; Gajęcki, M. The effect of experimental fusarium mycotoxicosis on microbiota diversity in porcine ascending colon contents. *Toxins* **2014**, *6*, 2064–2081. [CrossRef] [PubMed]

25. Jia, J.; Frantz, N.; Khoo, C.; Gibson, G.R.; Rastall, R.A.; McCartney, A.L. Investigation of the faecal microbiota associated with canine chronic diarrhea. *FEMS Microbiol. Ecol.* **2010**, *71*, 304–312. [CrossRef] [PubMed]

26. Swanson, S.P.; Helaszek, C.; Buck, W.B.; Rood, H.D., Jr.; Haschek, W.M. The role of intestinal microflora in the metabolism of trichothecene mycotoxins. *Food Chem. Toxicol.* **1988**, *26*, 823–829. [CrossRef]

27. McCormick, S.P. Microbial detoxification of mycotoxins. *J. Chem. Ecol.* **2013**, *39*, 907–918. [CrossRef] [PubMed]

28. Kabak, B.; Dobson, A.D.; Var, I. Strategies to prevent mycotoxins contamination of food and animal feed: A review. *Crit. Rev. Food Sci. Nutr.* **2006**, *46*, 593–619. [CrossRef] [PubMed]

29. Kabak, B.; Dobson, A.D.W. Biological strategies to counteract the effects of mycotoxins. *J. Food Protect.* **2009**, *72*, 2006–2016. [CrossRef]

30. Saint-Cyr, M.J.; Perrin-Guyomard, A.; Houée, P.; Rolland, J.G.; Laurentie, M. Evaluation of an oral subchronic exposure of deoxynivalenol on the composition of human gut microbiota in a model of human microbiota associated rats. *PLoS ONE* **2013**, *8*, e80578. [CrossRef] [PubMed]

31. Yang, J.; Zhao, Z.; Guo, W.; Guo, J. Effects of deoxynivalenol on intestinal microbiota of mice analyzed by Illumina-MiSeq high-throughput sequencing technology. *Chin. J. Anim. Nutr.* **2017**, *29*, 158–167.

32. Scaldaferri, F.; Gerardi, V.; Lopetuso, L.R.; Del Zompo, F.; Mangiola, F.; Boškoski, I.; Bruno, G.; Petito, V.; Laterza, L.; Cammarota, G.; et al. Gut microbial flora, prebiotics, and probiotics in IBD: Their current usage and utility. *BioMed Res. Int.* **2013**, *307*, 307–315. [CrossRef] [PubMed]

33. Arqués, J.L.; Rodríguez, E.; Langa, S.; Landete, J.M.; Medina, M. Antimicrobial activity of lactic acid bacteria in dairy products and gut: Effect on pathogens. *BioMed. Res. Int.* **2015**. [CrossRef] [PubMed]

34. Goyal, N.; Rishi, P.; Shukla, G. Lactobacillus rhamnosus GG antagonizes Giardia intestinalis induced oxidative stress and intestinal disaccharidases: An experimental study. *World J. Microbiol. Biotechnol.* **2013**, *29*, 1049–1057. [CrossRef] [PubMed]

35. Konstantinov, S.R.; Awati, A.; Smidt, H.; Williams, B.A.; Akkermans, A.D.L.; de Vos, W.M. Specific response of a novel and abundant *Lactobacillus amylovorus*-like phylotype to dietary prebiotics in the guts of weaning piglets. *Appl. Environ. Microbiol.* **2004**, *70*, 3821–3830. [CrossRef] [PubMed]

36. Hill, J.E.; Hemmingsen, S.M.; Goldade, B.G.; Dumonceaux, T.J.; Klassen, J.; Zijlstra, R.T.; Goh, S.H.; Van Kessel, A.G. Comparison of ileum microflora of pigs fed corn-, wheat, or barley-based diets by chaperonin–60 sequencing and quantitative PCR. *Appl. Environ. Microbiol.* **2005**, *71*, 867–875. [CrossRef] [PubMed]

37. El-Nezami, H.S.; Mykkänen, H.; Kankaanpää, P.E.; Suomalainen, T.; Ahokas, J.T.; Salminen, S. The ability of a mixture of *Lactobacillus* and *Propionibacterium* examining to influence the fecal recovery of aflatoxins in healthy Egyptian volunteers: A pilot clinical study. *Biosci. Microflora* **2000**, *19*, 41–45. [CrossRef]

38. Pieridis, M.; El-Nezami, H.; Peltonen, K.; Salminen, S.; Ahokas, J. Ability of dairy strains of lactic acid bacteria to bind aflatoxin M_1 in a food model. *J. Food Prot.* **2000**, *63*, 645–650. [CrossRef]

39. Sonnenburg, J.L.; Backhed, F. Diet-microbiota interactions as moderators of human metabolism. *Nature* **2016**, *535*, 56–64. [CrossRef] [PubMed]

40. El-Nezami, H.S.; Chrevatidis, A.; Auriola, S.; Salminen, S.; Mykkanen, H. Removal of common *Fusarium* toxins in vitro by strains of *Lactobacillus* and *Propionibacterium*. *Food Addit. Contam.* **2002**, *19*, 680–686. [CrossRef] [PubMed]

41. Yang, W.C.; Hsu, T.C.; Cheng, K.C.; Liu, J.R. Expression of the *Clonostachys rosea* lactonohydrolase gene by *Lactobacillus reuteri* to increase its zearalenone-removing ability. *Microb. Cell Fact.* **2017**, *16*. [CrossRef]

42. El-Nezami, H.; Polychronaki, N.; Salminen, S.; Mykkänen, H. Binding rather than metabolism may explain the interaction of two food-grade *Lactobacillus* strains with zearalenone and its derivative α-zearalenol. *Appl. Environ. Microbiol.* **2002**, *68*, 3545–3549. [CrossRef] [PubMed]

43. Haskard, C.; El-Nezami, H.S.; Kankaanpää, P.; Salminen, S.; Ahokas, J. Surface binding of aflatoxin B1 by lactic acid bacteria. *Appl. Environ. Microbiol.* **2001**, *67*, 3086–3091. [CrossRef] [PubMed]

44. Zhou, T.; He, J.; Gong, J. Microbial transformation of trichothecene mycotoxins. *World Mycotoxin J.* **2008**, *1*, 23–30. [CrossRef]

45. Rajendran, R.; Ohta, Y. Binding of heterocyclic amines by lactic acid bacteria from miso, a fermented Japanese food. *Can. J. Microbiol.* **1998**, *44*, 109–115. [CrossRef] [PubMed]

46. Yoshizawa, T.; Takeda, H.; Ohi, T. Structure of a novel metabolite from deoxynivalenol, a trichothecene mycotoxin, in animals. *Agric. Biol. Chem.* **1983**, *47*, 2133–2135. [CrossRef]

47. Cote, L.M.; Dahlem, A.M.; Yoshizawa, T.; Swanson, S.P.; Buck, W.B. Excretion of deoxynivalenol and its metabolite in milk, urine and feces of lactating cows. *J. Dairy Sci.* **1986**, *69*, 2416–2423. [CrossRef]

48. Shima, J.; Takase, S.; Takahashi, Y.; Iwai, Y.; Fujimoto, H.; Yamazaki, M.; Ochi, K. Novel detoxification of the trichothecene mycotoxin deoxynivalenol by a soil bacterium isolated by enrichment culture. *Appl. Environ. Microbiol.* **1997**, *63*, 3825–3830. [PubMed]

49. Robert, H.; Payros, D.; Pinton, P.; Théodorou, V.; Mercier-Bonin, M.; Oswald, I.P. Impact of mycotoxins on the intestine: Are mucus and microbiota new targets? *J. Toxicol. Environ. Health* **2017**, *20*, 249–275. [CrossRef] [PubMed]

50. Pinton, P.; Graziani, F.; Pujol, A.; Nicoletti, C.; Paris, O.; Ernouf, P.; Di Pasquale, E.; Perrier, J.; Oswald, I.P.; Maresca, M. Deoxynivalenol inhibits the expression by goblet cells of intestinal mucins through a PKR and MAP kinase dependent repression of the resistin-like molecule β. *Mol. Nutr. Food Res.* **2015**, *59*, 1076–1087. [CrossRef] [PubMed]

51. Gratz, S.; Mykkanen, H.; Ouwehand, A.C.; Juvonen, R.; Salminen, S.; El-Nezami, H. Intestinal mucus alters the ability of probiotic bacteria to bind aflatoxin B1 in vitro. *Appl. Environ. Microbiol.* **2004**, *70*, 6306–6308. [CrossRef] [PubMed]

52. Rotter, B.A.; Prelusky, D.B.; Pestks, J.J. Toxicology of deoxynivalenol (vomitoxin). *J. Toxicol. Environ. Health* **1996**, *48*, 1–34. [CrossRef] [PubMed]

53. Lessard, M.C.; Savard, K.; Deschene, K.; Lauzon, V.A.; Pinilla, C.A.; Gagnon, J.; Lapointe, F.; Chorfi, Y. Impact of deoxynivalenol (DON) contaminated feed on intestinal integrity and immune response in swine. *Food Chem. Toxicol.* **2015**, *80*, 7–16. [CrossRef] [PubMed]

54. Klieve, A.V.; Hennessy, D.; Ouwerkerk, D.; Forster, R.J.; Mackie, R.I.; Attwood, G.T. Establishing populations of *Megasphaera elsdenii* YE 34 and *Butyrivibrio fibrisolvens* YE 44 in the rumen of cattle fed high grain diets. *J. Appl. Microbiol.* **2003**, *95*, 621–630. [CrossRef] [PubMed]

55. Shetty, S.A.; Marathe, N.P.; Lanjekar, V.; Ranade, D.; Shouche, Y.S. Comparative genome analysis of *Megasphaera* sp. reveals niche specialization and its potential role in the human gut. *PLoS ONE* **2013**, *8*, e79353. [CrossRef] [PubMed]

56. Barnett, A.M.; Roy, N.C.; McNabb, W.C.; Cookson, A.L. The interactions between endogenous bacteria, dietary components and the mucus layer of the large bowel. *Food Funct.* **2012**, *3*, 690–699. [CrossRef] [PubMed]

57. Osselaere, A.M.; Devreese, J.; Goossens, V.; Vandenbroucke, S.; De Baere, P.; Croubels, S. Toxicokinetic study and absolute oral bioavailability of deoxynivalenol, T-2 toxin and zearalenone in broiler chickens. *Food Chem. Toxicol.* **2013**, *51*, 350–355. [CrossRef] [PubMed]

58. Frey, J.C.; Pell, A.N.; Berthiaume, R.; Lapierre, H.S.; Lee, J.K.; Ha, J.E.; Angert, E.R. Comparative studies of microbial populations in the rumen, duodenum, ileum and faeces of lactating dairy cows. *J. Appl. Microbiol.* **2010**, *108*, 1982–1993. [CrossRef] [PubMed]

59. Prelusky, D.B.; Veira, D.M.; Trenholm, H.L. Plasma pharmacokinetics of the mycotoxin deoxynivalenol following oral and intravenous administration to sheep. *J. Environ. Sci. Health* **1985**, *20*, 603–624. [CrossRef] [PubMed]

60. Eriksen, G.S.; Pettersson, H.; Johnsen, K.; Lindberg, J.E. Transformation of trichothecenes in ileal digesta and faeces from pigs. *Arch. Anim. Nutr.* **2002**, *56*, 263–274. [CrossRef]

61. National Research Council (NRC). *Nutrition Requirements of Swine*, 11th ed.; National Academy Press: Washington, DC, USA, 2012.

62. Yu, Z.; Morrison, M. Improved extraction of PCR-quality community DNA from digesta and fecal samples. *Biotechniques* **2004**, *36*, 808–812. [CrossRef] [PubMed]
63. Magoc, M.; Salzberg, S. FLASH: Fast length adjustment of short reads to improve genome assemblies. *Bioinformatics* **2011**, *27*, 2957–2963. [CrossRef] [PubMed]
64. Caporaso, J.G.; Kuczynski, J.; Stombaugh, J.; Bittinger, K.; Bushman, F.D.; Costello, E.K.; Fierer, N.; Pena, A.G.; Goodrich, J.K.; Gordon, J.I.; et al. QIIME allows analysis of high-throughput community sequencing data. *Nat. Methods* **2010**, *7*, 335–336. [CrossRef] [PubMed]
65. DeSantis, T.Z.; Hugenholtz, P.; Larsen, N.; Rojas, M.; Brodie, E.L.; Keller, K.; Huber, T.; Dalevi, D.; Hu, P.; Andersen, G.L. Greengenes, a chimera-checked 16S rRNA gene database and workbench compatible with ARB. *Appl. Environ. Microbiol.* **2006**, *72*, 5069–5072. [CrossRef] [PubMed]
66. Edgar, R.C. Search and clustering orders of magnitude faster than BLAST. *Bioinformatics* **2010**, *26*, 2460–2461. [CrossRef] [PubMed]

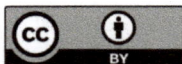

toxins

MDPI

Article

Fumonisin-Exposure Impairs Age-Related Ecological Succession of Bacterial Species in Weaned Pig Gut Microbiota

Ivan Mateos [1,2], Sylvie Combes [1,*], Géraldine Pascal [1], Laurent Cauquil [1], Céline Barilly [1], Anne-Marie Cossalter [3], Joëlle Laffitte [3], Sara Botti [4], Philippe Pinton [3] and Isabelle P. Oswald [3,*]

[1] GenPhySE, Université de Toulouse, INRA, INPT, ENVT, 31326 Castanet-Tolosan, France; ivan.mateos-alvarez@inra.fr (I.M.); geraldine.pascal@inra.fr (G.P.); laurent.cauquil@inra.fr (L.C.); celine.barilly@inra.fr (C.B.)
[2] Lallemand SAS, 19 rue des Briquetiers, BP 59, 31702 Blagnac CEDEX, France
[3] Toxalim (Research Center in Food Toxicology), Université de Toulouse, INRA, INP-Purpan, ENVT, UPS, 31027 Toulouse, France; anne-marie.cossalter@inra.fr (A.-M.C.); joelle.laffitte@inra.fr (J.L.); philippe.pinton@inra.fr (P.P.)
[4] PTP Science Park, via Einstein, loc. Cascina Codazza, 26900 Lodi, Italy; sara.botti@ptp.it
[*] Correspondence: sylvie.combes@inra.fr (S.C.); isabelle.oswald@inra.fr (I.P.O.); Tel.: +33-(0)5-61-28-51-06 (S.C.); +33-(0)5-82-06-63-66 (I.P.O.)

Received: 18 April 2018; Accepted: 31 May 2018; Published: 5 June 2018

Abstract: Pigs are highly affected by dietary mycotoxin contamination and particularly by fumonisin. The effects of fumonisin on pig intestinal health are well documented, but little is known regarding its impact on gut microbiota. We investigate the effects of the fumonisin (FB1, 12 mg/kg feed) on the fecal microbiota of piglets ($n = 6$) after 0, 8, 15, 22, and 29 days of exposure. A control group of six piglets received a diet free of FB1. Bacterial community diversity, structure and taxonomic composition were carried out by V3–V4 16S rRNA gene sequencing. Exposure to FB1 decreases the diversity index, and shifts and constrains the structure and the composition of the bacterial community. This takes place as early as after 15 days of exposure and is at a maximum after 22 days of exposure. Compared to control, FB1 alters the ecological succession of fecal microbiota species toward higher levels of *Lactobacillus* and lower levels of the Lachnospiraceae and Veillonellaceae families, and particularly OTUs (Operational Taxonomic Units) of the genera *Mitsuokella*, *Faecalibacterium* and *Roseburia*. In conclusion, FB1 shifts and constrains age-related evolution of microbiota. The direct or indirect contribution of FB1 microbiota alteration in the global host response to FB1 toxicity remains to be investigated.

Keywords: fumonisin; microbiota; pigs; MiSeq 16S rDNA sequencing

Key contribution: Dietary fumonisin (FB1) exposure in pigs hinders age-related dynamic of fecal microbiota. FB1 shifts and constrains the structure, the diversity and the taxonomic composition of the fecal bacterial community as early as after 15 days of exposure.

1. Introduction

Food safety is a major issue throughout the world. Therefore, much attention needs to be paid to the possible contamination of food and feed by fungi and the potential risk of mycotoxin production. Mycotoxins are fungal secondary metabolites, potentially hazardous to human and animal health following consumption of contaminated food or feed. These metabolites are very resistant to technological treatments and difficult to remove. Therefore, they can be present in human food and animal feed [1]. Feed materials are often contaminated with fungi and their metabolites, which pose a potential threat to human and animal health [2,3]. Contamination of cereals with mycotoxin is a worldwide problem leading to important economic losses for the agricultural industry. Cereals and soybean are the main components of pig diets and due to the high ingestion of cereals and their sensitivity, pigs are highly impacted by the presence of mycotoxins [4]. The toxicological syndromes caused by ingestion of mycotoxins range from sudden death to reproductive disorders and growth impairment. Consumption of fungal toxins may also decrease resistance to infectious diseases. Pigs are considered to be the farm animals that are the most affected by mycotoxins in general and horses and pigs are the animals that are the most sensitive to fumonisins in particular [5]. Mycotoxin contamination levels in pig feedstuffs are usually not high enough to cause a clinical disease but may result in economic loss through changes in growth, production and immunosuppression [4].

From an intestinal health perspective, the most notorious mycotoxins are fumonisins, especially fumonisin B1 (FB1), and trichothecenes, deoxynivalenol and zearalenone [6]. FB1 is the diester of propane-1,2,3-tricarboxylic acid and 2-amino-12,16-dimethyl-3,5,10,14,15-pentahydro xyeicosane. Pierron et al. [5], reported the toxicity of FB1 and the effects of this mycotoxin on pig intestine, because the intestinal tract is the first barrier and, consequently, the first target of mycotoxins ingested with food. The toxicity of FB1 differs according to several parameters such as the dose, the duration of exposure, the age and the sex of the animal, in additional to nutritional factors. Performances and health are most impacted in young animals and males [7]. The main effects of FB1 are a reduction of feed intake and animal growth, an alteration of the absorptive functionality of the intestine, histological damages on intestinal tissue, an impairment of intestinal barrier functions, a systemic decrease and/or local immune response, as well as lung and liver damages [8].

Gut microbiota plays a key role in physiological, developmental, nutritional and immunological processes of the host, and impacts host health and performance [9]. An appropriate composition of the intestinal microbiota of animals, as well as the quantitative and qualitative stability of that ecosystem, is an essential factor to guarantee animal health. Microbiota provides nutritional and protective functions to animals, by stimulating of host immunity, producing fermentation outputs, and preventing colonization by pathogens [10].

The effect of mycotoxins on the intestinal microbiota is gaining interest [11–13]. Nevertheless, the effect of mycotoxins, especially FB1 on the intestinal microbiota is poorly documented [14,15]. The aim of this work was to study the impact of adding FB1 (12 mg/kg) in the diet of piglets on their fecal microbiota during a four-week period of time using high throughput Illumina MiSeq 16S V3–V4 amplicon sequencing. These results complete the data previously published on fumonisin diet contamination host response [8].

2. Results

2.1. Diversity and Structure Dynamics of the Fecal Bacterial Community

The effect of fumonisin (FB1) on the gut microbiota of piglets was first assessed on the fecal bacterial community diversity using the Shannon and the InvSimpson indexes (Table 1 and Figure 1). After 4 weeks of exposure to a control diet or a fumonisin-contaminated diet (12 mg/kg) the Shannon and the InvSimpson diversity indexes tended ($p = 0.057$) or was ($p = 0.003$) lower, respectively, in feces from fumonisin-exposed animals compared to those in the Control group. However, for both indexes, significant interaction between age and treatment reveals a differential evolution with age according to groups. In contrast to the Control group where bacterial community diversity is stable over the 4 weeks, the InvSimpson and Shannon indexes decreases after 15 and 22 days of exposure respectively (Figure 1) in fumonisin-exposed piglets.

Table 1. Effect of FB1 exposure in the diet on piglet fecal microbiota Shannon and InvSimpson diversity indexes.

Diversity Index	Treatment			*p* Value		
	Control	FB1	SEM	Group	Day	Group × Day
Shannon	4.00	3.67	0.062	0.057	0.067	0.010
InvSimpson	21.9	11.0	1.28	0.003	0.052	0.037

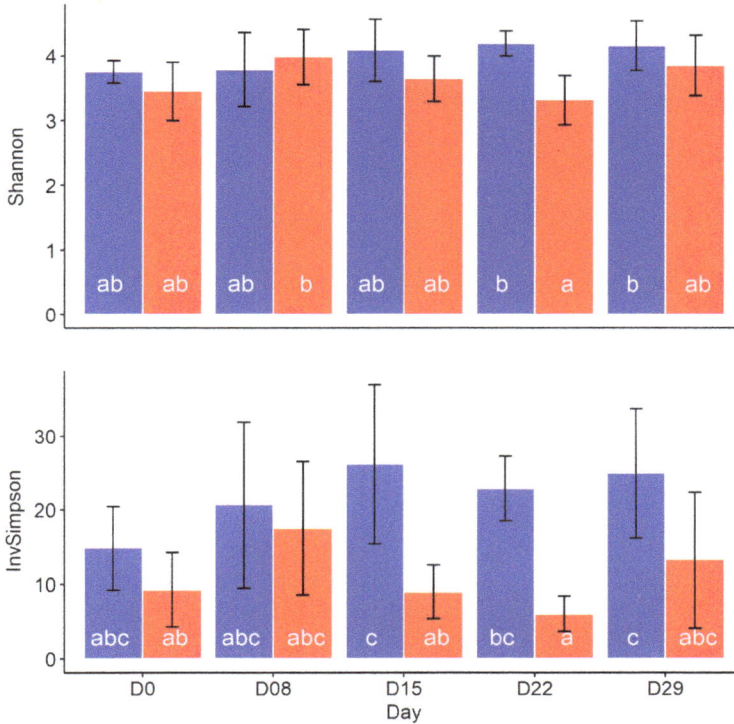

Figure 1. Time effect of dietary FB1 exposure on piglet fecal microbiota Shannon and InvSimpson diversity indexes. In blue, control animals (*n* = 6) and in red, FB1-exposed piglets. (Mean ± SD). LS-means with a common superscript did not differ at *p* = 0.05 level according to linear mixed model analysis of variance.

The principal coordinate analysis (PCoA) based on the Bray–Curtis distance (Figure 2a) segregates samples into two groups corresponding to the treatment. Percentages of variance explained by the principal coordinates 1, 2 and 3 are 32.7%, 12.7% and 8.3% respectively. Pairwise ADONIS tests performed on the Bray-Curtis distance matrix (Table S1) indicate that the bacterial community evolves slightly throughout the days of the experiment in both groups of piglets (R^2-ADONIS < 0.27, $p < 0.05$). When the PCoA axis 1 is plotted against age (Figure 2b) a complete separation of FB1 and Control group can be observed after 22 days of treatment (ADONIS-R^2 = 0.51, $p < 0.01$, Table S1). To compare the stability of the bacterial community, the distance within two consecutive ages for both groups is calculated (Figure 2c). Except for the 0–8 day interval, the distance between two consecutive ages is lower in the FB1 group than in Control one, suggesting that ingestion of fumonisin contaminated diet hinders the normal rate of age-related evolution of microbiota. Moreover, in the FB1 group, the lowest variation between two consecutive ages is observed for the intervals 15–22 and 22–29 days ($p < 0.05$) suggesting a constraint effect of FB1 on microbiota evolution. Finally, we calculated within-group dispersion, which is the variation of the distance between piglets within an age group (Figure 2d). Individual variations within the group remain unchanged with age in the Control group whereas they sharply decrease in the FB1 group. After 15 days of treatment, the FB1 group exhibits lower within-group distance compared to the Control group. The highest similarity between individuals in the FB1 group is observed at 22 days of age. This result demonstrates that fumonisin exposure exerts a constraint on piglet fecal microbiota evolution that strongly decreases inter-individual variability.

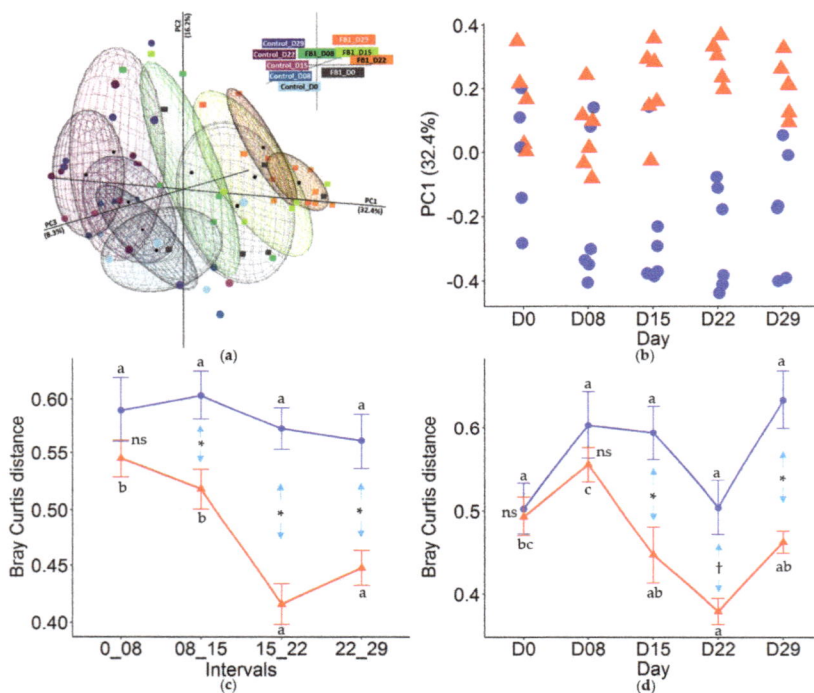

Figure 2. (a) Principal coordinate analysis (PCoA) ordination 3D-plot based on the Bray-Curtis distance matrix. Circles and squares are for samples from FB1–exposed and Control animals, respectively. (b) PCoA axis1 coordinates plotted against days of treatment. (c) Stability between two consecutive age groups calculated from the Bray-Curtis distance for pairwise comparison. (d) Age evolution of the individual dispersion within each group using the Bray-Curtis distance. Red triangles: FB1-exposed animals; blue circles: Control animals. * = ($p < 0.05$), † = ($p < 0.1$) and ns = ($p > 0.1$) between groups. a,b = mean with unlike superscripts in a group are significantly different from each other ($p < 0.05$) ($n = 6$ pigs per group, mean ± SEM).

2.2. Taxonomic Assignation

Concerning the taxonomic composition of the bacterial community, the Firmicutes phylum is the most abundant one in the microbiota of animals from both groups, with 82% of relative abundance (Figure 3 and Table S2). Bacteroidetes is the second most abundant phylum (14%) followed by Proteobacteria (1.8%) Spirochaetes (1.5%) and Actinobacteria (0.7%). Tenericutes and Fibrobacteres are detected at abundances lower than 0.05% below a quantitative statistical analysis threshold. Actinobacteria and Proteobacteria tend to be observed in higher proportion in Control fecal microbiota than in that of FB1 (1.12% vs. 0.25% and 2.29% vs. 1.18%, respectively, *p*-adjusted < 0.10). Spirochaetes tends to be higher in FB1 than in Control (2.03% vs. 1.01%, *p*-adjusted < 0.10).

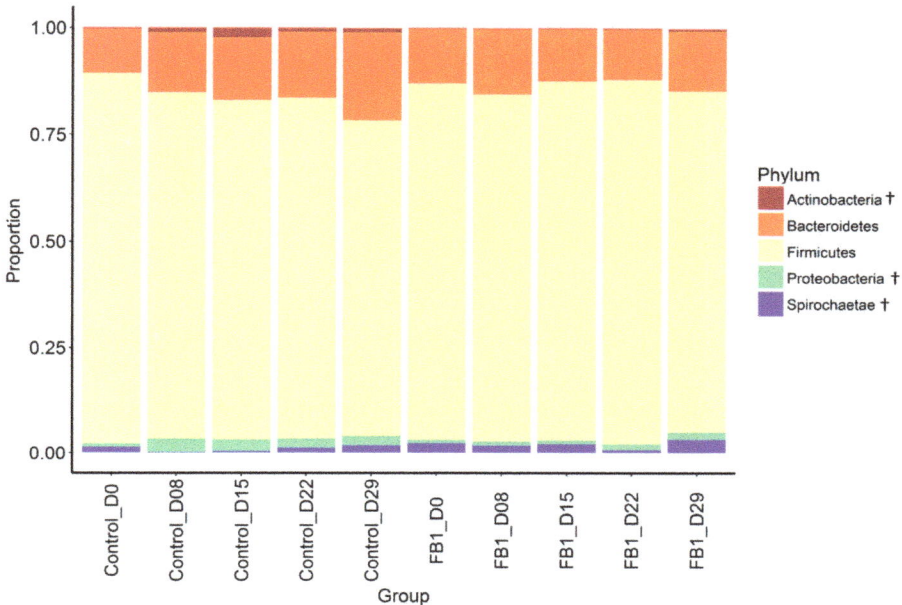

Figure 3. Relative abundance of main phyla in fecal microbiota from Control vs. FB1-exposed pigs. Between treatments: † = *p*-adjusted < 0.10.

The most abundant families in the samples are Lactobacillaceae, Lachnospiraceae, Ruminococcaceae and Prevotellaceae with more than 10%, Clostridiaceae (4.38%), Peptostreptococcaceae (4.37%) and Veillonellaceae (4.21%) (Figure 4 and Table S3). Compared to Control piglets, fumonisin exposure increases the relative abundance of Lactobacillaceae (*p*-adjusted = 0.031), Peptococcaceae (*p*-adjusted = 0.001), the Bacteroidales RF16 group (*p*-adjusted < 0.001) and the Rickettsiales Incertae Sedis (*p*-adjusted < 0.001) families, and decrases Lachnopiraceae (*p*-adjusted = 0.006), Veillonaceae (*p*-adjusted = 0.005) Eubacteriaceae (*p*-adjusted = 0.009), Succinivibrionaceae (*p*-adjusted = 0.006) and Coriobacteriaceae (*p*-adjusted = 0.031) in fecal microbiota. Among the most abundant families, there is an effect of day on the proportion of Lachnospiraceae that decreases with time, respectively, whereas Veillonaceae increases until day 15 and return to initial values afterward in control group (Figure S1, *p*-adjusted < 0.05).

The 10 most abundant genera (Figure 5) are *Lactobacillus* with (30.3%), *Prevotella* (7.5%), *Blautia* (5.3%), *Terrisporobacter* (3.5%), *Mitsuokella* (3.3%), *Faecalibacterium* (3.0%), *Roseburia* (2.7%), the Prevotellaceae NK3B31 group (2.4%), *Sarcina* (2.4%) and Ruminococcaceae UCG-008 (2.3%), respectively. Out of the 20 genera whose proportions are affected by FB1 exposure (*p*-adjusted < 0.05; Table S4), *Lactobacillus* and Ruminococcaceae UCG-005 are increased while *Mitsuokella*, *Succinivibrio*, *Roseburia* and *Ruminococcus* proportions are depressed (*p* < 0.05).

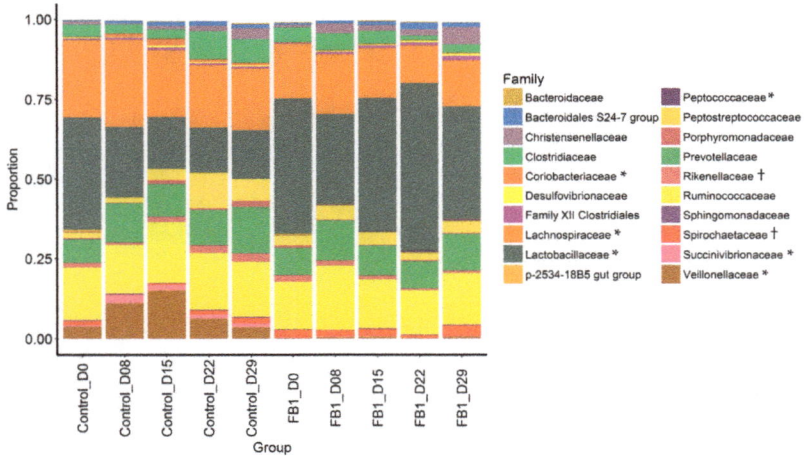

Figure 4. Relative abundance of main families in fecal microbiota from Control vs. FB1-exposed pigs. Between treatments: † = *p* adjusted < 0.10 and * = *p* adjusted < 0.05.

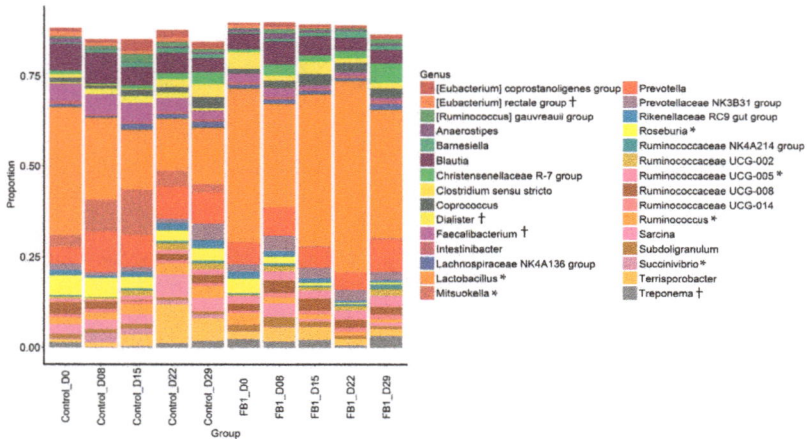

Figure 5. Relative abundance of main genera in fecal microbiota from Control vs. FB1-exposed pigs. Between treatments: † = *p* adjusted < 0.10 and * = *p* adjusted < 0.05.

2.3. OTU Differential Abundance

To further investigate the FB1-related shift effect on the fecal bacterial community structure, we explored the differential abundance at the OTU (Operational Taxonomic Unit) level. Of the 765 OTUs detected, in the three last days of sampling, 220, 249 and 197 OTUs were differentially abundant between feces from Control and fumonisin-exposed animals (*p* < 0.05, Figure 6). A total of 70 differential abundant OTUs are common to the three days of sampling. Among the 30 most abundant OTUs (Figure 7), consecutive to FB1 exposure, the relative abundance of three of them (OTUs 6, 11 and 17 assigned to the genera *Lactobacillus*, *Prevotella* and *Treponema*, respectively) was increased, whereas the relative abundance of six others was decreased (OTUs 5, 9 12, 13, 16 and 19, assigned to the genera *Faecalibacterium*, *Roseburia*, *Prevotella*, *Mitsuokella* and *Dialister*, respectively). On day 22, the OTU 1 assigned to the *Lactobacillus* genus, reached more than 40% of abundance in FB1 samples (Figure 7b). Thus, the FB1-related shift effect on the fecal bacterial community is mainly explained by the significant abundance changes in the major OTUs that make up fecal bacterial community and that leads to the installation of some dominant OTUs which at least include the two main OTUs assigned to the *Lactobacillus* genera.

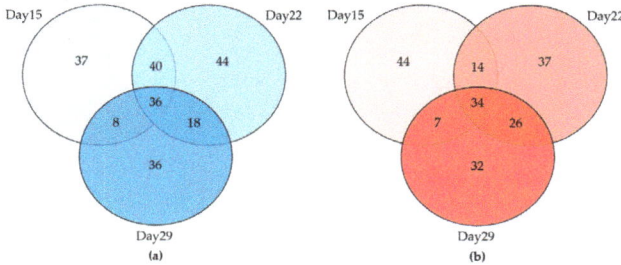

Figure 6. Venn diagram of the number of Operational Taxonomic Units (OTUs) with (**a**) differential lower abundance and (**b**) higher abundance after 15, 22 and 29 days of FB1exposure compared to control.

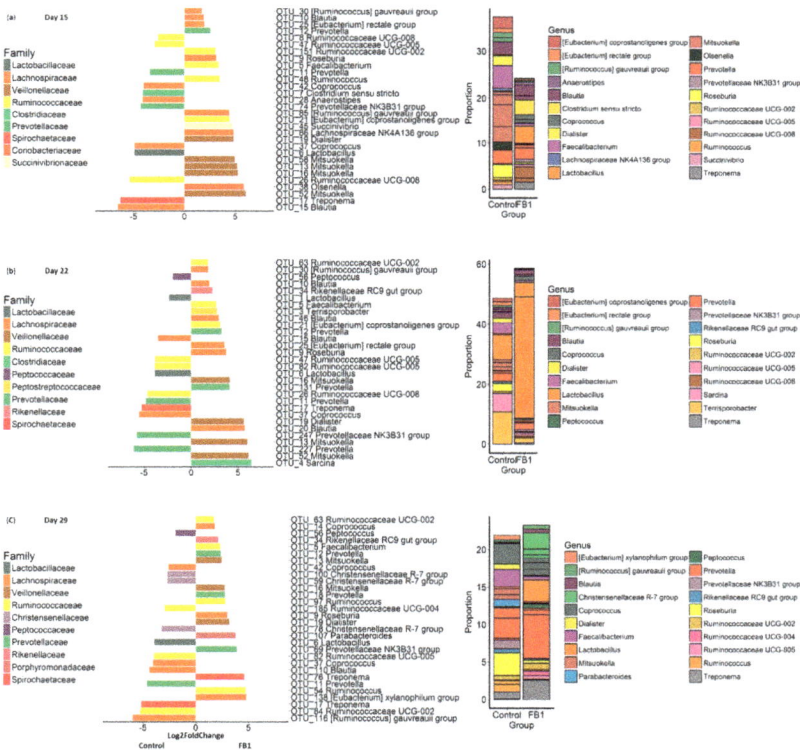

Figure 7. Differential abundance of the 30 most abundant OTUs, (**a**) for day 15, (**b**) for day 22 and (**c**) for day 29. Left panel: log2Fold change abundance, bar color of each OTU are given according to their family assignation, right panel: stacked barplot of the differential abundant OTUs. Each box represent one OTU abundance and color of each OTU are given according to their genus assignation.

In total, the taxonomic composition analysis of the fecal bacterial community reveals that FB1 alters the ecological succession of fecal microbiota species toward higher levels of *Lactobacillus* and lower levels of the Lachnospiraceae and Veillonellaceae families and, particularly OTUs of genera *Roseburia*, *Mitsuokella* and *Faecalibacterium*.

3. Discussion

In spite of the economic and health impact of fumonisin diet contamination on livestock and particularly in pigs, to our knowledge, this study is the first to investigate the dynamic effect of FB1 exposure in feed on fecal microbiota in young weaned pigs. In a companion paper, the detrimental effect of FB1 on the same animals was demonstrated, decreasing the growth rate, increasing the ratio Sa/So (which is a marker of the exposure to this mycotoxin in the liver) and decreasing villi length [8]. In the present study, we clearly demonstrate that FB1 exposure in feed impairs age-related evolution of gut microbiota.

In agreement with the literature [16–20], Firmicutes and Bacteroidetes phyla represent more than 90% of the bacterial community OTUs. The bacterial community is dominated by the Lactobacillaceae, Lachnospiraceae, Ruminococcaceae and Prevotellaceae families and *Lactobacillus*, *Prevotella* and *Blautia* genera. Over the time of the experiment (from 35 to 57 days of age), Lachnospiraceae decreased corresponding mainly to a decrease in *Blautia* and *Roseburia* genera. Over the 4 weeks of the experiment, the diversity indexes were stable in the Control group and the structure of the community evolved slightly with high inter-individual variations. Indeed, major changes in diversity occur at birth when the colonization process takes place in neonates in contact with a microbial metacommunity provided by the mother during and after the passage through the birth canal and the surrounding environment [21]. The gut microbiota then undergoes a progressive species age-related succession [17,19,22] driven by both extrinsic factors and intrinsic factors [23]. The extrinsic factors concern surrounding conditions such as housing [24,25], congener proximity [26] and nutritional factors that act throughout the development of the animal. The most impacting one is related to the feed transition from milk to solid feed [19]. The intrinsic factors are those related to the host physiological state, the qualitative and quantitative availability of endogenous nutrients, the motility of the intestinal tract, bile salts and other endogenous secretions, immune tolerance and host-microbiota interactions through PRR and PAMPs (Pattern-Recognition Receptors and Pathogen Associated Molecular Pattern) [27]. All these extrinsic and intrinsic factors shape each individual gut microbial pattern, explaining the inter and intra-individual variability of gut microbiota.

Studies on mycotoxin actions on gut microbiota are rare [11,13] and they mainly concern the effect of deoxynivalenol [12,28–30] and aflatoxins [31,32]. After two weeks of dietary exposure to FB1, the diversity of the fecal bacterial community decreases. Concomitantly, a shift in the structure together with a decrease in the rate of the evolution of the bacterial community is observed. In agreement, exposure to FB1 for 29 days in 11 week-old specific pathogen-free pigs modifies the CE-SCCP (Capillary Electrophoresis Single Strand Conformation Polymorphism) bacterial community profiles [14]. Additionally, exposure to FB1 constrains the bacterial community evolution, driving it in a new extremely homogenous equilibrium with low inter-individual variations. Altogether, these results indicate the establishment of some dominant species in the fecal bacterial community that adapt to FB1-related conditions. Considering taxonomic composition of major genera, exposure to FB1 leads to a sharp increase in *Lactobacillus* and Ruminococcaceae UCG-005 and a decrease in *Mitsuokella*, *Roseburia*, *Ruminococcus* and *Succinivibrio*. Several hypothesis might explain solely or in combination these microbiota modifications following FB1 exposure: a direct effect of FB1 on gut microbiota, and/or a direct or an indirect host mediated effect.

One hypothesis to explain the constraint effect of FB1 on piglet fecal microbiota would be an intrinsic antimicrobial effect of mycotoxin. The addition of FB1 to *in vitro* incubation of cecal chime decreased the anaerobic bacteria, whereas *Lactobacillus* and total bacteria increased [15]. In contrast, 20 years ago, Becker et al. [33] used culture techniques and observed no inhibition of bacterial growth including *Lactobacillus acidophilus*, *Lactobacillus johnsoni*, *Lactobacillus plantarum* and *Lactobacillus reuteri*. Finally, two independent studies [34,35] found no antibiotic effect of FB1, thus excluding an antimicrobial effect to explain a fumonisin-related shaping action on gut microbiota.

Considering bacterial community structure evolution and inter individual dispersion criteria and the number of OTUs found to be differentially abundant, the greatest effect of fumonisin on fecal microbiota seems to occur after 22 days of exposure in the diet, whereas at 29 days of exposure, this effect seems to be alleviated, although taxa relative abundance has not yet recovered to levels similar to those observed in the Control group. It may be speculated that the bacterial community might evolve toward a new equilibrium adapted to the exposure to fumonisin. In this latter perspective, microorganisms might metabolize this mycotoxin. Although, 20 years ago, under culture conditions, there was no indication that fumonisin was metabolized by intestinal bacteria [33], it is now admitted that some bacteria isolated from soil and plants are known to degrade and thereby detoxify fumonisins [36]. It was recently reported in pigs that an oral single dose exposure of fumonisin leads to a 47% fumonisin degradation into their partially hydrolyzed forms in the gastro-intestinal tract, thus indicating the ability of the microbiota to hydrolyze fumonisin [37]. The capacity to degrade or remove FB1 *in vitro* was emphasized for *Lactobacillus brevis*, *L. plantarum L. pentosus* and some yeasts [38,39]. The mechanism of action of *Lactobacillus* to remove FB1 was related to a process of physical adsorption involving various components of cell wall [39]. Peptidoglycans was the main binding sites, and its structural integrity was necessary. Therefore, the high proportion of *Lactobacillus* in our work might result from a competitive advantage linked to their ability to metabolize FB1.

In addition to a direct effect on gut microbiota, FB1 might shape microbial composition through its well-known actions on the host. In pigs, exposure to mycotoxins reduces feed intake [1]. Reducing feed intake has been shown to affect both functioning and composition of microbiota [40]. Indeed, reduction of nutrient supply decreases short-chained fatty acid concentration which in turn affect the microbiota composition. In pigs, a favorable effect of feed restriction was observed on *Lactobacillus* abundance [24]. Although, after oral exposure, FB1 is poorly absorbed in the intestine and feces is the main excretory route [37], it induces abdominal pain and diarrhea [1]. In piglets in the present study, it reduced villi length [8]. Impairment of the intestinal barrier function [41] has also been reported. In the jejunum and the ileum of piglets fed deoxynivalenol alone or with fumonisin, the number of goblet cells that synthesize and secrete mucins decreased significantly [42]. Mucins can be an important factor in the shaping of the bacterial community since mucins provide attachment sites and are an endogenous carbon and energy source for intestinal bacteria [43]. Altogether, the reduced feed intake of host and alteration of its intestinal barrier function following exposure to FB1 might modify host control of its symbiotic microbial community.

4. Conclusions

The present study investigated the effects of a 4-week dietary exposure to fumonisin on piglet fecal microbiota. We demonstrate that dietary exposure to fumonisin in pigs hinders age-related dynamics of fecal microbiota. Fumonisin decreases the diversity, and shifts and constrains the structure and taxonomic composition of the fecal bacterial community as early as after 15 days of exposure and is at a maximum at 22 days. Dietary exposure to fumonisin promotes the installation of an ecological dominance since it decreases diversity and increases the abundance of *Lactobacillus* at the expense of the abundance of Lachnospiraceae groups, *Roseburia* and *Mitsuokella* genera. The action mechanisms of fumonisin that drive microbiota to this new equilibrium are not known and need further investigations.

5. Materials and Methods

5.1. Animals, Housing and Experimental Design

This work was done at the same time and with the same animals as the experiment made by Régnier et al. [8]. The study was carried out with twelve 7-week-old weaned castrated male pigs.

Animals were obtained from a local farm (Gaec de Calvignac, St. Vincent d'Autejac, France). They were individually identified and divided into two groups and were acclimatized for one week in the animal facility of the INRA ToxAlim Unit (Toulouse, France) prior to being used in experimental protocols. The two groups of six animals, were housed in a separate block of the housing unit with free access to feed and water. Pigs were randomly distributed within pens in order to avoid the effect of the lineage (11.8 ± 1.0 kg and 13.9 ± 1.0 kg, $p < 0.05$, for FB1 and control pigs respectively). Pigs were examined daily for body temperature and feces aspect. No morbidity or mortality was recorded during the study. Room temperature and air velocity were automatically controlled, and pens were cleaned daily. The experiments were carried out in accordance with European Guidelines for the Care and Use of Animals for Research Purposes (accreditation number APAFIS#5917-2016070116429578 v3).

5.2. Experimental Diet, Growth Rate and Sample Collection

Diets were formulated as already described [44]. The detailed composition is provided in Table S5. A control diet, and a diet supplemented with fumonisin enriched extract were prepared [8]. Fumonisin extract was obtained from Dr Bailly at the Veterinary School of Toulouse. In brief, *F. verticillioides* strain NRRL 34281 was cultured on maize grains for 4 weeks at 25 °C. After incubation culture material was dried and grounded into powder and fumonisin extract content was determined by HPLC/MS-MS. Required quantity of powder was then included in the premix before its inclusion in the final diet. After an acclimation week, pigs were fed with the control or the experimentally contaminated diet (10.2 mg FB1 + 2.5 mg FB2 + 1.5 mg FB3/kg), which constituted day 0 of the trial. Because deoxynivalenol and zearalenone were naturally present in the cereals used, this results in concentrations of 0.12 and 0.015 mg/kg feed, respectively. All other mycotoxins, including aflatoxins, T-2 toxin, HT-2 toxin, and ochratoxin A, were below the limits of detection. Mycotoxins were analyzed in the final diet in the Laboca laboratory (Ploufragan, France) with a LC-MS/MS method described [44].

5.3. DNA Extraction and PCR

Total genomic DNA was extracted from 0.5 g of fecal sample, combining a mechanical lysis with a TissueLyser II instrument (Qiagen, Hilden, Germany) and the Quick-DNA™ Fecal/Soil Microbe 96 Kit Zymo Research, Irvine, CA, USA), according to the manufacturer's instructions [45]. The quality and quantity of DNA extracts were checked using a NanoDrop ND-1000 spectrophotometer (NanoDrop Technologies, Wilmington, DE, USA).

The V3–V4 regions of 16S rRNA genes of samples were amplified from purified genomic DNA with the primers F343 (5′-CTTTCCCTACACGACGCTCTTCCGATCTTACGGRAGGCAGCAG-3′; [46]) and reverse R784 (5′-GGAGTTCAGACGTGTGCTCTTCCGATCTTACCAGGGTATCTAATC CT-3′; [47]). The PCR was carried out with an annealing temperature of 65 °C for 30 amplification cycles. Since MiSeq sequencing machine enables paired 250-bp reads, the ends of each read are overlapped and can be stitched together to generate high-quality, reads of the entire V3 and V4 region in a single run 412 ± 11 nucleotides. At the Genomic and Transcriptomic Platform (INRA, Toulouse, France) single multiplexing was performed using 6 bp index sequences, which were added to R784 during a second PCR with 12 cycles. The resulting PCR products were purified and loaded onto the Illumina MiSeq cartridge (Illumina, San Diego, CA, USA) according to the manufacturer's instructions. Each pair-end sequence was assigned to its sample with the help of the previously integrated index. Sequencing reads were deposited in the National Center for Biotechnology Information Sequence Read Archive (NCBI SRA; SRP139897).

5.4. Sequence Analysis

A total of 1,810,933 16S ribosomal DNA amplicon sequences were sorted based on their respective barcodes, representing the 59 fecal samples. Using FROGS [48], in keeping with the SOP, sequences were filtered by removing sequences that did not match both proximal PCR primer sequences (no mismatch allowed), erroneous sequencing length (<400 or >500 nucleotides), with at least one ambiguous base. Chimeric DNA sequences were detected using VSEARCH and removed. Reads were clustered into OTUs using SWARM [49]. OTU taxonomic assignment was performed using the BLAST algorithm against the SILVA SSU Ref NR 128 database [50]. A phyloseq R package [51] object was generated to perform further statistical analysis.

5.5. Statistical Analyses

All statistical analyses were carried out using R software, version 3.4.2 [52] in RStudio software, version 1.1.383 [53]. Shannon and InvSimpson diversity indexes were calculated and the structure of the bacterial community was investigated after calculation of a Bray-Curtis distance matrix that was plot using a Principal Coordinate Analysis, after matrix rarefaction normalization. Using a pairwise Bray Curtis distance calculation, bacterial community stability and inter-individual variability within a group were evaluated between two consecutive day group using the principle of moving window analysis and within each day group respectively [54]. To check group differences an ADONIS pairwise test with the Bray-Curtis distance was carried out. The differential abundance analysis for sequence count data between groups was performed using the DESeq package [55]. Venn diagrams were obtained with the jvenn plug-in [56]. The linear model used had treatment, time and the interaction treatment x time as fixed effects and animal as the random effect.

Supplementary Materials: The following are available online at http://www.mdpi.com/2072-6651/10/6/230/s1, Table S1. Pairwise ADONIS tests between treatments for each day of sampling. Table S2. Phylum relative abundance (%) in fecal microbiota from Control and FB1-exposed piglets. Table S3. Percentage (%) of main bacterial families in fecal microbiota from Control vs. FB1-exposed pigs. Table S4. Percentage (%) of main genera in fecal microbiota from Control vs. FB1-exposed pigs. Table S5. Diet composition in percentage (%). Figure S1 Relative abundance of main bacterial families in fecal microbiota from Control (blue) vs. FB1-exposed pigs (red). Figure S2. Relative abundance of main bacterial genera in fecal microbiota from Control (blue) vs. FB1-exposed pigs (red).

Author Contributions: I.P.O. and P.P. conceived and designed the experiments; A.-M.C., J.L., C.B., S.B. and S.C. performed the experiments; I.M., S.C., L.C. and G.P. processed and analyzed the data; I.M., S.C. and I.P.O. wrote the paper.

Funding: This study was supported by projects from the Agence Nationale de la Recherche ANR Fumolip (ANR-16-CE21-0003), ANR LipoReg (ANR-15-Carn0016), ANR ExpoMycoPig (ANR-17-Carn012) and by project from region Occitanie CLE2014 (funded by the Occitanie Region and Lallemand).

Acknowledgments: We thank GeT-PlaGe Genotoul platform for performing the MiSeq sequencing. We are grateful to the genotoul bioinformatics platform Toulouse Midi-Pyrenees and Sigenae group for providing computing and storage ressources thanks to Galaxy instance http://sigenae-workbench.toulouse.inra.fr.

Conflicts of Interest: The authors declare no conflict of interest.

References

1. Karlovsky, P.; Suman, M.; Berthiller, F.; De Meester, J.; Eisenbrand, G.; Perrin, I.; Oswald, I.P.; Speijers, G.; Chiodini, A.; Recker, T.; et al. Impact of food processing and detoxification treatments on mycotoxin contamination. *Mycotoxin Res.* **2016**, *32*, 179–205. [CrossRef] [PubMed]
2. Okorski, A.; Polak-Sliwinska, M.; Karpiesiuk, K.; Pszczolkowska, A.; Kozera, W. Real time pcr: A good tool to estimate mycotoxin contamination in pig diets. *World Mycotoxin J.* **2017**, *10*, 219–228. [CrossRef]
3. Wu, F.; Groopman, J.D.; Pestka, J.J. Public health impacts of foodborne mycotoxins. *Annu. Rev. Food Sci. Technol.* **2014**, *5*, 351–372. [CrossRef] [PubMed]
4. Pierron, A.; Alassane-Kpembi, I.; Oswald, I.P. Impact of two mycotoxins deoxynivalenol and fumonisin on pig intestinal health. *Porc. Health Manag.* **2016**, *2*, 21. [CrossRef] [PubMed]
5. Pierron, A.; Alassane-Kpembi, I.; Oswald, I.P. Impact of mycotoxin on immune response and consequences for pig health. *Anim. Nutr.* **2016**, *2*, 63–68. [CrossRef] [PubMed]
6. Vardon, P.; McLaughlin, C.; Nardinelli, C. Potential economic costs of mycotoxins in the United States. In *Council for Agricultural Science and Technology (CAST): Mycotoxins: Risks in Plant, Animal, and Human Systems*; Task Force Report No. 139; Council for Agricultural Science and Technology: Ames, IA, USA, 2003; Volume 139, pp. 136–142.

7. Marin, D.E.; Taranu, I.; Pascale, F.; Lionide, A.; Burlacu, R.; Bailly, J.D.; Oswald, I.P. Sex-related differences in the immune response of weanling piglets exposed to low doses of fumonisin extract. *Br. J. Nutr.* **2006**, *95*, 1185–1192. [CrossRef] [PubMed]

8. Régnier, M.; Gourbeyre, P.; Pinton, P.; Napper, S.; Laffite, J.; Cossalter, A.M.; Bailly, J.D.; Lippi, Y.; Bertrand-Michel, J.; Bracarense, A.P.F.R.L.; et al. Identification of signaling pathways targeted by the food contaminant fb1: Transcriptome and kinome analysis of samples from pig liver and intestine. *Mol. Nutr. Food Res.* **2017**, *61*, 1700433. [CrossRef] [PubMed]

9. Sommer, F.; Backhed, F. The gut microbiota—Masters of host development and physiology. *Nat. Rev. Microbiol.* **2013**, *11*, 227–238. [CrossRef] [PubMed]

10. Piotrowska, M.; Slizewska, K.; Nowak, A.; Zielonka, L.; Zakowska, Z.; Gajecka, M.; Gajecki, M. The effect of experimental fusarium mycotoxicosis on microbiota diversity in porcine ascending colon contents. *Toxins* **2014**, *6*, 2064–2081. [CrossRef] [PubMed]

11. Liew, W.-P.; Mohd-Redzwan, S. Mycotoxin: Its impact on gut health and microbiota. *Front. Cell. Infect. Microbiol.* **2018**, *8*, 60. [CrossRef] [PubMed]

12. Payros, D.; Dobrindt, U.; Martin, P.; Secher, T.; Bracarense, A.P.F.L.; Boury, M.; Laffitte, J.; Pinton, P.; Oswald, E.; Oswald, I.P. The food contaminant deoxynivalenol exacerbates the genotoxicity of gut microbiota. *mBio* **2017**, *8*, e00007–e00017. [CrossRef] [PubMed]

13. Robert, H.; Payros, D.; Pinton, P.; Theodorou, V.; Mercier-Bonin, M.; Oswald, I.P. Impact of mycotoxins on the intestine: Are mucus and microbiota new targets? *J. Toxicol. Environ. Health. Part B Crit. Rev.* **2017**, *20*, 249–275. [CrossRef] [PubMed]

14. Burel, C.; Tanguy, M.; Guerre, P.; Boilletot, E.; Cariolet, R.; Queguiner, M.; Postollec, G.; Pinton, P.; Salvat, G.; Oswald, I.P.; et al. Effect of low dose of fumonisins on pig health: Immune status, intestinal microbiota and sensitivity to salmonella. *Toxins* **2013**, *5*, 841–864. [CrossRef]

15. Dang, H.A.; Zsolnai, A.; Kovacs, M.; Bors, I.; Bonai, A.; Bota, B.; Szabo Fodor, J. In vitro interaction between fumonisin b1 and the intestinal microflora of pigs. *Pol. J. Microbiol.* **2017**, *66*, 245–250. [CrossRef] [PubMed]

16. Isaacson, R.; Kim, H.B. The intestinal microbiome of the pig. *Anim. Health Res. Rev.* **2012**, *13*, 100–109. [CrossRef] [PubMed]

17. Kim, H.B.; Borewicz, K.; White, B.A.; Singer, R.S.; Sreevatsan, S.; Tu, Z.J.; Isaacson, R.E. Longitudinal investigation of the age-related bacterial diversity in the feces of commercial pigs. *Vet. Microbiol.* **2011**, *153*, 124–133. [CrossRef] [PubMed]

18. Looft, T.; Allen, H.K.; Cantarel, B.L.; Levine, U.Y.; Bayles, D.O.; Alt, D.P.; Henrissat, B.; Stanton, T.B. Bacteria, phages and pigs: The effects of in-feed antibiotics on the microbiome at different gut locations. *ISME J.* **2014**, *8*, 1566. [CrossRef] [PubMed]

19. Mach, N.; Berri, M.; Estellé, J.; Levenez, F.; Lemonnier, G.; Denis, C.; Leplat, J.-J.; Chevaleyre, C.; Billon, Y.; Doré, J.; et al. Early-life establishment of the swine gut microbiome and impact on host phenotypes. *Environ. Microbiol. Rep.* **2015**, *7*, 554–569. [CrossRef] [PubMed]

20. Yang, H.; Huang, X.; Fang, S.; He, M.; Zhao, Y.; Wu, Z.; Yang, M.; Zhang, Z.; Chen, C.; Huang, L. Unraveling the fecal microbiota and metagenomic functional capacity associated with feed efficiency in pigs. *Front. Microbiol.* **2017**, *8*, 1555. [CrossRef] [PubMed]

21. Katouli, M.; Lund, A.; Wallgren, P.; Kühn, I.; Söderlind, O.; Möllby, R. Metabolic fingerprinting and fermentative capacity of the intestinal flora of pigs during pre- and post-weaning periods. *J. Appl. Microbiol.* **1997**, *83*, 147–154. [CrossRef] [PubMed]

22. Mann, E.; Schmitz-Esser, S.; Zebeli, Q.; Wagner, M.; Ritzmann, M.; Metzler-Zebeli, B.U. Mucosa-associated bacterial microbiome of the gastrointestinal tract of weaned pigs and dynamics linked to dietary calcium-phosphorus. *PLoS ONE* **2014**, *9*, e86950. [CrossRef] [PubMed]

23. Mackie, R.I.; Sghir, A.; Gaskins, H.R. Developmental microbial ecology of the neonatal gastrointestinal tract. *Am. J. Clin. Nutr.* **1999**, *69*, 1035S–1045S. [CrossRef] [PubMed]

24. Le Floc'h, N.; Knudsen, C.; Gidenne, T.; Montagne, L.; Merlot, E.; Zemb, O. Impact of feed restriction on health, digestion and faecal microbiota of growing pigs housed in good or poor hygiene conditions. *Animal* **2014**, *8*, 1632–1642. [CrossRef] [PubMed]

25. Mulder, I.E.; Schmidt, B.; Stokes, C.R.; Lewis, M.; Bailey, M.; Aminov, R.I.; Prosser, J.I.; Gill, B.P.; Pluske, J.R.; Mayer, C.-D.; et al. Environmentally-acquired bacteria influence microbial diversity and natural innate immune responses at gut surfaces. *BMC Biol.* **2009**, *7*, 79. [CrossRef] [PubMed]

26. Thompson, C.L.; Holmes, A.J. A window of environmental dependence is evident in multiple phylogenetically distinct subgroups in the faecal community of piglets. *FEMS Microbiol. Lett.* **2009**, *290*, 91–97. [CrossRef] [PubMed]

27. Peterson, L.W.; Artis, D. Intestinal epithelial cells: Regulators of barrier function and immune homeostasis. *Nat. Rev. Immunol.* **2014**, *14*, 141. [CrossRef] [PubMed]

28. Gratz, S.W.; Currie, V.; Richardson, A.J.; Duncan, G.; Holtrop, G.; Farquharson, F.; Louis, P.; Pinton, P.; Oswald, I.P. Porcine small and large intestinal microbiota rapidly hydrolyze the masked mycotoxin deoxynivalenol-3-glucoside and release deoxynivalenol in spiked batch cultures in vitro. *Appl. Environ. Microbiol.* **2018**, *84*, e02106–e02117. [CrossRef] [PubMed]

29. Saint-Cyr, M.J.; Perrin-Guyomard, A.; Houée, P.; Rolland, J.-G.; Laurentie, M. Evaluation of an oral subchronic exposure of deoxynivalenol on the composition of human gut microbiota in a model of human microbiota-associated rats. *PLoS ONE* **2013**, *8*, e80578. [CrossRef] [PubMed]

30. Wache, Y.J.; Valat, C.; Postollec, G.; Bougeard, S.; Burel, C.; Oswald, I.P.; Fravalo, P. Impact of deoxynivalenol on the intestinal microflora of pigs. *Int. J. Mol. Sci.* **2009**, *10*, 1–17. [CrossRef] [PubMed]

31. Ishikawa, A.T.; Weese, J.S.; Bracarense, A.P.F.R.L.; Alfieri, A.A.; Oliveira, G.G.; Kawamura, O.; Hirooka, E.Y.; Itano, E.N.; Costa, M.C. Single aflatoxin b1 exposure induces changes in gut microbiota community in c57bl/6 mice. *World Mycotoxin J.* **2017**, *10*, 249–254. [CrossRef]

32. Wang, J.; Tang, L.; Glenn, T.C.; Wang, J.S. Aflatoxin b1 induced compositional changes in gut microbial communities of male f344 rats. *Toxicol. Sci.* **2016**, *150*, 54–63. [CrossRef] [PubMed]

33. Becker, B.; Bresch, H.; Schillinger, U.; Thiel, P.G. The effect of fumonisin b1 on the growth of bacteria. *World J. Microbiol. Biotechnol.* **1997**, *13*, 539–543. [CrossRef]

34. Ali-Vehmas, T.; Rizzo, A.; Westermarck, T.; Atroshi, F. Measurement of antibacterial activities of t-2 toxin, deoxynivalenol, ochratoxin a, aflatoxin b-1 and fumonisin b-1 using microtitration tray-based turbidimetric techniques. *J. Vet. Med. Ser. A Physiol. Pathol. Clin. Med.* **1998**, *45*, 453–458. [CrossRef]

35. Sondergaard, T.E.; Fredborg, M.; Oppenhagen Christensen, A.-M.; Damsgaard, S.K.; Kramer, N.F.; Giese, H.; Sørensen, J.L. Fast screening of antibacterial compounds from fusaria. *Toxins* **2016**, *8*, 355. [CrossRef] [PubMed]

36. Vanhoutte, I.; Audenaert, K.; De Gelder, L. Biodegradation of mycotoxins: Tales from known and unexplored worlds. *Front. Microbiol.* **2016**, *7*, 561. [CrossRef] [PubMed]

37. Schertz, H.; Kluess, J.; Frahm, J.; Schatzmayr, D.; Dohnal, I.; Bichl, G.; Schwartz-Zimmermann, H.; Breves, G.; Dänicke, S. Oral and intravenous fumonisin exposure in pigs—A single-dose treatment experiment evaluating toxicokinetics and detoxification. *Toxins* **2018**, *10*, 150. [CrossRef] [PubMed]

38. Tuppia, C.M.; Atanasova-Penichon, V.; Chéreau, S.; Ferrer, N.; Marchegay, G.; Savoie, J.M.; Richard-Forget, F. Yeast and bacteria from ensiled high moisture maize grains as potential mitigation agents of fumonisin b1. *J. Sci. Food Agric.* **2017**, *97*, 2443–2452. [CrossRef] [PubMed]

39. Zhao, H.; Wang, X.; Zhang, J.; Zhang, J.; Zhang, B. The mechanism of lactobacillus strains for their ability to remove fumonisins b1 and b2. *Food Chem. Toxicol.* **2016**, *97*, 40–46. [CrossRef] [PubMed]

40. Morishita, Y. Effect of food restriction on caecal microbiota and short-chain fatty acid concentrations in rats. *Microb. Ecol. Health Dis.* **1995**, *8*, 35–39. [CrossRef]

41. Loiseau, N.; Polizzi, A.; Dupuy, A.; Therville, N.; Rakotonirainy, M.; Loy, J.; Viadere, J.L.; Cossalter, A.M.; Bailly, J.D.; Puel, O.; et al. New insights into the organ-specific adverse effects of fumonisin b1: Comparison between lung and liver. *Arch. Toxicol.* **2015**, *89*, 1619–1629. [CrossRef] [PubMed]

42. Bracarense, A.P.; Lucioli, J.; Grenier, B.; Drociunas Pacheco, G.; Moll, W.D.; Schatzmayr, G.; Oswald, I.P. Chronic ingestion of deoxynivalenol and fumonisin, alone or in interaction, induces morphological and immunological changes in the intestine of piglets. *Br. J. Nutr.* **2012**, *107*, 1776–1786. [CrossRef] [PubMed]

43. Derrien, M.; van Passel, M.W.; van de Bovenkamp, J.H.; Schipper, R.G.; de Vos, W.M.; Dekker, J. Mucin-bacterial interactions in the human oral cavity and digestive tract. *Gut Microbes* **2010**, *1*, 254–268. [CrossRef] [PubMed]

44. Souto, P.; Jager, A.; Tonin, F.G.; Petta, T.; Di Gregório, M.; Cossalter, A.; Pinton, P.; Oswald, I.; Rottinghaus, G.; Oliveira, C. Determination of fumonisin b1 levels in body fluids and hair from piglets fed fumonisin b1-contaminated diets. *Food Chem. Toxicol.* **2017**, *108*, 1–9. [CrossRef] [PubMed]

45. Verschuren, L.M.G.; Calus, M.P.L.; Jansman, A.J.M.; Bergsma, R.; Knol, E.F.; Gilbert, H.; Zemb, O. Fecal microbial composition associated with variation in feed efficiency in pigs depends on diet and sex1. *J. Anim. Sci.* **2018**, *96*, 1405–1418. [CrossRef] [PubMed]

46. Liu, Z.; Lozupone, C.; Hamady, M.; Bushman, F.D.; Knight, R. Short pyrosequencing reads suffice for accurate microbial community analysis. *Nucleic Acids Res.* **2007**, *35*, e120. [CrossRef] [PubMed]

47. Andersson, A.F.; Lindberg, M.; Jakobsson, H.; Bäckhed, F.; Nyrén, P.; Engstrand, L. Comparative analysis of human gut microbiota by barcoded pyrosequencing. *PLoS ONE* **2008**, *3*, e2836. [CrossRef] [PubMed]

48. Escudié, F.; Auer, L.; Bernard, M.; Mariadassou, M.; Cauquil, L.; Vidal, K.; Maman, S.; Hernandez-Raquet, G.; Combes, S.; Pascal, G. FROGS: Find, rapidly, OTUs with galaxy solution. *Bioinformatics* **2018**, *34*, 1287–1294. [CrossRef]

49. Mahé, F.; Rognes, T.; Quince, C.; de Vargas, C.; Dunthorn, M. Swarm: Robust and fast clustering method for amplicon-based studies. *PeerJ* **2014**, *2*, e386v381. [CrossRef] [PubMed]

50. Quast, C.; Pruesse, E.; Yilmaz, P.; Gerken, J.; Schweer, T.; Yarza, P.; Peplies, J.; Glöckner, F.O. The silva ribosomal rna gene database project: Improved data processing and web-based tools. *Nucleic Acids Res.* **2013**, *41*, D590–D596. [CrossRef] [PubMed]

51. McMurdie, P.J.; Holmes, S. Phyloseq: An r package for reproducible interactive analysis and graphics of microbiome census data. *PLoS ONE* **2013**, *8*, e61217. [CrossRef] [PubMed]

52. Team, R.C. *R: A Language and Environment for Statistical Computing*; R Foundation for Statistical Computing: Vienna, Austria, 2017.

53. Team, R. *Rstudio: Integrated Development for R. Rstudio*; RStudio, Inc.: Boston, MA, USA, 2016.

54. Combes, S.; Michelland, R.J.; Monteils, V.; Cauquil, L.; Soulie, V.; Tran, N.U.; Gidenne, T.; Fortun-Lamothe, L. Postnatal development of the rabbit caecal microbiota composition and activity. *FEMS Microbiol. Ecol.* **2011**, *77*, 680–689. [CrossRef] [PubMed]

55. Anders, S.; Huber, W. Differential expression analysis for sequence count data. *Genome Biol.* **2010**, *11*, R106. [CrossRef] [PubMed]

56. Bardou, P.; Mariette, J.; Escudié, F.; Djemiel, C.; Klopp, C. Jvenn: An interactive venn diagram viewer. *BMC Bioinform.* **2014**, *15*, 293. [CrossRef] [PubMed]

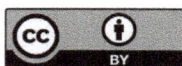

Article

Ergot Alkaloids at Doses Close to EU Regulatory Limits Induce Alterations of the Liver and Intestine

Viviane Mayumi Maruo [1,4], Ana Paula Bracarense [2], Jean-Paul Metayer [3], Maria Vilarino [3], Isabelle P. Oswald [4,*] and Philippe Pinton [4]

[1] Universidade Federal do Tocantins, Araguaína 77824-838, Brazil; vmmaruo@hotmail.com
[2] Laboratory of Animal Pathology, Universidade Estadual de Londrina, Londrina 86057-970, Brazil; ana.bracarense29@gmail.com
[3] ARVALIS-Institut du Végétal, Station expérimentale, 41100 Villerable, France; jp.mj.metayer@free.fr (J.-P.M.); M.Vilarino@arvalis.fr (M.V.)
[4] Toxalim (Research Centre in Food Toxicology), Université de Toulouse, INRA, ENVT, INP-Purpan, UPS, 31027 Toulouse, France; philippe.pinton@inra.fr
*   Correspondence: isabelle.oswald@inra.fr; Tel.: +33-582-066-366

Received: 21 March 2018; Accepted: 17 April 2018; Published: 1 May 2018

Abstract: An increase in the occurrence of ergot alkaloids (EAs) contamination has been observed in North America and Europe in recent years. These toxins are well known for their effects on the circulatory and nervous systems. The aim of this study was to investigate the effect of EAs on the liver and on the intestine using the pig both as a target species and as a non-rodent model for human. Three groups of 24 weaned piglets were exposed for 28 days to control feed or feed contaminated with 1.2 or 2.5 g of sclerotia/kg, i.e., at doses close to EU regulatory limits. Contaminated diets significantly reduced feed intake and consequently growth performance. In the liver, alteration of the tissue, including development of inflammatory infiltrates, vacuolization, apoptosis and necrosis of hepatocytes as well as presence of enlarged hepatocytes (megalocytes) were observed. In the jejunum, EAs reduced villi height and increased damage to the epithelium, reduced the number of mucus-producing cells and upregulated mRNA coding for different tight junction proteins such as claudins 3 and 4. In conclusion, in term of animal health, our data indicate that feed contaminated at the regulatory limits induces lesions in liver and intestine suggesting that this limit should be lowered for pigs. In term of human health, we establish a lowest observed adverse effect level (LOAEL) of 100 µg/kg body weight (bw) per day, lower than the benchmark dose limit (BMDL) retained by European Food Safety Authority (EFSA) to set the tolerable daily intake, suggesting also that regulatory limit should be revised.

Keywords: *Claviceps*; liver; digestive tract; mycotoxin; sclerotia; ergot alkaloids; toxicity

Key contribution: In term of pig, our data indicate that feed contaminated at the regulatory limits (1 g sclerotia/kg) induces liver and intestine suggesting that the limit should be lowered. In term of human health; the present experiment established a LOAEL of 100 µg EAs/kg bw per day; lower than the BMDL associated with a 10% response of 330 µg/kg bw per day retained by EFSA to set the tolerable daily intake.

1. Introduction

Ergot is a parasitic fungus that belongs to the *Claviceps* genus. It forms on various grains and grasses a dark mass of mycelium called sclerotia producing toxic secondary metabolites, the ergot alkaloids (EAs). These mycotoxins gained notoriety in the Middle Ages because of mass poisonings in Europe, characterized by gangrene and convulsions [1].

More than 50 different EAs have been identified so far. The main EAs produced by *Claviceps* species are ergometrine, ergotamine, ergosine, ergocristine, ergocryptine and ergocornine. Their toxicity is linked to their structural similarity with dopamine, noradrenaline, adrenaline and serotonin, enabling binding to the biogenic amine receptor and the interruption of neurotransmission [2]. Typical clinical symptoms of ergot poisoning are vasoconstriction, which may progress into gangrene, disruption of reproduction, abortion, neurotoxic signs including feed refusal, dizziness and convulsions, agalactia and adverse effects to the cardiovascular system [1,3–5]. Although acute poising has become rare, EAs are still a source of concern because they continue to be detected in cereals and cereal products in Europe and North America [6,7]. Moreover, the occurrence of *Claviceps purpurea* (*C. purpurea*) infections has been increasing in the last few years [8–11].

Currently, regulations are based on the quantities of ergot sclerotia. Codex Alimentarius established maximum levels for sclerotia of *C. purpurea* in wheat and durum wheat intended for processing for human consumption at 0.5 g/kg and 5 g/kg, respectively [12]. In animal feed, the European Commission fixed the maximum content at 1 g/kg of feed stuff containing unground cereals [13]. Recently, the EFSA Panel on Contaminants in the Food Chain conducted a risk assessment and proposed a tolerable daily intake (TDI) of 0.6 µg total EA/kg body weight (bw) per day [1] for humans.

The aim of this study was to investigate the effects of ingestion of EA-contaminated feed at concentrations close to the regulatory limits. We chose to perform the experiment in pigs as they may be exposed to EAs. In addition, they represent a choice species as a biomedical model for human toxicology, due to their similarities in anatomy, genetics and pathophysiology [14].

We mainly focused on the effects of EAs on the intestine and the liver. The intestine is of particular importance since it represents the first barrier against food contaminants and foreign antigens. The jejunum is one of the major intestinal sites of absorption, including the absorption of toxins. Intestinal epithelium integrity plays a critical role in the maintenance of the physical and immune barrier that is achieved by an ensemble of well-organized structural and secretory components including tight junctions, mucus and cytokines [15]. Most of the metabolization processes for xenobiotics, including mycotoxins, occur in the liver [16]. The metabolizing enzymes of the cytochrome P450 family are involved in and induced by ergot metabolism [17]. Moreover, certain hepatic enzymatic activities were found to be inhibited by ergotamine and ergometrine [18]. Reports in the literature on the effects of ergot on the intestine and the liver are rare, especially concerning biochemical and morphological parameters.

2. Results

2.1. Effects of Ergot Alkaloids on Clinical Signs, Growth and Feed Intake

The effects of ergot were first investigated in pigs exposed for 28 days at doses of 1.2 and 2.5 g sclerotia/kg feed, which are just above the European regulatory limit. When assessing clinical signs, no typical symptoms of acute toxicity, such as convulsions or muscle spasms, or necrosis of the extremities were observed. Similarly, no vomiting or fever was observed in animals exposed to ergot.

The effects of ergot on feed intake were already detected the second week in animal exposed to the highest dose. For animals exposed to the lower dose of ergot, this reduction only appeared in the last 14 days of treatment (Figure 1). During the experimental period, the daily feed intake of animals exposed to the higher dose of ergot was reduced by about 18% in comparison with control group (Figure 1). Taking into account the whole period of treatment, the daily feed intake was significantly reduced as a function of ergot content (Figure 1).

The reduction in feed ingestion led to a decrease of animal weight gain that was significant in the group exposed to the higher dose of EA (data not shown).

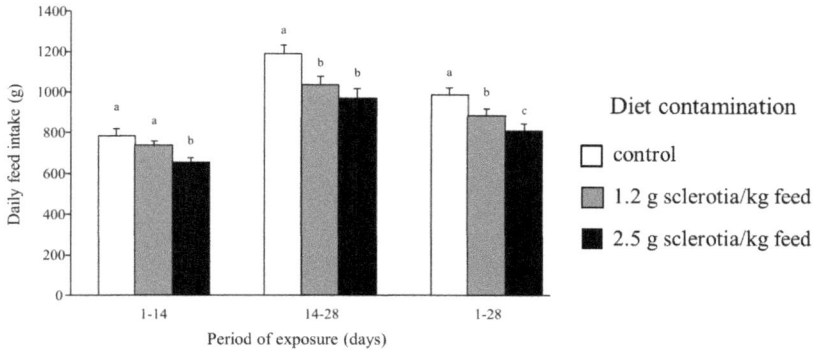

Figure 1. Daily feed intake of piglets fed ergot sclerotia for 28 days (n = 24/group). Values are means with standard errors of the mean represented by vertical bars. [a, b, c] mean values with different letters are statistically different ($p < 0.05$).

2.2. Effects of Ergot Alkaloids on Hematology and Blood Chemistry

Hematology and serum biochemical analysis were performed at the end of the experiment. When animals were exposed to ergot, the percentage of neutrophils was reduced and the decrease was significant in the group exposed to the lower dose (Table 1). The percentage of lymphocytes also increased in animals exposed to ergot, with a significant difference in animals exposed to the higher dose (Table 1).

Table 1. Hematological analysis of pigs fed 1.2 or 2.5 g ergot sclerotia/kg feed (n = 24/group).

Parameters	Contamination of the Diet (g of Sclerotia/kg Feed)		
	0	1.2	2.5
Red blood cells (T/L)	7.75 ± 0.12	7.80 ± 0.13	8.08 ± 0.13
Hemoglobin (g/dL)	10.45 ± 0.22 [a,b]	10.09 ± 0.21 [a]	10.97 ± 0.19 [b]
Hematocrit (%)	36.6 ± 0.70 [a,b]	35.52 ± 0.87 [a]	38.31 ± 0.63 [b]
Mean corpuscular volume (fL)	47.46 ± 0.93	45.67 ± 0.93	47.58 ± 0.91
White blood cells (10^3/mm^3)	14.5 ± 0.6	14.2 ± 0.9	16.5 ± 0.9
Neutrophils (%)	40.92 ± 2.51 [a]	30.67± 1.84 [b]	36.17 ± 2.55 [a,b]
Eosinophils (%)	0.38 ± 0.15	0.54 ± 0.30	0.29 ± 0.14
Basophils (%)	0.08 ± 0.08	0.08 ± 0.08	0.00 ± 0.00
Lymphocytes (%)	53.96 ± 2.66 [a]	63.96 ± 1.95 [b]	58.79 ± 2.77 [a,b]
Monocytes (%)	4.67 ± 0.42	4.75 ± 0.68	4.75 ± 0.63
Platelets/mm^3	521.58 ± 32.67	465.00 ± 28.08	533.04 ± 32.39

[a, b] mean values with different letters are statistically different ($p < 0.05$).

Biochemical analysis revealed a significant dose-dependent reduction in the levels of creatine kinase in animals exposed to ergot. In addition, the level of cholesterol decreased and that of glucose increased upon exposure to ergot (Table 2).

Table 2. Serum biochemical analysis of pigs fed 1.2 or 2.5 g ergot sclerotia/kg feed (n = 24/group).

Parameters	Contamination of the Diet (g of Sclerotia/kg Feed)		
	0	1.2	2.5
Alkaline phosphatase (U/L)	275.7 ± 24.5	237.6 ± 16.7	228.6 ± 16.1
Alanine aminotransferase (U/L)	37.3 ± 1.9	31.74 ± 1.5	33.32 ± 1.6
Amylase (U/L)	1783 ± 123	1815 ± 99	2074 ± 122
Aspartate aminotransferase (U/L)	56.0 ± 6.8	42.6 ± 5.4	44.4 ± 3.94
Creatine kinase (U/L)	3377 ± 396 [a]	1924 ± 297 [b]	1300 ± 252 [b]

Table 2. *Cont.*

Parameters	Contamination of the Diet (g of Sclerotia/kg Feed)		
	0	1.2	2.5
Lactate dehydrogenase (U/L)	962.8 ± 50.5	968.3 ± 57.7	1013.3 ± 72.5
Lipase (U/L)	6.45 ± 0.5	6.9 ± 0.3	5.9 ± 0.8
Albumin (μmol/L)	533.0 ± 9.7	530.4 ± 11.7	522.4 ± 13.3
T bilirubine (μmol/L)	11.2 ± 1.2	11.0 ± 1.2	7.4 ± 1.3
Cholesterol (mmol/L)	3.0 ± 0.1 [a]	2.6 ± 0.1 [b]	2.8 ± 0.1 [a]
Creatinine (μmol/L)	61.9 ± 6.2	63.3 ± 6.5	71.7 ± 6.4
Glucose PAP (mmol/L)	4.4 ± 0.2 [a]	4.7 ± 0.3 [a]	5.4 ± 0.3 [b]
Phosphorus (mmol/L)	3.1 ± 0.1	3.2 ± 0.1	3.0 ± 0.1
Total proteins (g/L)	63.5 ± 7.8	59.1 ± 7.4	62.5 ± 8.2
Urea (mmol/L)	4.7 ± 0.4	4.3 ± 0.3	3.5 ± 0.4

[a,b] mean values with different letters are statistically different ($p < 0.05$).

2.3. Alterations of Tissue Morphology Caused by Ergot Alkaloids

The effects of ergot on the liver and the intestine were investigated through histological analyses. Exposure to ergot led to mild to moderate lesions of the liver (Figure 2) and the jejunum (Figure 3) of pigs.

In the liver, tissue disorganization of hepatic cords, inflammation and vacuolation of hepatocytes, megalocytosis and necrosis were the main morphological alterations (Figure 2B). Furthermore, animals fed the contaminated diets presented a significant increase in the lesion liver score (Figure 2C).

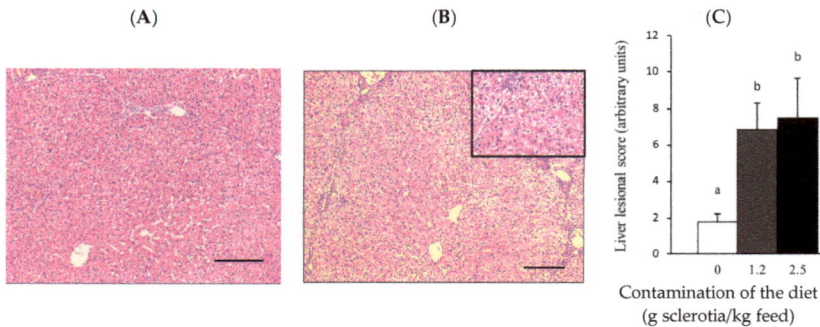

(A)   **(B)**   **(C)**

Figure 2. Liver of piglets fed ergot diets. (**A**) Control piglet. Normal liver. HE. Objective 10×; (**B**) Piglet fed 2.5 g ergot sclerotia/kg feed. Disorganization of hepatic cords and periportal hepatocyte vacuolation. HE. Objective 10×. Insert: Hepatocyte vacuolation. HE. Objective 40×; (**C**) Liver lesion score. Values are means with their standard errors of mean represented by vertical bars (*n* = 6 animals). Mean values with different letters are significantly different ($p < 0.05$). Bar = 100 μm.

The main histological changes observed in the jejunum were villi atrophy, edema of lamina propria and cytoplasmic vacuolation of enterocytes. As shown in Figure 3C, animals exposed to the higher dose of ergot displayed a significant increase of the lesion score in the jejunum compared to control animals (3.4 fold increase, $p < 0.005$). Morphometrical analysis revealed a significant decrease in villi height (1.2 fold decrease at both doses) (Figure 3D). The number of goblet cells decreased significantly in the jejunum (mean 1.6 fold decrease, $p < 0.001$) of piglets exposed to ergot (Figure 3E). Similar effects were observed in jejunum areas with Peyer's patches (data not shown).

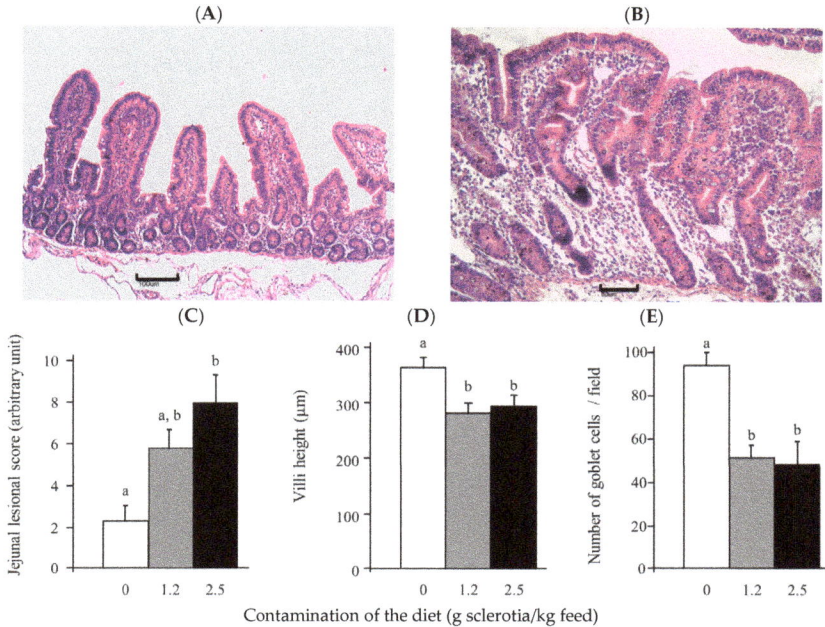

Figure 3. Effect of ergot exposure on jejunum of pigs receiving a control diet or a diet contaminated with 1.2 or 2.5 g ergot sclerotia/kg feed for 28 days. Jejunal section with hematoxylin-eosin (HE), Objective 10×: (**A**) Control piglet; (**B**) Piglet fed 2.5 g ergot sclerotia/kg feed; (**C**) Lesion score according to the occurrence and severity of lesions observed on formalin-fixed tissue sections stained with HE; (**D**) Villi height measured on formalin-fixed tissue sections stained with HE; (**E**) Number of goblet cells observed on formalin-fixed tissue sections stained with Schiff's periodic acid. Values are means of the score, villi height and number of goblet cells/field respectively, with standard errors of the mean represented by vertical bars ($n = 6$ animals). [a,b] mean values with different letters are statistically different ($p < 0.05$).

2.4. Effects of Ergot Alkaloids on mRNA Expression in the Jejunum

Given the lesions induced by ergot exposure in the jejunum and due to the lack of studies on the toxicity of EAs in this organ, the expression of 34 genes coding for junctional proteins, inflammatory and immunological mediators was evaluated by real-time-quantitative PCR (RT-qPCR) in the jejunum. The expression profile of mRNA expression of different toll-like receptors (TLR) and cytokines (TLR4, nuclear factor kappa B (NFkB), interleukin (IL)-6, IL-8, tumor necrosis factor-α (TNFA)) showed a tendency to downregulation. In animals exposed to the higher dose of ergot, analysis of mRNA expression of junctional proteins revealed a significant increase in claudin-3 (CLDN3), claudin-4 (CLDN4), occludin (OCLN), zonula occludens-1 (ZO-1), junctional adhesion molecule (JAM-A) and E-cadherin (ECAD) (Figure 4). The expression of genes coding for mucin-1 (MUC1), alkaline phosphatase (ALP) and proliferating cell nuclear antigen (PCNA) was also significantly increased. Altogether, the overexpression of the genes involved in maintaining the structure of the intestinal mucosa may reflect an attempt by the tissue to reestablish its function.

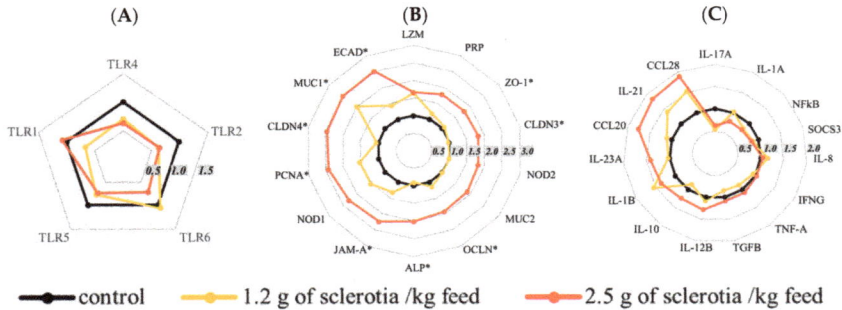

Figure 4. Expression of selected genes in the jejunum of pigs fed with a control diet or a diet including ergot alkaloids for 28 days. mRNA levels were measured by RT-qPCR. The three panels present different groups: TLR-encoding genes (**A**), junctional protein-encoding genes (**B**) and immune mediator-encoding genes (**C**). The gene expression levels for the control group are shown in black (mean value adjusted to 1 for this group) and those for the groups exposed to 1.2 and 2.5 g sclerotia/kg feed ergot are shown in orange and red, respectively (*n* = 6 animals/group). * statistical difference in gene expression between control animals and pigs exposed to the highest dose of ergot (*p* < 0.05).

3. Discussion

The aim of this study was to investigate the effects of ingestion of EA-contaminated feed on the liver and intestine in pig. The levels of sclerotia in the feed were 1.2 g sclerotia or 2.4 mg total ergot alkaloids/kg. Using these concentrations that were close to the regulatory limits for 28 days, we observed not only effects on animal performances but also lesions in the liver and the intestine. This study shows that the regulation of 1 g sclerotia/kg of feed materials is probably not protective enough for pigs and deserves to be re-evaluated. In terms of human health, a LOAEL of 100 µg/kg bw per day could be established from the present data. This is lower than the BMDL associated with a 10% response of 330 µg/kg bw per day, which is set by EFSA as the tolerable daily intake for human. The present experiment thus provides evidence of the necessity to re-examine the current TDI for humans.

Considering the mean feed intake of these animals (1163 and 962 g/day after respectively, two and four weeks of exposure) and their mean weight (17.5 and 27.8 kg after respectively, two and four weeks of exposure), it represents an exposure to ergot alkaloids of 159 and 83 µg/kg bw per day after two and four weeks of exposure, respectively. The lowest observed adverse effect level (LOAEL) is lower than the benchmark dose limit (BMDL) associated with a 10% response of 330 µg/kg bw per day retained by EFSA to set the tolerable daily intake (TDI) of 0.6 µg/kg bw per day [1], based on the vasoconstrictive effects observed in a rat model exposed to ergotamine for 13 weeks [19]. Given the interspecies differences in the observed effects, pig could be considered as a relevant species for ergot alkaloids risk assessments. These data reinforce the need to increase the knowledge on the effects of EAs and suggest a revision of the TDI for EAs.

As already reported in other studies, we observed that the ingestion of EAs damages the zootechnical parameters as measured by feed intake and average daily gain [17,20]. Reduction of weight gain appears to be caused by the reduction in feed intake, which in turn may be explained by the action of the EAs on serotoninergic receptors in the gut, thereby affecting motility [2]. The composition and proportion of EAs in sclerotia can vary but the total EA content appears to be more important than the composition of EA for the alteration of animal performances [21].

The consumption of ergot also affected intestinal integrity, as revealed by histological and molecular analyses, and might have contributed to growth impairment of the animals. Histological and morphometric evaluation of the intestinal tissue revealed a sensitive endpoint for the evaluation of the effects of mycotoxin exposure. Modifications in villi height reflect changes in the balance between enterocyte proliferation and apoptosis. The increase in the lesion score and villi flattening in the intestine of animals exposed to EAs could be explained by their action on serotoninergic receptors present in epithelial intestinal cells, primary afferent neurons and secretor motor neurons of the intestine [22]. In addition to the action of EAs on the serotoninergic system, recent in vitro studies demonstrated that EAs also cause cytotoxicity and apoptosis in intestinal HT-29 and liver HepG2 cell lines, providing evidence for an intricate mode of action [23]. Additionally, the number of goblet cells was reduced in animals exposed to EAs, revealing impairment in the intestinal barrier function [15,24]. Taken together, these alterations could lead to a compensatory upregulation of mRNA levels of CLDN3, CLDN4, OCLN, ZO-1, JAM-A, ECAD, ALP and PCNA, as already described in the intestine of mice [25] or in intestinal epithelial cells exposed to deoxynivalenol [26]. Immunoregulatory mechanisms in the intestine play a crucial role in the defense of the organism [27]. The pattern recognition receptors (PRR) are membrane-bound receptors that specifically bind to pathogen-associated molecular patterns (PAMPs) shared by various microorganisms. PRR are highly expressed in the jejunum and ileum of pigs and trigger an inflammatory response, involving the activation of myeloid differentiation 88 and NFkB [28]. In the present work, mRNA expression of TLR-1 2, 4, 5 and 6 as well as TNF-A, IL-1A, IL-8 and IFNG tended to be downregulated in the jejunum of animals exposed to EAs. This could reduce tolerance to commensal microbiota and the organism's ability to trigger inflammation response against pathogens, thereby increasing susceptibility to infections [29].

Besides the action of EAs on the intestine, their effects were also studied on the liver where tissue disorganization, inflammation and necrosis were observed and assessed by a significant increase of the lesion liver score. We observed that the consumption of EA-contaminated feed affected the levels of cholesterol, glucose and creatine kinase, parameters correlated with adiposity and muscle growth [30]. Hypocholesterolemia could correlate with the malabsorption of nutrients as well as with an altered lipid metabolism that often accompanies hepatic disease [31]. Glucose levels were elevated in the group that received the higher ergot content. In the post-absorptive phase, glucose is transported from its site of uptake in the gut to the sites of glycogen storage, principally the liver and muscles [32]. The increase in glucose level indicates glycogen mobilization from the storage sites to provide energy to the organism. In the present study, the morphological changes observed in hepatocytes could be associated with functional alterations such as lipid metabolism and glycogen storage. The reduction in creatine kinase may indicate hypoplasia, atrophy or the mild destruction of skeletal muscles [31,32]. EAs induce vasoconstriction through binding with serotoninergic receptors in the smooth muscle cells of vessels walls [5]. Therefore, an association between a relative ischemia and changes in creatine kinase could be hypothesized. In short, the biochemical alterations observed in animals exposed to ergot could be correlated to liver and mild muscle lesions [30].

4. Conclusions

The contamination of cereals by EAs has recently been shown to be increasing in different countries and is a source of concern for human and animal health. This study confirmed that EA reduces the performances of pigs, and demonstrated that EAs provoke hepatotoxicity, as revealed by deleterious effects on tissue morphology, and mild biochemical alterations. Moreover, EA alters the intestinal epithelium, reduces the number of goblet cells and modulates the expression of genes involved in immune response and barrier function. This suggests that ingestion of EA-contaminated feed may alter the intestinal barrier function, predisposing animals to enteric infections and potentially causing hepatotoxicity.

From the point of view of pig health, our data indicate that feed contaminated at the regulatory limits induces deleterious effects in the liver and intestine in pigs, suggesting that the regulatory limit is not adequately protective. From the point of view of human health, this study reveals the sensitivity of pigs to EAs with a LOAEL lower than the BMDL obtained in rats, which is employed by EFSA to set the tolerable daily intake for human. The present data should be considered in a further assessment of human risk of exposure to EAs.

5. Materials and Methods

5.1. Experimental Diets

Experimental diets, based on wheat, corn and soybean and formulated according to the CORPEN (1996) norms are detailed in Table 3. Two batches of sclerotia obtained from contaminated wheat were used to prepare the contaminated diets. Levels of sclerotia of 0 (control), 1.2 g/kg (dose 1) and 2.5 g/kg (dose 2) were used, the first dose being close to the regulatory limit of 1 g/kg [13].

Table 3. Chemical composition of the diets (% of dry matter DM).

Parameters	Contamination of the Diet (g of Sclerotia/kg Feed)		
	0	1.2	2.5
Total nitrogen	20.1	20.2	20.3
Raw cellulose	2.6	2.7	2.8
Lipids	4.3	4.4	4.4
Minerals	6.0	6.1	6.0

5.2. Ergot Alkaloid Composition of the Diets

The quantities of EAs were determined by liquid chromatography coupled with a tandem mass spectrometry (LC/MS/MS) (TSQ Quantum Ultra, ThermoFisher Scientific, Villebon sur Yvette, France) at Qualtech laboratory (Vandœuvre, France).

After preparation, diets were analyzed four times and the mean EA concentrations were 2.36 and 5.05 mg/kg, for diets with ergot dose 1 and 2, respectively. The most abundant alkaloid was ergotamine, followed by ergosine, ergocristine and their corresponding-inine epimers (Table 4). The amount of the-ine isomers was approximately two-thirds of total alkaloids.

Contamination with other mycotoxins was investigated. Deoxynivalenol was naturally present in the wheat (19 µg/kg) and corn (171 µg/kg) but at an insignificant rate. Other mycotoxins, including DON acetylated, nivalenol, T2, HT-2, zearalenone and fumonisin were below the detection limit.

Table 4. Ergot alkaloid content in experimental feed (mg/kg).

Alkaloids (mg/kg Feed)	Contamination of the Diet (g of Sclerotia/kg Feed)	
	1.2	2.5
Ergotamine	0.52	1.03
Ergotaminine	0.24	0.58
Ergosine	0.29	0.58
Ergosinine	0.16	0.34
Ergocristine	0.26	0.47
Ergocristinine	0.18	0.40
Ergometrine	0.17	0.44
Ergometrinine	0.06	0.12
Ergocornine	0.15	0.30
Ergocorninine	0.11	0.29
Ergocryptine	0.13	0.30
Ergocryptinine	0.09	0.21
Total alkaloids	**2.4**	**5.1**

5.3. Animals

Animal experiments were carried out at ARVALIS—Institut du végétal facility (Villerable, France) in accordance with the guidelines for protection of animals used for scientific purposes issued by French Ministry of Higher Education and Research. Seventy-two castrated, 21 day-old crossbreed (P76 X Naïma) piglets (mean weight 10.7 ± 0.9 kg) were housed in the facility with free access to control starter feed and water. When they were 34 days old, they were housed in individual pens and assigned to three groups of 12 males and 12 females one group fed the control diet, another ergot dose 1 and the third ergot dose 2 diet. At the end of the experiment (62 days old) their mean weight was 27.9 ± 3.8 kg, 27.8 ± 2.6 kg, 25.6 ± 3.1 kg in the control group, ergot dose 1 and ergot dose 2 diet groups, respectively.

5.4. Experimental Setting and Sample Collection

Animals received experimental diets for a period of 28 days. Weight and consumption were measured on the first day of the experiment, 14 days later and on the last day of the experiment. The animals were observed daily to detect possible signs of ergot intoxication such as balance disorders or necrosis of the extremities.

At the end of the experiment, blood samples were taken from the external jugular vein of all the animals for biochemical and hematological analyses. In addition, six male animals in each group were euthanized and liver, jejunum and jejunum with Peyer's patches were sampled in 10% buffered formalin (Sigma, Saint-Quentin Fallavier, France) for histopathological analysis or immediately quick-frozen in liquid nitrogen and stored at $-80\,°C$ until RNA extraction [33].

5.5. Hematology and Blood Chemistry

Hematological parameters (white and red blood cells, hemoglobin and platelets) were analyzed at Medibiolab (Vendome, France), with a Sysmex XT2000i automated hematology analyzer (Sysmex, Villepinte, France). Serum biochemistry was determined with a Pentra 400 Clinical Chemistry benchtop analyzer (Horiba, Les Ulis, France) at GenoToul-Anexplo platform (Toulouse, France).

5.6. Histomorphometrical Analysis

Formalin-fixed tissue samples were dehydrated in ethanol and embedded in paraffin wax. Sections (3 µm) were stained with hematoxylin-eosin (HE, Sigma) for histopathological analysis. A lesion score per animal was established by taking into account the severity of the lesion and its extent (intensity or observed frequency; scored from 0 to 3) as described previously [34]. Morphometry was evaluated in the jejunum by measuring the height of 30 randomly chosen villi using a MOTIC Image Plus 2.0 ML 1 image analysis system (Richmond, Canada, 2003), as described previously. In addition, Schiff's periodic acid stain was used to evaluate goblet cell density (five fields/slide, objective 20×) [35].

5.7. Expression of mRNA by Real-Time PCR

Intestinal tissue was processed in lysing matrix D tubes (MP Biomedicals, Illkirch, France) containing Extract-All (Eurobio, Les Ulis, France) in a Fast-Prep FP120 instrument (MP Biomedicals) as described previously [36,37]. The concentrations and purity of RNA were determined using a Nanodrop nd1000 instrument (Labtech International, Paris, France). Total RNA samples were reverse-transcribed using a High Capacity cDNA-RT kit (Life Technologies, Saint Aubin, France). RT-qPCR was performed in 384-well plates in a ViiA 7 thermocycler (Life Technologies, Saint Aubin, France) as described previously [38]. All reactions were performed in duplicate and averages were used for further analysis. Primers for the real-time quantitative PCR are presented in Table 5. Among the different internal reference genes tested were Beta-2-microglobulin (B2M), peptidylprolyl isomerase A (PPIA—cyclophilin A) and ribosomal protein L32 (RPL32); the latter were selected for their stability of expression assessed with the NormFinder program [39]. Data from qPCR were analyzed with the LinRegPCR 2016. 2 program [40], enabling the determination of the starting concentrations (N0).

Table 5. Primer sequences of genes used for qRT-PCR analysis of the jejunum (F: forward; R: reverse).

Target Gene		Primer Sequence (5′–3′)	mRNA	Reference
Alkaline phosphatase (ALP)	F	AAGCTCCGTTTTTGGCCTG	ENSSSCT00000037252.1	[28]
	R	GGAGGTATATGGCTTGAGATCCA		
Beta-2-microglobulin (B2M)	F	TTCTACCTTCTGGTCCACACTGA	NM_213978.1	[41]
	R	TCATCCAACCCAGATGCA		
C-C Motif Chemokine Ligand 20 (CCL20)	F	GCTCCTGGCTGCTTTGATGTC	NM_001024589	Present study
	R	CATTGGCGAGCTGCTGTGTG		
C-C Motif Chemokine Ligand 28 (CCL28)	F	GGCTGCTGTCATCCTTCATGT	ENSSSCT00000018375	Present study
	R	TGAGGGCTGACACAGATTCTTCT		
Claudin 3 (CLDN3)	F	CTGCTCTGCTGCTCGTGCCC	AY625258.1	Present study
	R	TCATACGTAGTCCTTGCGGTCGTAG		
Claudin 4 (CLDN4)	F	CTGCTTTGCTGCAACTGCC	NM_001161637.1	[26]
	R	TCAACGGTAGCACCTTACACGTAGT		
E-cadherin (ECAD)	F	ACCACCGCCATCAGGACTC	NM_001163060.1	Present study
	R	TGGGAGCTGGGAAACGTG		
Interferon gamma (IFNG)	F	TGGTAGCTCTGGGAAACTGAATG	NM_213948	[28]
	R	GGCTTTGCGCTGGGATCTG		
Interleukin 1A (IL-1A)	F	TCAGCCGCCCATCCA	NM_214029.1	[38]
	R	AGCCCCCGGTGCCATGT		
Interleukin 1B (IL-1B)	F	ATGCTGAAGGCTCTCCACCTC	NM_214055	[28]
	R	TTGTTGCTATCATCTCCTTGCAC		
Interleukin 8 (IL-8)	F	GCTCTCTGTGAGGCTGCAGTTC	NM_213867.1	[38]
	R	AAGGTGTGGAATGCGTATTTATGC		
Interleukin 10 (IL-10)	F	GGCCCAGTGAAGAGTTTCTTTC	NM_214041	[38]
	R	CAACAAGTCGCCCATCTGGT		
Interleukin 12B (IL-12B)	F	GGTTTCAGACCCGACGAACTCT	NM_214013.1	[38]
	R	CATATGGCCACAATGGGAGATG		
Interleukin 17A (IL-17A)	F	CCAGACGGCCCTCAGATTAC	NM_001005729.1	[38]
	R	GGTCCTCGTTGCGTTGGA		
Interleukin 21 (IL-21)	F	GGCACAGTGGCCCATAAATC	NM_214415	Present study
	R	GCAGCAATTCAGGGTCCAAG		
Interleukin 23A (IL-23A)	F	TTCTCTACACCCTGATGGCTCTG	ENSSSCT00000047550.1	Present study
	R	TCGGGCTGCAAGAGTTGC		
Junctional adhesion molecule A (JAM-A)	F	CGTGCCTTCATCAACTCTTCCTAT	NM_001128444.1	Present study
	R	CACAAGTGTAATCTCCAGCATCAGA		
Lysozyme (LZM)	F	GGTCTATGATCGGTGCGAGTTC	NM_214392.2	[28]
	R	TCCATGCCAGACTTTTTCAGAAT		
Mucin 1 (MUC1)	F	GCATTACAAACCTCCAGTTTACCT	AY243508.1	[42]
	R	CCCAGAAGCCCGTCTTCTTT		
Mucin 2 (MUC2)	F	GCAGCCTGTGCGAGGAA	XM_003122394.1	[42]
	R	TGTCATCATACACAGTGCCTTCTG		
Occludin (OCLN)	F	AGCTGGAGGAAGACTGGATCAG	U79554.1	[43]
	R	TGCAGGCCACTGTCAAAATT		
Nuclear Factor Kappa B (NFkB)	F	CCTCCACAAGGCAGCAAATAG	ENSSSCT00000033438	Present study
	R	TCCACACCGCTGTCACAGA		
Nuclear oligomerization domain 1 (NOD1)	F	TGGGCTGCGTCCTGTTCA	AB_187219.1	[28]
	R	GGTGACCCTGACCGATGT		
Nuclear oligomerization domain 2 (NOD2)	F	GAGCGCATCCTCTTAACTTTC	AB426547.1	[28]
	R	ACGCTCGTGATCCGTGAAC		
Proliferating cell nuclear antigen (PCNA)	F	GTTGATAAAGAGGAGGAAGCAGTT	NM_001291925.1	[28]
	R	TGGCTTTTGTAAAGAAGTTCAGGTAC		
Peptidylprolyl isomerase A (cyclophilin A)	F	CCCACCGTCTTCTTCGACAT	NM_214353.1	[38]
	R	TCTGCTGTCTTTGGAACTTTGTCT		
Prion protein (PRP)	F	TTTGTGCATGACTGCGTCAAC	NM_001008687.1	Present study
	R	CGTGGTCACTGTGTGCTGCT		
Ribosomal protein L32 (RPL32)	F	AGTTCATCCGGCACCAGTCA	NM_001001636.1	[26]
	R	GAACCTTCTCCGCACCCTGT		
Suppressor of Cytokine Signaling 3 (SOCS3)	F	CTTCACGCTCAGCGTCAAG	HM045422.1	Present study
	R	CTTGAGCACGCAGTCGAAG		
Transforming growth factor beta (TGFB)	F	GAAGCGCATCGAGGCCATTC	NM_214015	[28]
	R	GGCTCCGGTTCGACACTTTC		

Table 5. *Cont.*

Target Gene		Primer Sequence (5′–3′)	mRNA	Reference
Toll-like receptor 1 (TLR1)	F	TGCTGGATGCTAACGGATGTC	AB219564.1	[28]
	R	AAGTGGTTTCAATGTTGTTCAAAGTC		
Toll-like receptor 2 (TLR2)	F	TCACTTGTCTAACTTATCATCCTCTTG	AB085935.1	[28]
	R	TCAGCGAAGGTGTCATTATTGC		
Toll-like receptor 4 (TLR4)	F	GCCATCGCTGCTAACATCATC	AB188301.2	[28]
	R	CTCATACTCAAAGATACACCATCGG		
Toll-like receptor 5 (TLR5)	F	CCTTCCTGCTTCTTTGATGG	NM_001348771	[28]
	R	CTGTGACCGTCCTGATGTAG		
Toll-like receptor 6 (TLR6)	F	AACCTACTGTCATAAGCCTTCATTC	AB085936.1	[28]
	R	GTCTACCACAAATTCACTTTCTTCAG		
Tumor Necrosis Factor alpha (TNF-A)	F	ACTGCACTTCGAGGTTATCGG	NM_214022	[28]
	R	GGCGACGGGCTTATCTGA		
Zonula occludens 1 (ZO-1)	F	ATAACATCAGCACAGTGCCTAAAGC	AJ318101.1	Present study
	R	GTTGCTGTTAAACACGCCTCG		

5.8. Statistical Analysis

The zootechnical parameters (daily feed intake and average weight gain) were measured on 24 piglets per group, and the differences in variance analysis were assessed with the Newman et Keuls post hoc test.

Histological data were measured on 6 animals per group and statistically analyzed by the free software Action 2.3 (Estatcamp, Campinas, SP, Brazil, 2003) using normality (Shapiro-Wilk's test) and homogeneity (Bartlett) tests. When these two assumptions were met, the lesional score, the intestinal morphometry and the number of goblet cells were analyzed by ANOVA followed by Tukey's test. For gene expression, quantification by qPCR and statistical analysis, the mRNA expression of target genes was normalized to the expressed housekeeping genes using REST© 2009 software (Qiagen, Valencia, CA, USA) which uses the pair-wise fixed reallocation randomization test as statistical model [44]. *P* values below 0.05 ($p \leq 0.05$) were considered significant.

Author Contributions: J.-P.M., M.V., P.P. and I.P.O. supervised the study and the design of the experiments. V.M.M., J.-P.M., A.P.B. and P.P. performed the experiments and analyzed the data. V.M.M., A.P.B., I.P.O., P.P. wrote the paper.

Acknowledgments: The authors are grateful to A.M. Cossalter and J. Laffitte (INRA Toxalim) for sample collection and to Y. Lippi (TRiX Facility, INRA Toxalim) for assistance in PCR data handling.

Conflicts of Interest: The authors declare no conflict of interest.

References

1. EFSA. Scientific opinion on ergot alkaloids in food and feed. *EFSA J.* **2012**, *10*, 2798.
2. Klotz, J.L. Activities and effects of ergot alkaloids on livestock physiology and production. *Toxins* **2015**, *7*, 2801–2821. [CrossRef] [PubMed]
3. Canty, M.J.; Fogarty, U.; Sheridan, M.K.; Ensley, S.M.; Schrunk, D.E.; More, S.J. Ergot alkaloid intoxication in perennial ryegrass (Lolium perenne): An emerging animal health concern in Ireland? *Ir. Vet. J.* **2014**, *67*, 21. [CrossRef] [PubMed]
4. Korn, A.K.; Gross, M.; Usleber, E.; Thom, N.; Köhler, K.; Erhardt, G. Dietary ergot alkaloids as a possible cause of tail necrosis in rabbits. *Mycotoxin Res.* **2014**, *30*, 241–250. [CrossRef] [PubMed]
5. Strickland, J.R.; Looper, M.L.; Matthews, J.C.; Rosenkrans, C.F., Jr.; Flythe, M.D.; Brown, K.R. Board-invited review: St. Anthony's Fire in livestock: Causes, mechanisms, and potential solutions. *J. Anim. Sci.* **2011**, *89*, 1603–1626. [CrossRef] [PubMed]
6. Di Mavungu, J.D.; Malysheva, S.V.; Sanders, M.; Larionova, D.; Robbens, J.; Dubruel, P.; Van Peteghem, C.; De Saeger, S. Development and validation of a new LC-MS/MS method for the simultaneous determination of six major ergot alkaloids and their corresponding epimers. Application to some food and feed commodities. *Food Chem.* **2012**, *135*, 292–303. [CrossRef]

7.   Scott, P. Ergot alkaloids: Extent of human and animal exposure. *World Mycotoxin J.* **2009**, *2*, 141–149. [CrossRef]

8.   Krska, R.; Crews, C. Significance, chemistry and determination of ergot alkaloids: A review. *Food Addit. Contam. Part A Chem. Anal. Control Expo. Risk Assess.* **2008**, *25*, 722–731. [CrossRef] [PubMed]

9.   Tittlemier, S.A.; Drul, D.; Roscoe, M.; McKendry, T. Occurrence of Ergot and Ergot Alkaloids in Western Canadian Wheat and Other Cereals. *J. Agric. Food Chem.* **2015**, *63*, 6644–6650. [CrossRef] [PubMed]

10. Topi, D.; Jakovac-Strajn, B.; Pavsic-Vrtac, K.; Tavcar-Kalcher, G. Occurrence of ergot alkaloids in wheat from Albania. *Food Addit. Contam. Part A Chem. Anal. Control. Expo. Risk Assess.* **2017**, *34*, 1333–1343. [CrossRef] [PubMed]

11. Orlando, B.; Maumené, C.; Piraux, F. Ergot and ergot alkaloids in French cereals: Occurrence, pattern and agronomic practices for managing the risk. *World Mycotoxin J.* **2017**, *10*, 327–338. [CrossRef]

12. Codex Alimentarius. Codex standard for wheat and durum wheat. *Codex Stand.* **1995**, 199–1995.

13. European-Union Directive 2002/32/EC. *Off. J. Eur. Communities* **2002**, 10–21.

14. Walters, E.M.; Wolf, E.; Whyte, J.J.; Mao, J.; Renner, S.; Nagashima, H.; Kobayashi, E.; Zhao, J.; Wells, K.D.; Critser, J.K.; et al. Completion of the swine genome will simplify the production of swine as a large animal biomedical model. *BMC Med. Genomics* **2012**, *5*, 55. [CrossRef] [PubMed]

15. Robert, H.; Payros, D.; Pinton, P.; Theodorou, V.; Mercier-Bonin, M.; Oswald, I.P.; Théodorou, V.; Mercier-Bonin, M.; Oswald, I.P. Impact of mycotoxins on the intestine: Are mucus and microbiota new targets? *Crit. Rev. Toxicol.* **2017**, *20*, 249–275. [CrossRef] [PubMed]

16. Ingawale, D.K.; Mandlik, S.K.; Naik, S.R. Models of hepatotoxicity and the underlying cellular, biochemical and immunological mechanism(s): A critical discussion. *Env. Toxicol Pharmacol* **2014**, *37*, 118–133. [CrossRef] [PubMed]

17. Danicke, S.; Diers, S. Effects of ergot alkaloids on liver function of piglets as evaluated by the (13)C-methacetin and (13)C-alpha-ketoisocaproic acid breath test. *Toxins* **2013**, *5*, 139–161. [CrossRef] [PubMed]

18. Moubarak, A.; Rosenkrans, C.J.; Johnson, Z.B. Modulation of cytochrome P450 metabolism by ergonovine and dihydroergotamine. *Vet. Hum. Toxicol.* **2003**, *45*, 6–9. [PubMed]

19. Speijers, G.J.A. *Subchronic Toxicity Experiment with Rats Fed a Diet Containing Ergotamine-Tartrate*; RIVM-report n°618312002; National Institute for Public Health the Environment Protection: Bilthoven, The Netherlands, 1993.

20. Mainka, S.; Dänicke, S.; Böhme, H.; Ueberschär, K.-H.; Polten, S.; Hüther, L.; Danicke, S.; Bohme, H.; Ueberschar, K.H.; Polten, S.; et al. The influence of ergot-contaminated feed on growth and slaughtering performance, nutrient digestibility and carry over of ergot alkaloids in growing-finishing pigs. *Arch. Anim. Nutr.* **2005**, *59*, 377–395. [CrossRef] [PubMed]

21. Mainka, S.; Danicke, S.; Bohme, H.; Ueberschar, K.H.; Liebert, F.; Dänicke, S.; Böhme, H.; Ueberschär, K.H.; Liebert, F.; Danicke, S.; et al. On the composition of ergot and the effects of feeding two different ergot sources on piglets. *Anim. Feed Sci. Technol.* **2007**, *139*, 52–68. [CrossRef]

22. Spiller, R. Recent advances in understanding the role of serotonin in gastrointestinal motility in functional bowel disorders: Alterations in 5-HT signalling and metabolism in human disease. *Neurogastroenterol. Motil.* **2007**, *19* (Suppl. 2), 25–31. [CrossRef] [PubMed]

23. Mulac, D.; Lepski, S.; Ebert, F.; Schwerdtle, T.; Humpf, H.U. Cytotoxicity and fluorescence visualization of ergot alkaloids in human cell lines. *J. Agric. Food Chem.* **2013**, *61*, 462–471. [CrossRef] [PubMed]

24. McGuckin, M.A.; Linden, S.K.; Sutton, P.; Florin, T.H.; Lindén, S.K.; Sutton, P.; Florin, T.H. Mucin dynamics and enteric pathogens. *Nat. Rev. Microbiol.* **2011**, *9*, 265–278. [CrossRef] [PubMed]

25. Akbari, P.; Braber, S.; Gremmels, H.; Koelink, P.J.; Verheijden, K.A.; Garssen, J.; Fink-Gremmels, J. Deoxynivalenol: A trigger for intestinal integrity breakdown. *FASEB J.* **2014**, *28*, 2414–2429. [CrossRef] [PubMed]

26. Pinton, P.; Braicu, C.; Nougayrede, J.-P.P.; Laffitte, J.; Taranu, I.; Oswald, I.P.P. Deoxynivalenol Impairs Porcine Intestinal Barrier Function and Decreases the Protein Expression of Claudin-4 through a Mitogen-Activated Protein Kinase-Dependent Mechanism. *J. Nutr.* **2010**, *140*, 1956–1962. [CrossRef] [PubMed]

27. Ramiro-Puig, E.; Pérez-Cano, F.J.; Castellote, C.; Franch, A.; Castell, M. The bowel: A key component of the immune system. *Rev. Esp. Enferm. Dig.* **2008**, *100*, 29–34. [PubMed]

28. Gourbeyre, P.; Berri, M.; Lippi, Y.; Meurens, F.; Vincent-Naulleau, S.; Laffitte, J.; Rogel-Gaillard, C.; Pinton, P.; Oswald, I.P.P. Pattern recognition receptors in the gut: Analysis of their expression along the intestinal tract and the crypt/villus axis. *Physiol. Rep.* **2015**, *3*. [CrossRef] [PubMed]

29. Kumar, H.; Kawai, T.; Akira, S. Pathogen recognition by the innate immune system. *Int. Rev. Immunol.* **2001**, *30*, 16–34. [CrossRef] [PubMed]

30. Cooper, C.A.; Moraes, L.E.; Murray, J.D.; Owens, S.D. Hematologic and biochemical reference intervals for specific pathogen free 6-week-old Hampshire-Yorkshire crossbred pigs. *J. Anim. Sci. Biotechnol.* **2014**, *5*, 5. [CrossRef] [PubMed]

31. Meyer, D.; Harvey, J.W. *Veterinary Laboratory Medicine: Interpretation and Diagnosis*, 2nd ed.; W. B. Saunders Co.: Philadelphia, Pennsylvania, 1998; pp. 157–186.

32. Kerr, M. *Veterinary Laboratory Medecine*, 2nd ed.; Blackwell Science Ltd.: London, UK, 2002; p. 392. [CrossRef]

33. Lucioli, J.; Pinton, P.; Callu, P.; Laffitte, J.; Grosjean, F.; Kolf-Clauw, M.; Oswald, I.P.P.; Bracarense, A.P.F.R.L.P. The food contaminant deoxynivalenol activates the mitogen activated protein kinases in the intestine: Interest of ex vivo models as an alternative to in vivo experiments. *Toxicon* **2013**, *66*, 31–36. [CrossRef] [PubMed]

34. Grenier, B.; Bracarense, A.P.; Schwartz, H.E.; Trumel, C.; Cossalter, A.M.; Schatzmayr, G.; Kolf-Clauw, M.; Moll, W.D.; Oswald, I.P. The low intestinal and hepatic toxicity of hydrolyzed fumonisin B(1) correlates with its inability to alter the metabolism of sphingolipids. *Biochem. Pharmacol.* **2012**, *83*, 1465–1473. [CrossRef] [PubMed]

35. Gerez, J.R.R.; Pinton, P.; Callu, P.; Grosjean, F.; Oswald, I.P.P.; Bracarense, A.P.F.L.P. Deoxynivalenol alone or in combination with nivalenol andzearalenone induce systemic histological changes in pigs. *Exp. Toxicol. Pathol.* **2015**, *67*, 89–98. [CrossRef] [PubMed]

36. García, G.R.; Payros, D.; Pinton, P.; Dogi, C.A.; Laffitte, J.; Neves, M.; González Pereyra, M.L.; Cavaglieri, L.R.; Oswald, I.P. Intestinal toxicity of deoxynivalenol is limited by Lactobacillus rhamnosus RC007 in pig jejunum explants. *Arch. Toxicol.* **2018**, *92*, 983–993. [CrossRef] [PubMed]

37. Pierron, A.; Mimoun, S.; Murate, L.S.; Loiseau, N.; Lippi, Y.; Bracarense, A.F.L.; Schatzmayr, G.; He, J.W.; Zhou, T.; Moll, W.D.; et al. Microbial biotransformation of DON: Molecular basis for reduced toxicity. *Sci. Rep.* **2016**, *6*, 29105. [CrossRef] [PubMed]

38. Cano, P.M.; Seeboth, J.; Meurens, F.; Cognie, J.; Abrami, R.; Oswald, I.P.; Guzylack-Piriou, L. Deoxynivalenol as a new factor in the persistence of intestinal inflammatory diseases: An emerging hypothesis through possible modulation of Th17-mediated response. *PLoS ONE* **2013**, *8*, e53647. [CrossRef] [PubMed]

39. Andersen, C.; Jensen, J.; Orntoft, T. Normalization of Real Time Quantitative Reverse Transcription—PCR Data: A Model—Based Variance Estimation Approach to Identify Genes Suited for Normalization, Applied to Bladder and Colon Cancer Data Sets. *Cancer Res.* **2004**, *64*, 5245. [CrossRef] [PubMed]

40. Ruijter, J.M.; Ramakers, C.; Hoogaars, W.M.H.; Karlen, Y.; Bakker, O.; van den hoff, M.J.B.; Moorman, A.F.M. Amplification efficiency: Linking baseline and bias in the analysis of quantitative PCR data. *Nucleic Acids Res.* **2009**, *37*. [CrossRef] [PubMed]

41. Alassane-Kpembi, I.; Gerez, J.R.; Cossalter, A.-M.; Neves, M.; Laffitte, J.; Naylies, C.; Lippi, Y.; Kolf-Clauw, M.; Bracarense, A.P.L.; Pinton, P.; et al. Intestinal toxicity of the type B trichothecene mycotoxin fusarenon-X: Whole transcriptome profiling reveals new signaling pathways. *Sci. Rep.* **2017**, *7*, 7530. [CrossRef] [PubMed]

42. Pinton, P.; Graziani, F.; Pujol, A.; Nicoletti, C.; Paris, O.; Ernouf, P.; Di Pasquale, E.; Perrier, J.; Oswald, I.P.P.; Maresca, M.; et al. Deoxynivalenol inhibits the expression by goblet cells of intestinal mucins through a PKR and MAP kinase-dependent repression of the resistin-like molecule beta. *Mol. Nutr. Food Res.* **2015**, *59*, 1076–1087. [CrossRef] [PubMed]

43. Yamagata, K.; Tagami, M.; Takenaga, F.; Yamori, Y.; Itoh, S. Hypoxia-induced changes in tight junction permeability of brain capillary endothelial cells are associated with IL-1beta and nitric oxide. *Neurobiol. Dis.* **2004**, *17*, 491–499. [CrossRef] [PubMed]

44. Pfaffl, M.; Horgan, G.; Dempfle, L. Relative expression software tool (REST) for group-wise comparison and statistical analysis of relative expression results in real-time PCR. *Nucleic Acids Res.* **2002**, *30*, e36. [CrossRef] [PubMed]

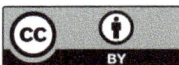

toxins

MDPI

Article

The Genotoxicity of Caecal Water in Gilts Exposed to Low Doses of Zearalenone

Katarzyna Cieplińska [1], Magdalena Gajęcka [2,*], Adriana Nowak [3], Michał Dąbrowski [2], Łukasz Zielonka [2] and Maciej T. Gajęcki [2]

[1] Microbiology Laboratory, Non-Public Health Care Centre, ul. Limanowskiego 31A, 10-342 Olsztyn, Poland; kasiacieplinska@gmail.com
[2] Department of Veterinary Prevention and Feed Hygiene, Faculty of Veterinary Medicine, University of Warmia and Mazury in Olsztyn, Oczapowskiego 13, 10-718 Olsztyn, Poland; michal.dabrowski@uwm.edu.pl (M.D.); lukaszz@uwm.edu.pl (Ł.Z.); gajecki@uwm.edu.pl (M.T.G.)
[3] Institute of Fermentation Technology and Microbiology, Lodz University of Technology, 90-924 Lodz, Poland; adriana.nowak@p.lodz.pl
* Correspondence: mgaja@uwm.edu.pl; Tel.: +48-89-523-3773; Fax: +48-89-523-3618

Received: 6 July 2018; Accepted: 28 August 2018; Published: 1 September 2018

Abstract: Zearalenone is a toxic low-molecular-weight molecule that is naturally produced by moulds on crops as a secondary metabolite. The aim of this study was to determine the genotoxicity of caecal water collected successively from the caecal contents of gilts exposed to low doses (LOAEL, NOAEL, and MABEL) of zearalenone. The experiment was performed on 60 clinically healthy gilts with average BW of 14.5 ± 2 kg, divided into three experimental groups and a control group. Group ZEN5 were orally administered ZEN at 5 μg/kg BW, group ZEN10—10 μg ZEN/kg BW and group ZEN15—15 μg ZEN/kg BW. Five gilts from every group were euthanized on analytical dates 1, 2, and 3. Caecal water samples for in vitro analysis were collected from the ileocaecal region. The genotoxicity of caecal water was noted, particularly after date 1 in groups ZEN10 and ZEN15 with a decreasing trend. Electrophoresis revealed the presence of numerous comets without tails in groups C and ZEN5 and fewer comets with clearly expressed tails in groups ZEN10 and ZEN15. The distribution of LLC-PK1 cells ranged from 15% to 20% in groups C and ZEN5, and from 30% to 60% in groups ZEN10 and ZEN15. The analysis of caecal water genotoxicity during exposure to very low doses of ZEN revealed the presence of a counter response and a compensatory effect in gilts.

Keywords: zearalenone; doses; caecal water; genotoxicity; pre-pubertal gilts

Key contribution: The extent of DNA damage was proportional to the ingested mycotoxin dose. Therefore, the proposed MABEL dose could be considered as a preventive dose for pre-pubertal gilts.

1. Introduction

The symptoms and health (toxicological) consequences of exposure to high doses of most mycotoxins, in particular, zearalenone (ZEN), are generally well known [1,2]. Research conducted in the past decade demonstrated that exposure to low doses of the parent compound without modified mycotoxins can also lead to health problems [3]. Similar findings had been reported previously by members of the EFSA Panel on Contaminants in the Food Chain [4,5]. The above is confirmed by the hormesis paradigm [6,7]. Doses below the lowest observed adverse effect level (LOAEL) values [8,9] that produce subclinical symptoms of disease are referred to as no observed adverse effect levels (NOAEL) doses [10]. The lowest measurable dose that enters positive interactions with the host's body in various stages of life is known as the minimal anticipated biological effect level (MABEL) dose [11]. The dose-response paradigm has been undermined by the low dose hypothesis.

The above applies particularly to hormonally active compounds [12], including mycosteroids such as ZEN. The dose-response relationship is ambiguous, and it does not support direct and monotone extrapolation or meta-analysis of the risks (clinical symptoms or laboratory results) associated with the shift from a high to a low dose [13]. The concept of a minimal dose (MABEL) that induces a counter-intuitive response is garnering increasing interest in biomedical sciences. The mechanisms associated with the MABEL dose must be researched to quantify the relevant risks and final outcomes [14] in the decision-making process.

Most *Fusarium* mycotoxins are absorbed primarily in the proximal segment of the small intestine [15]. Intestinal fragments are characterized by high physiological variability. The duodenum and the jejunum have the lowest content of mucus glycoproteins, which maximizes the availability of digesta for intestinal walls [16] and, consequently, the body. Most carbohydrates are also absorbed in the proximal segment of the small intestine [17], which promotes absorption, accumulation, and, probably, biotransformation of mycotoxins in enterocytes [18,19].

The highest percentage content of ZEN was observed in the small intestine in early stages of exposure. On successive days of exposure, ZEN was also accumulated in the duodenum and the descending colon. During exposure to the parent compound (ZEN) only, biotransformation processes were not observed or were significantly inhibited in the porcine gastrointestinal tract [20]. The accumulation of ZEN in intestinal tissues began already in the first week of exposure.

According to research into the changes that accompany exposure to small ZEN doses [21], the mycotoxin can produce side effects that are difficult to predict. This uncertainty is associated with both the dose and the duration of exposure. The exposure to small doses often produces surprising effects: (i) The body fails to recognize the presence of undesirable substances, such as mycotoxins [22], and the underlying principle is similar to the T-regs theory [23], postulating that these cells do not respond to small amounts of infectious factors; (ii) Mycotoxin absorption increases during prolonged *per os* exposure to ZEN [20]; (iii) The compensatory effect [24] inhibits the analysed factors, and homeostasis is restored [13] despite ongoing exposure.

Minimal doses of undesirable substances such as ZEN can be used for preventive or even therapeutic purposes. The genotoxicity of various (perhaps threshold) doses of the administered compound should be studied to determine their mutagenic effects. Fleck et al. [25] and Pfeiffer et al. [26] compared the genotoxicity of estradiol (E_2), estrone (E_1), ZEN, and α-zearalenol in a cell-free system and found that these compounds had similar DNA-damaging potential to endogenous steroids, and that they enhanced the carcinogenic effects of endogenous estrogens. These results are difficult to apply to the results of in vivo studies, which investigate the correlations between the dose and DNA-damaging potential.

De Ruyck et al. [27] observed that various substances, including carcinogenic compounds, are accumulated in the bodily tissues of animals exposed to ZEN. The epithelium of the digestive tract is exposed first to the ingested low doses of ZEN [28–31]. The intestinal mucosa prevents antigens, including undesirable substances such as ZEN, commensal bacteria, and pathogens from penetrating deeper tissues [32]. In a study by Nowak et al. [33], ZEN administered *per os* at 40 µg/kg BW increased the genotoxicity of caecal water (CW), mainly in the sixth week of the experiment, in the proximal and distal segments of the large intestine. Genotoxicity also increased in the proximal part of the colon. The authors suggested that the slow transit of intestinal contents after exposure to ZEN [34] increased the risk of adverse changes, including carcinogenic changes, in tissues containing estrogen receptors [35].

Genotoxins such as ZEN can damage DNA [36]. In somatic cells, DNA damage can lead to somatic mutations and, consequently, malignant transformations. There is a wide variety of in vitro and in vivo genotoxicity tests supporting the detection of many terminal points of DNA damage or its biological consequences for eukaryotic cells, including in mammals [37]. These tests should be used to evaluate the safety of feedstuffs and detect the presence of undesirable substances, including mycotoxins, in animal feed.

The comet assay is one of the most popular techniques for detecting DNA damage. The test is highly sensitive, and it can be performed on a small number of cells. Several modifications of the comet assay have been proposed to detect various types of DNA damage. The alkaline comet assay detects a combination of DNA changes, including single- and double-strand breaks, and alkali-labile sites [37]. Several indicators are used in the comet test, but the percentage of DNA damage in the comet tail (%DNAT) is regarded as the most reliable indicator, because it covers the broadest range of DNA damage and is linearly correlated with the frequency of DNA breaks [37]. For this reason, %DNAT was the indicator of choice in this study.

The above arguments indicate that prolonged oral administration of a natural parent compound such as ZEN increases carry-over values in successive segments of the gastrointestinal tract and increases the concentration of ZEN in digesta [20]. The degree of exposure can be evaluated by analysing the contents of the distal fragment of the digestive tract. The results of such analyses constitute valuable inputs for dietary intervention studies [33]. Biological markers are used to detect the DNA-damaging potential and/or mutagenic effects in digesta sampled from different intestinal segments. The aim of this study was to evaluate the genotoxicity of CW collected successively from the caecal contents of gilts exposed to low (LOAEL, NOAEL, and MABEL) doses of ZEN.

2. Results

2.1. Experimental Feed

The analysed feed did not contain mycotoxins, or its mycotoxin content was below the sensitivity of the method (VBS). The concentrations of modified and masked mycotoxins were not analysed.

2.2. Clinical Observations

Clinical signs of ZEN mycotoxicosis were not observed throughout the experiment. However, changes in specific tissues or cells were frequently observed in analyses of selected biochemical parameters in samples collected from the same animals and in those animals' growth performance. The results of these analyses were published in a different paper [38].

2.3. General Information

The percentage of DNA damage in the comet tail (%DNAT) of non-exposed cells (negative control, LLC-PK1 cells in DMEM/Ham's F12 medium) was determined at 4.1% ± 0.7%. In cells exposed to 25 µM hydrogen peroxide (positive control), %DNAT reached 86.3% ± 2.3%.

2.4. Single Cell Gel Electrophoreses (Comet Assay)

The genotoxicity of CW (Figure 1) obtained from gilts exposed to different ZEN doses was determined on three analytical dates. On every date, CW genotoxicity was lowest in group C (control group) with mean values of 19.5% to 22.0% and standard error of the mean (S.E.M.) of 2.7% and 1.9%, respectively.

No significant differences (Figure 1) were observed on analytical date 1 between groups C and ZEN5 (5 µg ZEN/kg BW), whereas the differences between groups ZEN10 (10 µg ZEN/kg BW) and ZEN15 (15 µg ZEN/kg BW) were significant. Similar differences were noted on date 2. On date 3, significant differences were observed between group C and groups ZEN5 and ZEN15 and between groups C and ZEN10 and groups ZEN5 and ZEN15.

Significant differences (Figure 1) between analytical dates were noted between groups ZEN10 and ZEN15 on date 1 vs. group ZEN10 on date 3 and group ZEN15 on date 2, and between group ZEN5 values on analytical dates 2 and 3.

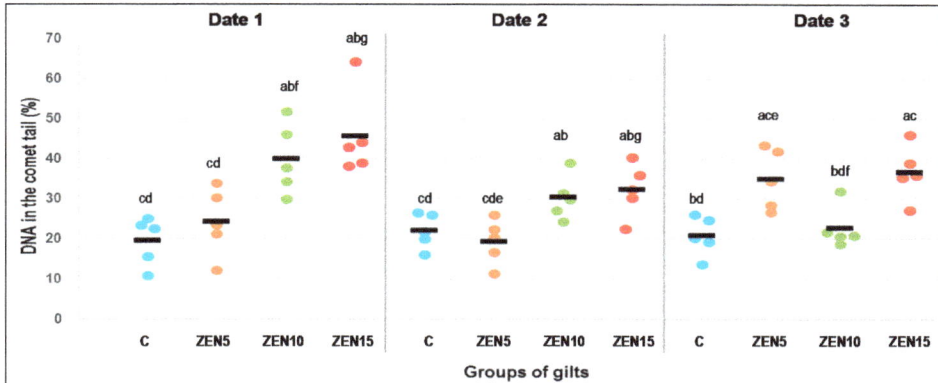

Figure 1. DNA damage expressed by the mean number of DNA breaks in the LLC-PK1 porcine kidney epithelial cell line of control gilts and gilts administered ZEN doses of 5, 10, and 15 µg ZEN/kg BW. Samples were collected on analytical dates 1, 2, and 3. A total of 100 cells was scored for each individual. Mean results differ significantly from: [a] control group, [b] ZEN5 group, [c] ZEN10 group, and [d] ZEN15 group values in a given week and [e,f,g] between the same concentrations of ZEN on different dates; ANOVA ($p \leq 0.05$).

Significant differences ($p \leq 0.05$) are indicative of genotoxicity (Figure 2—clear comet tail). On analytical date 1, an increase was observed in groups ZEN10 and ZEN15, in which mean values reached 40.0% ± 7.5% and 45.6% ± 7.4%, respectively, relative to groups C and ZEN5 (Figure 1), in which mean values were determined 19.8% ± 5.44% and 24.1% ± 6.26%, respectively.

On analytical date 2, %DNAT values were significantly less scattered across groups, but they were significantly more scattered in groups ZEN10 and ZEN15 (30.2% ± 3.9% and 32.2% ± 4.7%, respectively) relative to group C (21.8% ± 3.15%) and even more scattered relative in group ZEN5 (19.2% ± 4.25%) ($p \leq 0.05$). These data indicate that genotoxic processes took place in groups ZEN10 and ZEN15, but not in groups C or ZEN5.

On analytical date 3, %DNAT was determined at 20.7% ± 3.67% in group C. In the LLC-PK1 cell line, %DNAT values in group ZEN5 increased in the range of 26.5% ± 3.3% to 43.3% ± 3.3%, with a mean value of 34.9% ± 6.2%. In group ZEN10, mean genotoxicity was determined at 22.6% ± 3.7% %DNAT, and it was lower than on dates 1 and 2 (40.0% ± 7.5% and 30.2% ± 3.9%, respectively) ($p \leq 0.05$). In group ZEN15, %DNAT ranged from 27.0% ± 9.6% to 45.9% ± 9.34% (Figure 1), with a mean value 36.6% ± 4.7%.

The values of correlation coefficients (Pearson's *r*) (Table 1) were calculated based on the relationship between the percentage of cells with damaged DNA and the percentage of DNA damage in a cell on different analytical dates and in different groups.

Table 1. Correlation coefficients (Pearson's *r*).

Analytical Date	Group C	Group ZEN5	Group ZEN10	Group ZEN15
1	0.29	0.29	0.52	0.61
2	0.45	0.16	0.41	0.08
3	0.26	0.07	0.44	0.46

Key: Ratio between the percentage of cells with damaged DNA and the percentage of DNA damage in a cell on different analytical dates and in different groups: Group C—placebo; Group ZEN5—5 µg ZEN/kg BW, administered once daily before morning feeding; Group ZEN10—10 µg ZEN/kg BW, administered once daily before morning feeding; Group ZEN15—15 µg ZEN/kg BW, administered once daily before morning feeding. Samples were collected immediately after euthanasia on three analytical dates (exposure days 7, 21, and 42).

The results presented in Table 1 should be analysed in view of the strength of the observed correlations [39]. The correlation is positive when $r > 0$. The strength of correlations is evaluated on the following scale: $r < 0.2$—absence of a linear correlation; $r = 0.2$–0.4—weak correlation; $r = 0.4$–0.7—moderate correlation; $r = 0.7$–0.9—relatively strong correlation; and $r > 0.9$—very strong correlation. A weak correlation and a moderate correlation were noted in group C on two dates (very low %DNAT, which is natural). In group ZEN5, a weak correlation was observed initially, followed by an absence of linear correlations on two successive dates (very low %DNAT, which could suggest that the analysed ZEN dose has protective effects). A moderate correlation was noted in group ZEN10 and in group ZEN15, but an absence of a linear correlation was noted on date 2 in group ZEN15. Very low values of r in groups C and ZEN5 point to the presence of certain trends with some outliers. Genotoxicity was confirmed when the values of r were closer to 1. The above was noted in group ZEN15, but the observed trend was highly variable.

The electrophoresis of exposed cells revealed an absence of comet tails (even short tails) and nearly symmetrical comets in groups C and ZEN5 (Figure 2A). Groups ZEN10 and ZEN15 were characterized by comets with relatively long and long tails with damaged DNA, respectively (Figure 2B). These comets had very long tails and small heads. Their density (number of comets per slide) was considerably lower than in group C.

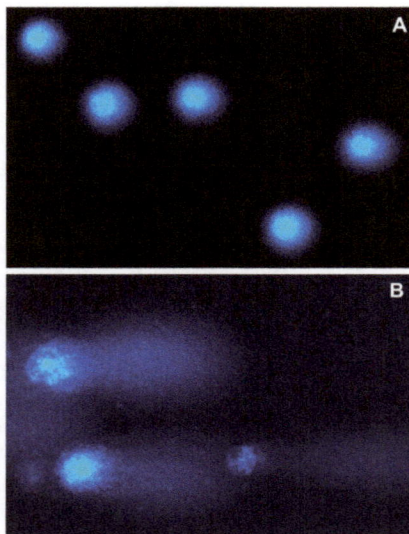

Figure 2. Typical images of DAPI-stained (4′,6-diamidino-2-phenylindole) comets: (**A**) group C; and (**B**) group ZEN15 on analytical date 1.

2.5. Histograms of Endogenous DNA Damage

The distribution of LLC-PK1 cells based on the percentage of damaged DNA in the comet tail is presented in Figure 3. In group C, maximum %DNAT values were distributed in columns 5% or 10% on date 1 (Figure 3A), in columns 5% or 15% on date 2 (Figure 3E), and in columns 10% or 15% on date 3 (Figure 3I). The maximum percentage of cells with damaged DNA was relatively low (below 20%).

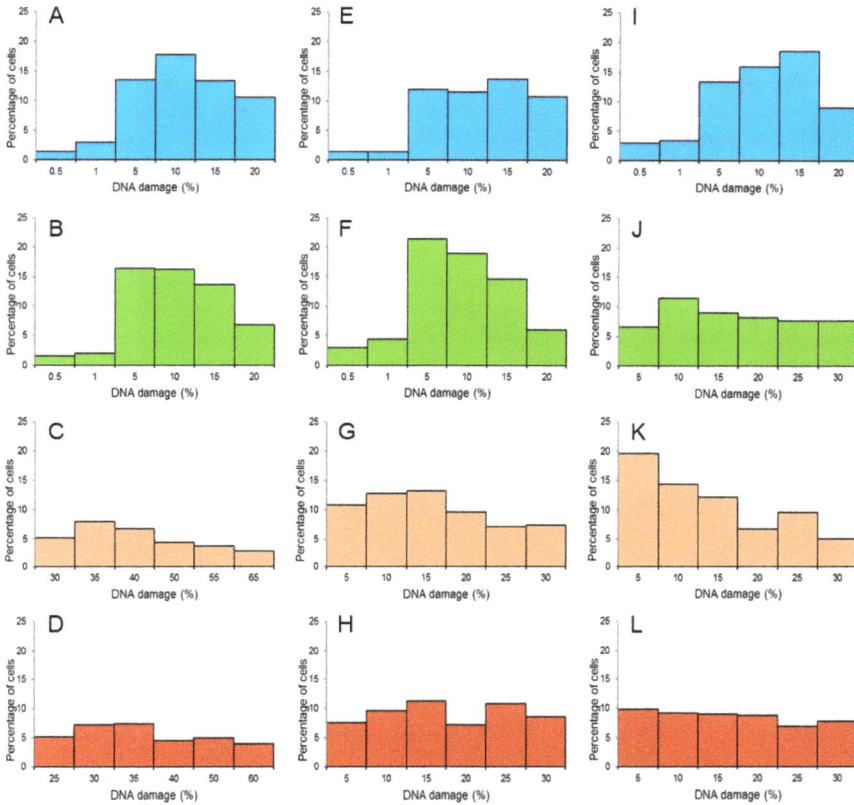

Figure 3. Histograms illustrating the distribution of endogenous DNA damage, measured as the mean %DNAT of porcine kidney epithelial cells (LLC-PK1 cell line) in: group C (**A,E,I**), CW of gilts fed with group ZEN5 (**B,F,J**), group ZEN10 (**C,G,K**) and group ZN15 (**D,H,L**). Analytical dates—date 1 (**A–D**), date 2 (**E–H**) and date 3 (**I–L**). A total of 100 cells were scored for each individual.

The distribution of cells with damaged DNA was similar in group ZEN5, in columns 5–15% (Figure 3B,F,J). On the first two analytical dates, %DNAT values were distributed in columns 5% or 10% (Figure 3B,F), and on date 3–in columns 10% or 15% (Figure 3J). On date 2, the maximum number of cells with damaged DNA exceeded 20% (Figure 3F), but it was noted in column 5%.

In groups ZEN10 and ZEN15, the maximum percentage of cells was very low (<10) on analytical date 1 (Figure 3C,D), but maximum %DNAT was distributed in columns 35% or 40% in group ZEN10 and in columns 30% or 35% in group ZEN15 (Figure 3C,D, respectively). In group ZEN10, the maximum percentage of cells with damaged DNA increased to 14% on date 2 (Figure 3G) and to nearly 20% on date 3 (Figure 3K). The maximum %DNAT values were distributed in columns 10% or 15% on date 2 (Figure 3G) and in columns 5% or 10% on date 3 (Figure 3K). In group ZEN15, the maximum percentage of cells with damaged DNA was estimated at 10% on analytical dates 2 and 3 (Figure 3H,L, respectively). The maximum %DNAT values were distributed in columns 15% or 25% on date 2 (Figure 3H) and in columns 5% or 10% on date 3 (Figure 3L).

3. Discussion

Zearalenone ingested with feed can lead to endocrinological disorders in humans and animals. Zearalenone is a macrocyclic β-resorcylic acid lactone with distinctive estrogen activity. Previous studies into the metabolism of ZEN revealed the presence of reducing metabolites, in particular α-zearalenol and its stereoisomer β-zearalenol. During the synthesis of these catechol metabolites, ZEN activity becomes similar to that of endogenous estrogens E_2 and E_1. These promiscuous steroids [40] and steroid-like substances are associated with the risk of bowel cancer [41], breast cancer [35], uterine cancer [9], and malignant changes in other estrogen-sensitive organs [21]. There is evidence to indicate that E_2/E_1 catechol metabolites are weak genotoxins that contribute to malignant transformations by producing quinones that generate DNA adducts [42]. Catechol production is the main metabolic pathway of ZEN and its metabolites in many mammals [43], including humans [44]. The above could suggest that even small doses of ZEN contribute to CW genotoxicity [25].

In this experiment, the tested ZEN doses confirmed that dose plays an important role during exposure to undesirable compounds. The above is validated by the results of the statistical analysis, which revealed a significant increase ($p < 0.05$) in CW genotoxicity on different analytical dates. The only exception was date 1 (exposure day 7) when maximum %DNAT values reached 39.8% ± 4.0% in group ZEN10 and 45.6% ± 4.8% in group ZEN15. The above results were among the highest %DNAT values noted in the experiment. The distribution of LLC-PK1 cells in groups C and ZEN5 based on their %DNAT values in comet tails ranged from 15% to 20%, which is a very low result when negative control values are subtracted (4.1%). These findings could point to the absence of genotoxicity in group ZEN5.

Similar observations were made in an analysis of the correlations between the percentage of cells with damaged DNA to the percentage of DNA damage in a cell (Pearson's r) (Table 1). On analytical date 1, r values were equally low in group ZEN5 and in group C, which could validate the hypothesis that small amounts of undesirable substances are not detected by the body (similarly to the T-regs theory, which postulates that T-regs do not respond to small amounts of infectious factors) [23]. Zearalenone was recognised by the body only on analytical date 3, as in group C. The proposed MABEL dose probably approximated threshold values [25,26]. It should also be noted that pre-pubertal gilts are characterised by physiological hypoestrogenism [21] when the demand for estrogens exceeds supply. As an exogenous estrogen, ZEN (mycoestrogen) can be utilized by the body to exert protective effects. Interestingly, r values in group ZEN5 continued to decrease on successive analytical dates (Table 1), which could indicate that the MABEL dose (5 µg ZEN/kg BW) exerted a protective effect on gilts throughout the experiment.

In contrast, the values of r observed in groups ZEN10 (10 µg/kg BW—NOAEL) and ZEN15 (15 µg/kg BW—LOAEL) on date 1 point to hyperestrogenism, namely, the presence of "free" ZEN in the body. Hyperestrogenism increases %DNAT values, namely, the percentage of comets with much longer tails and small heads (Figure 2B) whose density was significantly lower than in group C (Figure 2A). The above suggests that CW genotoxicity, preceded by oxidative damage and mitotic spindle dysfunction, is induced already by the NOAEL dose (10 µg ZEN/kg BW) [42]. The above is generally accompanied by a host of genotoxic effects in CW, including intensified Ca^{2+} transfer to cells [45] and changes in the activity of selected hydroxysteroid dehydrogenase enzymes [46], which can lead to steroidogenesis disorders [19].

The ZEN doses administered to groups ZEN10 and ZEN15 induced CW genotoxicity, but the observed correlations were moderate ($r = 0.4$ to 0.7, Table 1) with a decreasing trend (Figure 3). According to Błasiak et al. [47], the results of the comet assay should be analysed based on the distribution of cells based on damage to their DNA (histograms) to determine the susceptibility of individual cells to DNA damage. The histograms illustrating the distribution of damage to endogenous DNA (Figure 3G,H,K,L) in the experimental cells differ significantly between groups. On analytical date 1, the histograms for groups ZEN10 and ZEN15 (Figure 3C,D) were very strongly shifted toward higher values (from 20% to 65%). On date 2, the extent of DNA damage decreased 1.3- to 1.4-fold relative to date 1. On the last two analytical dates, the histograms for groups ZEN10 and ZEN15 were significantly flattened and shifted toward higher values in comparison with the histograms for groups C and ZEN5 (Figure 3H,L). This could imply that under exposure to higher ZEN doses, genotoxic processes in CW are initially more expressed and can provoke clinical symptoms. On successive days of exposure, genotoxic processes in CW were still more pronounced than in groups C and ZEN5. The above could be attributed to the fact that in gilts exposed to ZEN, the carry-over of ZEN to tissues other than the intestines [20], the initiation of biotransformation processes in the liver, the detoxifying activity of gut microbiota [48], and the conversion of modified mycotoxins to a free form in the colon [3] proceeded at a faster rate than the destruction of DNA in the caecal epithelium.

The results of this study suggest that ZEN has a damaging effect on cells cultured in vitro and, most importantly, on cells on the organism of gilts. The values corresponding to the percentage of DNA breaks in cells were highly scattered. On successive days of exposure to ZEN, damage histograms were flattened and shifted toward lower values in groups C and ZEN5 and were shifted toward higher values in groups ZEN10 and ZEN15, which indicates that the counter response in the porcine model is influenced by the amount of ZEN ingested with feed.

The present results support the formulation of two hypotheses. The first hypothesis postulates the presence of a compensatory effect based on the values of r in groups ZEN10 and ZEN15, which were higher on analytical date 1 than on successive days of exposure. The second hypothesis states that the proposed MABEL dose is not genotoxic, but further research is needed to confirm this observation.

4. Conclusions

The results of this study, which investigated CW genotoxicity, indicate that very small doses of ZEN (LOAEL, NOAEL, and MABEL) induce a counter response and a compensatory effect in the porcine model. The extent of DNA damage was proportional to the administered mycotoxin dose. Our findings suggest that the MABEL dose could be used for preventive purposes in pre-pubertal gilts.

5. Materials and Methods

5.1. In Vivo Study

5.1.1. General Information

All experimental procedures involving animals were carried out in compliance with Polish regulations setting forth the terms and conditions of animal experimentation (Opinions No. 12/2016 and 45/2016/DLZ of the Local Ethics Committee for Animal Experimentation of 27 April 2016 and 30 November 2016).

5.1.2. Experimental Animals and Feed

The in vivo experiment was performed at the Department of Veterinary Prevention and Feed Hygiene of the Faculty of Veterinary Medicine at the University of Warmia and Mazury in Olsztyn on 60 clinically healthy pre-pubertal gilts with initial BW of 14.5 ± 2 kg. The animals were housed in pens with free access to water. All groups of gilts received the same feed throughout the experiment. They were randomly assigned to three experimental groups (group ZEN5, group ZEN10, and group ZEN15; n = 15) and a control group (group C; n = 15) [49,50]. Group ZEN5 gilts were orally administered ZEN (Z2125-26MG, Sigma-Aldrich, St. Louis, MO, USA) at 5 µg ZEN/kg BW, group ZEN10 pigs–10 µg ZEN/kg BW, and group ZEN15 pigs–15 µg ZEN/kg BW. Analytical samples of ZEN were dissolved in 96 µL of 96% ethanol (SWW 2442-90, Polskie Odczynniki SA, Poland) in weight-appropriate doses. Feed containing different doses of ZEN in an alcohol solution was placed in gel capsules. The capsules were stored at room temperature before administration to evaporate the alcohol. In the experimental groups, ZEN was administered daily in gel capsules before morning feeding. The animals were weighed at weekly intervals, and the results were used to adjust individual mycotoxin doses. Feed was the carrier, and group C pigs were administered the same gel capsules but without mycotoxins.

The feed administered to all experimental animals was supplied by the same producer. Friable feed was provided *ad libitum* twice daily, at 8:00 a.m. and 5:00 p.m., throughout the experiment. The composition of the complete diet, as declared by the manufacturer, is presented in Table 2.

Table 2. Declared composition of the complete diet.

Parameters	Composition Declared by the Manufacturer (%)
Soybean meal	16
Wheat	55
Barley	22
Wheat bran	4.0
Chalk	0.3
Zitrosan	0.2
Vitamin-mineral premix [1]	2.5

[1] Composition of the vitamin-mineral premix per kg: vitamin A–500.000 IU; iron–5000 mg; vitamin D3–100.000 IU; zinc–5000 mg; vitamin E (alpha-tocopherol)–2000 mg; manganese–3000 mg; vitamin K–150 mg; copper ($CuSO_4 \cdot 5H_2O$)–500 mg; vitamin B_1–100 mg; cobalt–20 mg; vitamin B_2–300 mg; iodine–40 mg; vitamin B_6–150 mg; selenium–15 mg; vitamin B_{12}–1500 µg; L-lysine–9.4 g; niacin–1200 mg; DL-methionine+cystine–3.7 g; pantothenic acid–600 mg; L-threonine–2.3 g; folic acid–50 mg; tryptophan–1.1 g; biotin–7500 µg; phytase+choline–10 g; ToyoCerin probiotic+calcium–250 g; antioxidant + mineral phosphorus and released phosphorus–60 g; magnesium–5 g; sodium; calcium–51 g.

The proximate chemical composition of diets fed to pigs in groups C, ZEN5, ZEN10, and ZEN15 was determined using the NIRS™ DS2500 F feed analyser (FOSS, Hillerød, Denmark), a monochromator-based NIR reflectance and transflectance analyser with a scanning range of 850–2500 nm.

5.1.3. Toxicological Analysis

Feed was analysed for the presence of ZEN and DON by high-performance liquid chromatography with UV–vis detection (HPLC-UV). The obtained values did not exceed the limits of quantitation (LOQ) of 2 ng/g for ZEN and 5 ng/g for DON based on the validation of chromatographic methods for the determination of ZEN and DON levels in feed materials and feeds, which was performed at the Department [51].

5.1.4. Sampling for In Vitro Tests

Five gilts from every group were euthanized on analytical date 1 (exposure day 7), date 2 (exposure day 21), and date 3 (exposure day 42) by intravenous administration of pentobarbital sodium (Fatro, Ozzano Emilia BO, Italy) and bleeding. Sections of intestinal tissues were collected immediately after cardiac arrest and were prepared for analyses. Caecal water samples for in vitro analysis were collected from a 10-cm-long intestinal fragment resected from the ileocecal region and the colon. Intestinal segments were tied at both ends before resection to avoid tissue damage. The resected fragments were transported to the laboratory, and CW samples were analysed.

5.2. In Vitro Study

The in vitro experiment was performed at the Institute of Fermentation Technology and Microbiology, Lodz University of Technology in Lodz.

5.2.1. Caecal Water Preparation

Caecal water samples were collected in plastic containers. Freshly obtained caecal contents (20%) were mixed with sterile phosphate-buffered saline (PBS, pH 7.2) (80%), homogenised for 2 min, and centrifuged (10,700× g, 40 min, 4 °C). The supernatant fractions were filtered (0.45 μm pore size, Merck–Millipore, Darmstadt, Germany) and stored at −20 °C until analysis.

5.2.2. Cell Culture and Treatment

The LLC-PK1 porcine kidney epithelial cell line (Cell Lines Service, Eppelheim, Germany) from 38 passage was used in the research. This cell line is often used to test the genotoxicity and cytotoxicity of mycotoxins [36,52].

The cells were cultured in T75 flasks (Roux type) (Becton, Dickinson and Co., Franklin Lakes, NJ, USA) as a monolayer in Dulbecco's Modified Eagle's Medium/Ham's F12 (DMEM/Ham's F12, 1:1; Cell Lines Service, Eppelheim, Germany) with 5% foetal bovine serum (FBS, Cell Lines Service, Eppelheim, Germany), supplemented with 2 mM L-glutamine (Cell Lines Service, Eppelheim, Germany) and HEPES (Cell Lines Service, Eppelheim, Germany). The cells were incubated in a CO_2 incubator (Galaxy 48S, New Brunswick, UK) at 37 °C under 5% CO_2 atmosphere for 7 days, until confluence. The cells were sub-cultivated, and the medium was changed every 2–3 days. LLC-PK1 cells were detached with TrypLE™ Express (Gibco, Thermo Fisher Scientific, Waltham, MA, USA) for 20 min and gently shaken off the plastic flask. According to the manufacturer's instructions, neutralisation with FBS is not required for reagents of the plant origin. After detaching, the cell suspension in PBS (Sigma-Aldrich, St. Louis, MO, USA) was transferred to a Falcon tube, centrifuged (182× g, 5 min), decanted, and resuspended in fresh medium. Cell counts and viability were determined by trypan blue exclusion assay (min. 90%), and the cells were ready to use.

5.2.3. Comet Assay—Single Cell Gel Electrophoresis Assay (SCGE)

The final concentration of LLC-PK1 cells in each sample was adjusted to 10^5 cells/mL. The cells were incubated with CW (20%, v/v) at 37 °C for 1 h. The cells were incubated in a medium without FBS to avoid interactions between FBS and the mycotoxin.

The comet assay was performed under alkaline conditions (pH > 13) according to Błasiak and Kowalik [53], as described previously [33]. After incubation, the cells were centrifuged (182× g, 15 min, 4 °C), decanted, suspended in 0.75% low melting point (LMP) agarose (Sigma-Aldrich, St. Louis, MO, USA), layered onto slides precoated with 0.5% normal melting (NMP) agarose (Sigma-Aldrich, St. Louis, MO, USA), and lysed at 4 °C for 1 h in a buffer consisting of: 2.5 M NaCl, 1% Triton X-100, 100 mM EDTA and 10 mM Tris, pH 10. Next, the slides were placed in an electrophoresis unit, and DNA was allowed to unwind for 20 min in an unwinding buffer containing 300 mM NaOH and 1 mM EDTA. Electrophoresis was conducted at 4 °C for 20 min at field strength of 0.73 V/cm (300 mA) in electrophoretic buffer containing 30 mM NaOH and 1 mM EDTA. Then, the slides were neutralised (0.4 mol/L Tris), stained with 1 μg/mL 4′,6-diamidino-2-phenylindole (DAPI, Sigma-Aldrich, St. Louis, MO, USA), and covered with cover slips. The slides were analysed at 200× magnification under a fluorescence microscope (Nikon, Tokyo, Japan) connected to a digital camera (Nikon Digital Sight DS-U3, Tokyo, Japan) and the Lucia-Comet v. 7.0 digital image analysis system (Laboratory Imaging, Prague, Czech Republic). One hundred images were randomly selected from each sample, and %DNAT was determined as a measure of DNA damage.

5.2.4. Statistical Analysis

Comet assay data were analysed by two-way analysis of variance (ANOVA), and mode of interaction × time was used to compare the effects induced by the chemicals in the analysed mode of interaction. Differences between samples with normal distribution were evaluated. ANOVA was performed using OriginPro 6.1 software (OriginLab Corporation, Northampton, MA, USA). Dose–response relationships were determined by Pearson's correlation. Differences were regarded as significant at $p \leq 0.05$. The results were presented as means ± standard error of the mean (S.E.M.).

Author Contributions: Conceptualization, M.G. and M.T.G.; Methodology, K.C., A.N., M.G. and M.D.; Software, M.G., A.N. and M.D.; Validation M.D. and Ł.Z.; Formal Analysis A.N. and K.C.; Investigation K.C.; M.D., M.G. and A.N.; Resources A.N.; Writing-original draft K.C. and A.N.; Project administration Ł.Z.; Writing-review and editing K.C., M.G. and M.T.G.

Funding: This research was funded by the "Healthy Animal–Safe Food" Scientific Consortium of the Leading National Research Centre (KNOW) pursuant to a decision of the Ministry of Science and Higher Education No. 05-1/KNOW2/2015. Publication cost was covered by KNOW (Leading National Research Center) Scientific Consortium "Healthy Animal-Safe Food", which was decided by the Ministry of Science and Higher Education No. 05-1/KNOW2/2015.

Conflicts of Interest: The authors declare no conflict of interest.

References

1. Zachariasova, M.; Dzumana, Z.; Veprikova, Z.; Hajkovaa, K.; Jiru, M.; Vaclavikova, M.; Zachariasova, A.; Pospichalova, M.; Florian, M.; Hajslova, J. Occurrence of multiple mycotoxins in European feeding stuffs, assessment of dietary intake by farm animals. *Anim. Feed Sci. Technol.* **2014**, *193*, 124–140. [CrossRef]

2. EFSA CONTAM Panel (EFSA Panel on Contaminants in the Food Chain). Scientific opinion on the risks for animal health related to the presence of zearalenone and its modified forms in feed. *EFSA J.* **2017**, *15*, 4851. [CrossRef]

3. Freire, L.; Sant'Ana, A.S. Modified mycotoxins: An updated review on their formation, detection, occurrence, and toxic effects. *Food Chem. Toxicol.* **2018**, *111*, 189–205. [CrossRef] [PubMed]

4. EFSA CONTAM Panel (EFSA Panel on Contaminants in the Food Chain). Scientific Opinion on the risks for human and animal health related to the presence of modified forms of certain mycotoxins in food and feed. *EFSA J.* **2014**, *12*, 3916. [CrossRef]

5. EFSA CONTAM Panel (EFSA Panel on Contaminants in the Food Chain). Scientific opinion on the appropriateness to set a group health-based guidance value for zearalenone and its modified forms. *EFSA J.* **2016**, *14*, 4425. [CrossRef]

6. Calabrese, E.J. Paradigm lost, paradigm found: The re-emergence of hormesis as a fundamental dose response model in the toxicological sciences. *Environ. Pollut.* **2005**, *138*, 378–411. [CrossRef] [PubMed]

7. Dobrzyński, L.; Fornalski, K.W. Hormesis-Natural phenomenon of answer of organism on stress. In Proceeding of VII International Scientific Conference: Veterinary Feed Hygiene—The Effects of Mycotoxins on Gastrointestinal Function, Olsztyn, Poland, 23–24 September 2011; pp. 6–14.

8. Gajęcka, M.; Zielonka, Ł.; Gajęcki, M. The effect of low monotonic doses of zearalenone on selected reproductive tissues in pre-pubertal female dogs—A review. *Molecules* **2015**, *20*, 20669–20687. [CrossRef] [PubMed]

9. Stopa, E.; Babińska, I.; Zielonka, Ł.; Gajęcki, M.; Gajęcka, M. Immunohistochemical evaluation of apoptosis and proliferation in the mucous membrane of selected uterine regions in pre-pubertal bitches exposed to low doses of zearalenone. *Pol. J. Vet. Sci.* **2016**, *19*, 175–186. [CrossRef] [PubMed]

10. Kramer, H.J.; van den Ham, W.A.; Slob, W.; Pieters, M.N. Conversion Factors Estimating Indicative Chronic No-Observed-Adverse-Effect Levels from Short-Term Toxicity Data. *Regul. Toxicol. Pharm.* **1996**, *23*, 249–255. [CrossRef] [PubMed]

11. Zielonka, Ł.; Jakimiuk, E.; Obremski, K.; Gajęcka, M.; Dąbrowski, M.; Gajęcki, M. An evaluation of the proliferative activity of immunocompetent cells in the jejunal and iliac lymph nodes of prepubertal female wild boars diagnosed with mixed mycotoxicosis. *B. Vet. I. Pulawy* **2015**, *59*, 197–203. [CrossRef]

12. Vandenberg, L.N.; Colborn, T.; Hayes, T.B.; Heindel, J.J.; Jacobs, D.R.; Lee, D.-H.; Shioda, T.; Soto, A.M.; vom Saal, F.S.; Welshons, W.V.; et al. Hormones and endocrine-disrupting chemicals: Low-dose effects and nonmonotonic dose responses. *Endocr. Rev.* **2012**, *33*, 378–455. [CrossRef] [PubMed]

13. Grenier, B.; Applegate, T.J. Modulation of intestinal functions following mycotoxin ingestion: Meta-analysis of published experiments in animals. *Toxins* **2013**, *5*, 396–430. [CrossRef] [PubMed]

14. Hickey, G.L.; Craig, P.S.; Luttik, R.; de Zwart, D. On the quantification of intertest variability in ecotoxicity data with application to species sensitivity distributions. *Environ. Toxicol. Chem.* **2012**, *31*, 1903–1910. [CrossRef] [PubMed]

15. Gajęcka, M.; Jakimiuk, E.; Zielonka, Ł.; Obremski, K.; Gajęcki, M. The biotransformation of chosen mycotoxins. *Pol. J. Vet. Sci.* **2009**, *12*, 293–303. [PubMed]

16. Bakhru, S.H.; Furtado, S.; Morello, A.P.; Mathiowitz, E. Oral delivery of proteins by biodegradable nanoparticles. *Adv. Drug Deliver. Rev.* **2013**, *65*, 811–821. [CrossRef] [PubMed]

17. Carlson, S.J.; Chang, M.I.; Nandivada, P.; Cowan, E.; Puder, M. Neonatal intestinal physiology and failure. *Semin. Pediatr. Surg.* **2013**, *22*, 190–194. [CrossRef] [PubMed]

18. Hueza, I.M.; Raspantini, P.C.F.; Raspantini, L.E.R.; Latorre, A.O.; Górniak, S.L. Zearalenone, an estrogenic mycotoxin, is an immunotoxic compound. *Toxins* **2014**, *6*, 1080–1095. [CrossRef] [PubMed]

19. Lupescu, A.; Bissinger, R.; Jilani, K.; Lang, F. In vitro induction of erythrocyte phosphatidyloserine translocation by the natural. *Naphthoquinone Shikonin. Toxins* **2014**, *6*, 1559–1574. [CrossRef] [PubMed]

20. Zielonka, Ł.; Waśkiewicz, A.; Beszterda, M.; Kostecki, M.; Dąbrowski, M.; Obremski, K.; Goliński, P.; Gajęcki, M. Zearalenone in the Intestinal Tissues of Immature Gilts Exposed *per os* to Mycotoxins. *Toxins* **2015**, *7*, 3210–3223. [CrossRef] [PubMed]

21. Gajęcka, M.; Zielonka, Ł.; Gajęcki, M. Activity of zearalenone in the porcine intestinal tract. *Molecules* **2017**, *22*, 18. [CrossRef] [PubMed]

22. Dąbrowski, M.; Obremski, K.; Gajęcka, M.; Gajęcki, M.; Zielonka, Ł. Changes in the subpopulations of porcine peripheral blood lymphocytes induced by exposure to low doses of zearalenone (ZEN) and deoxynivalenol (DON). *Molecules* **2016**, *21*, 557. [CrossRef] [PubMed]

23. Silva-Campa, E.; Mata-Haro, V.; Mateu, E.; Hernández, J. Porcine reproductive and respiratory syndrome virus induces CD4$^+$ CD8$^+$ CD25$^+$ Foxp3$^+$ regulatory T cells (Tregs). *Virology* **2012**, *430*, 73–80. [CrossRef] [PubMed]

24. Bryden, W.L. Mycotoxin contamination of the feed supply chain: Implications for animal productivity and feed security. *Anim. Feed Sci. Technol.* **2012**, *173*, 134–158. [CrossRef]

25. Fleck, S.C.; Hildebrand, A.A.; Müller, E.; Pfeiffer, E.; Metzler, M. Genotoxicity and inactivation of catechol metabolites of the mycotoxin zearalenone. *Mycotoxin Res.* **2012**, *28*, 267–273. [CrossRef] [PubMed]

26. Pfeiffer, E.; Wefers, D.; Hildebrand, A.A.; Fleck, S.C.; Metzler, M. Catechol metabolites of the mycotoxin zearalenone are poor substrates but potent inhibitors of catechol-*O*-methyltransferase. *Mycotoxin Res.* **2013**, *29*, 177–183. [CrossRef] [PubMed]

27. De Ruyck, K.; De Bovre, M.; Huybrechts, I.; De Saeger, S. Dietary mycotoxins, co-exposure, and carcinogenesis in humans: Short review. *Mutat. Res.-Rev. Mutat.* **2015**, *766*, 32–41. [CrossRef] [PubMed]

28. Przybylska-Gornowicz, B.; Lewczuk, B.; Prusik, M.; Hanuszewska, M.; Petrusewicz-Kosińska, M.; Gajęcka, M.; Zielonka, Ł.; Gajęcki, M. The Effects of Deoxynivalenol and Zearalenone on the Pig Large Intestine. A Light and Electron Microscopic study. *Toxins* **2018**, *10*, 148. [CrossRef] [PubMed]

29. Przybylska-Gornowicz, B.; Tarasiuk, M.; Lewczuk, B.; Prusik, M.; Ziółkowska, N.; Zielonka, Ł.; Gajęcki, M.; Gajęcka, M. The Effects of Low Doses of Two Fusarium Toxins, Zearalenone and Deoxynivalenol, on the Pig Jejunum. A Light and Electron Microscopic Study. *Toxins* **2015**, *7*, 4684–4705. [CrossRef] [PubMed]

30. Lewczuk, B.; Przybylska-Gornowicz, B.; Gajęcka, M.; Targońska, K.; Ziółkowska, N.; Prusik, M.; Gajęcki, M. Histological structure of duodenum in gilts receiving low doses of zearalenone and deoxynivalenol in feed. *Exp. Toxicol. Pathol.* **2016**, *68*, 157–166. [CrossRef] [PubMed]

31. Van der Aar, P.J.; Molist, F.; van der Klis, J.D. The central role of intestinal health on the effect of feed additives on feed intake in swine and poultry. *Anim. Feed* **2016**. [CrossRef]

32. Antonissen, G.; Martel, A.; Pasmans, F.; Ducatelle, R.; Verbrugghe, E.; Vandenbroucke, V.; Li, S.; Haesebrouck, F.; Immerseel, F.V.; Croubels, S. The impact of *Fusarium* mycotoxins on human and animal host susceptibility to infectious diseases. *Toxins* **2014**, *6*, 430–452. [CrossRef] [PubMed]

33. Nowak, A.; Śliżewska, K.; Gajęcka, M.; Piotrowska, M.; Żakowska, Z.; Zielonka, Ł.; Gajęcki, M. The genotoxicity of cecal water from gilts following experimentally induced *Fusarium* mycotoxicosis. *Vet. Med.-Czech.* **2015**, *60*, 133–140. [CrossRef]

34. Gajęcka, M.; Stopa, E.; Tarasiuk, M.; Zielonka, Ł.; Gajęcki, M. The expression of type-1 and type-2 nitric oxide synthase in selected tissues of the gastrointestinal tract during mixed mycotoxicosis. *Toxins* **2013**, *5*, 2281–2292. [CrossRef] [PubMed]

35. Kuciel-Lisieska, G.; Obremski, K.; Stelmachów, J.; Gajęcka, M.; Zielonka, Ł.; Jakimiuk, E.; Gajęcki, M. Presence of zearalenone in blood plasma in women with neoplastic lesions in the mammary gland. *Bull. Vet. Inst. Pulawy* **2008**, *52*, 671–674.

36. Gutleb, A.C.; Morrison, E.; Murk, A.J. Cytotoxicity assays for mycotoxins produced by *Fusarium* strains: A review. *Environ. Toxicol. Pharmacol.* **2002**, *11*, 309–320. [CrossRef]

37. Pukalskienė, M.; Slapšytė, G.; Dedonytė, V.; Lazutka, J.R.; Mierauskienė, J.; Venskutonis, P.R. Genotoxicity and antioxidant activity of five *Agrimonia* and *Filipendula* species plant extracts evaluated by comet and micronucleus assays in human lymphocytes and Ames *Salmonella*/microsome test. *Food Chem. Toxicol.* **2018**. [CrossRef] [PubMed]

38. Rykaczewska, A.; Gajęcka, M.; Dąbrowski, M.; Wiśniewska, A.; Szcześniewska, J.; Gajęcki, M.T.; Zielonka, Ł. Growth performance, selected blood biochemical parameters and body weight of pre-pubertal gilts fed diets supplemented with different doses of zearalenone (ZEN). *Toxicon* **2018**, *152*, 84–94. [CrossRef] [PubMed]

39. Williams, M.S.; Ebel, E.D. Estimating correlation of prevalence at two locations in the farm-to-table continuum using qualitative test data. *Inter. J. Food Microbiol.* **2017**, *245*, 29–37. [CrossRef] [PubMed]

40. Lathe, R.; Kotelevtsev, Y.; Mason, J.I. Steroid promiscuity: Diversity of enzyme action. *J. Steroid Biochem.* **2015**, *151*, 1–2. [CrossRef] [PubMed]

41. Jarolim, K.; Wolters, K.; Woelflingseder, L.; Pahlke, G.; Beisl, J.; Puntscher, H.; Braun, D.; Sulyok, M.; Warth, B.; Marko, D. The secondary *Fusarium* metabolite aurofusarin induces oxidative stress, cytotoxicity and genotoxicity in human colon cells. *Toxicol. Lett.* **2018**, *284*, 170–183. [CrossRef] [PubMed]

42. Salah-Abbès, J.B.; Abbès, S.; Ouanes, Z.; Abdel-Wahhab, M.A.; Bacha, H.; Oueslati, R. Isothiocyanate from the Tunisian radish (*Raphanus sativus*) prevents genotoxicity of Zearalenone in vivo and in vitro. *Mutat. Res.* **2009**, *677*, 59–65. [CrossRef] [PubMed]

43. Jakimiuk, E.; Gajęcka, M.; Jana, B.; Brzuzan, P.; Zielonka, Ł.; Skorska-Wyszyńska, E.; Gajęcki, M. Factors determining sensitivity of prepubertal gilts to hormonal influence of zearalenone. *Pol. J. Vet. Sci.* **2009**, *12*, 149–158. [PubMed]

44. Tatay, E.; Espín, S.; García-Fernández, A.-J.; Ruiz, M.-J. Oxidative damage and disturbance of antioxidant capacity by zearalenone and its metabolites in human cells. *Toxicol. In Vitro* **2017**, *45*, 334–339. [CrossRef] [PubMed]

45. Gajęcka, M.; Przybylska-Gornowicz, B. The low doses effect of experimental zearalenone (ZEN) intoxication on the presence of Ca^{2+} in selected ovarian cells from pre-pubertal bitches. *Pol. J. Vet. Sci.* **2012**, *15*, 711–720. [CrossRef] [PubMed]

46. Gajęcka, M.; Otrocka-Domagała, I. Immunocytochemical expression of 3β- and 17β-hydroxysteroid dehydrogenase in bitch ovaries exposed to low doses of zearalenone. *Pol. J. Vet. Sci.* **2013**, *16*, 55. [CrossRef] [PubMed]

47. Błasiak, J.; Arabski, M.; Krupa, R.; Woźniak, K.; Rykała, J.; Kolacinska, A.; Morawiec, Z.; Drzewoski, J.; Zadrożny, M. Basal, oxidative and alkylative DNA damage, DNA repair efficacy and mutagen sensitivity in breast cancer. *Mut. Res.* **2004**, *554*, 139–148. [CrossRef] [PubMed]

48. Piotrowska, M.; Śliżewska, K.; Nowak, A.; Zielonka, Ł.; Żakowska, Z.; Gajęcka, M.; Gajęcki, M. The effect of experimental *Fusarium* mycotoxicosis on microbiota diversity in porcine ascending colon contents. *Toxins* **2014**, *6*, 2064–2081. [CrossRef] [PubMed]

49. Heberer, T.; Lahrssen-Wiederholt, M.; Schafft, H.; Abraham, K.; Pyrembel, H.; Henning, K.J.; Schauzu, M.; Braeunig, J.; Goetz, M.; Niemann, L.; et al. Zero tolerances in food and animal feed-Are there any scientific alternatives? A European point of view on an international controversy. *Toxicol. Lett.* **2007**, *175*, 118–135. [CrossRef] [PubMed]

50. Smith, D.; Combes, R.; Depelchin, O.; Jacobsen, S.D.; Hack, R.; Luft, J.; Lammens, L.; von Landenberg, F.; Phillips, B.; Pfister, R.; et al. Optimising the design of preliminary toxicity studies for pharmaceutical safety testing in the dog. *Regul. Toxicol. Pharmcol.* **2005**, *41*, 95–101. [CrossRef] [PubMed]

51. Gajęcki, M. *The Effect of Experimentally Induced Fusarium Mycotoxicosis on Selected Diagnostic and Morphological Parameters of the Porcine Digestive Tract*; Final Report; Development Project NR12-0080-10; National Centre for Research and Development: Warsaw, Poland, 2013; pp. 1–180.

52. Aichinger, G.; Beisl, J.; Marko, D. Genistein and delphinidin antagonize the genotoxic effects of the mycotoxin alternariol in human colon carcinoma cells. *Mol. Nutr. Food Res.* **2017**, *61*. [CrossRef] [PubMed]

53. Błasiak, J.; Kowalik, J. A comparison of the in vitro genotoxicity of tri- and hexavalent chromium. *Mut. Res.* **2000**, *469*, 135–145. [CrossRef]

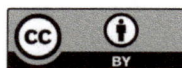

![toxins logo] *toxins*

MDPI

Article

Saccharomyces cerevisiae boulardii Reduces the Deoxynivalenol-Induced Alteration of the Intestinal Transcriptome

Imourana Alassane-Kpembi [1,2,*], **Philippe Pinton** [1], **Jean-François Hupé** [3], **Manon Neves** [1], **Yannick Lippi** [1], **Sylvie Combes** [4], **Mathieu Castex** [3] and **Isabelle P. Oswald** [1,*]

[1] Toxalim (Research Centre in Food Toxicology), Université de Toulouse, INRA, ENVT, INP-PURPAN, UPS, BP.93173 F-31027 Toulouse CEDEX 3, France; philippe.pinton@inra.fr (P.P.); manon.neves@inra.fr (M.N.); yannick.lippi@inra.fr (Y.L.)
[2] Hôpital d'Instruction des Armées—Centre Hospitalier Universitaire Cotonou Camp Guézo, Cotonou 01BP517, Benin
[3] Lallemand SAS, 19 rue des Briquetiers, BP 59, 31702 Blagnac CEDEX, France; jfhupe@lallemand.com (J.-F.H.); mcastex@lallemand.com (M.C.)
[4] GenPhySE, Université de Toulouse, INRA, ENVT, 31320 Castanet Tolosan, France; sylvie.combes@inra.fr
* Correspondence: imourana.alassane-kpembi@inra.fr (I.A.-K.); Isabelle.oswald@inra.fr (I.P.O.)

Received: 13 March 2018; Accepted: 11 May 2018; Published: 15 May 2018

Abstract: Type B trichothecene mycotoxin deoxynivalenol (DON) is one of the most frequently occurring food contaminants. By inducing trans-activation of a number of pro-inflammatory cytokines and increasing the stability of their mRNA, trichothecene can impair intestinal health. Several yeast products, especially *Saccharomyces cerevisiae*, have the potential for improving the enteric health of piglets, but little is known about the mechanisms by which the administration of yeast counteracts the DON-induced intestinal alterations. Using a pig jejunum explant model, a whole-transcriptome analysis was performed to decipher the early response of the small intestine to the deleterious effects of DON after administration of *S. cerevisiae* boulardii strain CNCM I-1079. Compared to the control condition, no differentially expressed gene (DE) was observed after treatment by yeast only. By contrast, 3619 probes—corresponding to 2771 genes—were differentially expressed following exposure to DON, and 32 signaling pathways were identified from the IPA software functional analysis of the set of DE genes. When the intestinal explants were treated with *S. cerevisiae* boulardii prior to DON exposure, the number of DE genes decreased by half (1718 probes corresponding to 1384 genes). Prototypical inflammation signaling pathways triggered by DON, including NF-κB and p38 MAPK, were reversed, although the yeast demonstrated limited efficacy toward some other pathways. *S. cerevisiae* boulardii also restored the lipid metabolism signaling pathway, and reversed the down-regulation of the antioxidant action of vitamin C signaling pathway. The latter effect could reduce the burden of DON-induced oxidative stress. Altogether, the results show that *S. cerevisiae* boulardii reduces the DON-induced alteration of intestinal transcriptome, and point to new mechanisms for the healing of tissue injury by yeast.

Keywords: deoxynivalenol; *Saccharomyces cerevisiae* boulardii CNCM I-1079; intestine; transcriptome; inflammation; oxidative stress; lipid metabolism

Key contribution: *Saccharomyces cerevisiae* boulardii reduces the transcriptional impact of deoxynivalenol on the intestine. The yeast strain is particularly effective in signaling pathways associated with (i) inflammation; (ii) oxidative stress; and (iii) lipid metabolism.

1. Introduction

The intestine has been identified as one of the critical targets of the food-borne mycotoxins [1,2]. Trichothecene (TCT) mycotoxin deoxynivalenol (DON) causes intestinal immune alterations which mimic inflammatory bowel diseases [3–5]. At the molecular level, the binding of DON or other TCTs to the ribosome activates mitogen-activated kinases (MAPKs), and also induces trans-activation of a number of pro-inflammatory cytokines, and an increase of the stability of their mRNA [6,7]. We showed that the frequently reported co-exposure to DON and other TCT could result in a synergistic inflammatory response of the intestinal tissue [8–10].

Among the ways to tackle the variety of factors threatening intestinal health, probiotics are considered good candidates, since they not only suppress the growth and binding of pathogenic bacteria, as well as improving the barrier function of the intestinal epithelium, but also tune the immune activity of the host [11,12]. Several yeast products are listed under the EC Regulation N.1831/2003 as feed additives for pigs in the EU; *Saccharomyces cerevisiae* in particular has demonstrated its potential for improving enteric health of piglets [13,14]. It was also recently shown that the yeast culture additive reduces immune and liver damage in pigs induced by a DON and aflatoxin contaminated diet [15].

Little is known about the mechanisms by which *S. cerevisiae* improves intestinal health. Preliminary in vitro data obtained in human monocytic, colonic, and gastric epithelial cells suggest that *S. cerevisiae* boulardii decreases inflammation by inhibiting NF-κB-mediated *IL-8* gene expression [16]. Regarding DON-induced alterations, *S. cerevisiae* boulardii decreases the activation of p38 MAPK pathway, and reduces the expression of downstream inflammatory cytokines; this yeast also promotes the expression of anti-apoptotic genes, and inhibits apoptosis in porcine alveolar macrophage cells [17].

In order to understand the early response of the small intestine to the administration of *S. cerevisiae* boulardii in response to the deleterious effects of DON, a whole transcriptome analysis of intestinal tissue was performed. Pre-treatment of the intestinal tissue with the yeast significantly reduced the global impact of DON on the transcriptome, and reversed prototypical inflammation signaling pathways including NF-κB and p38 MAPK. The yeast also restored the lipid metabolism signaling pathway and reverted the down-regulation of the antioxidant action of the vitamin C signaling pathway.

2. Results and Discussion

2.1. S. cerevisiae boulardii Reduces the Transcriptomic Impact of DON on the Intestine

To analyze the ability of *S. cerevisiae* boulardii to counteract the intestinal effect of DON, a pan genomic analysis of the transcriptomic fingerprint was conducted in control jejunal explants, explants treated with the yeast, and explants challenged with 10 μM DON in the presence, or absence, of *S. cerevisiae* boulardii. In human gut, concentrations of 0.16–2 μg DON/mL (0.5–7 μM) are considered realistic [8]. The lowest concentration value corresponds to the mean estimated daily intake of French adult consumers on a chronic basis. The highest concentration value simulates levels that can be reached after the consumption of heavily contaminated food, as can be occasionally encountered. Animals, especially pigs, can be exposed to higher concentrations of DON. Assuming that DON is ingested in one meal, diluted in 1 L of gastrointestinal fluid, and is totally bio accessible, the in vitro concentration of 10 μM used in this study corresponds to feed contaminated with 3 mg DON/Kg [18]. In a recent scientific opinion, EFSA reported levels of DON in feed grains of up to 9.5 mg/kg [19]. Regarding the use of *S. cerevisiae* boulardii, the EFSA expert panel concluded that the additive has the potential to be efficacious in weaned piglets at a dose of 2×10^9 CFU/kg feed [20]. The yeast concentration used in this study was chosen to reflect the recommended dose.

A total of 4398 transcripts, out of the 40,726 tested, were differentially expressed in at least one of the treatments when compared to control samples (adjusted *p* value < 0.05). As expected, and as shown on the heatmap (Figure 1), exposure of the intestinal tissue to DON resulted in clear alteration of the transcriptome. Hierarchical clustering indicated that control and *S. cerevisiae* boulardii-treated intestinal tissue samples separated from DON and DON + yeast treated groups. In comparison with the control, 3619 probes—corresponding to 2771 genes—were differentially expressed (DEG) (adjusted p value < 0.05) following exposure to DON, with fold-change values ranging from −3.43 to 11.44. No DEG was observed for the yeast condition (Figure 2A).

The top-regulated genes are listed in Table 1. As previously reported, the top-up regulated genes in intestinal explants exposed to DON were mainly related to inflammation [10,21,22]. The most up-regulated genes include interleukin 1 alpha and beta (*IL-1α* and *IL-1β*) and interleukin 22 (*IL-22*), the macrophage inflammatory proteins genes *MIP-2* alpha and *MIP-3* alpha (also known as *CXCL2* and *CCL20*), the receptor for MIP-3 beta chemokine gene (*CCR7*), the positive regulatory domain I-binding factor 1 gene (*PRDM1*) which drives the maturation of B-lymphocytes into Ig secreting cells, and the A disintegrin and metalloproteinase with thrombospondin motifs gene (*ADAMTS*) which may be associated with various inflammatory process. The amphiregulin gene (*AREG*), which can be expressed by multiple populations of activated immune cells under inflammatory conditions, was also up-regulated. Other genes in the top up-regulated category included *FOSL-1*, which regulates cell proliferation, differentiation, or transformation, *PLK-2*, which may play an important role in cells undergoing rapid cell division, and the transcriptional co-activator/repressor *IFRD1*, which controls the growth and differentiation of specific cell types.

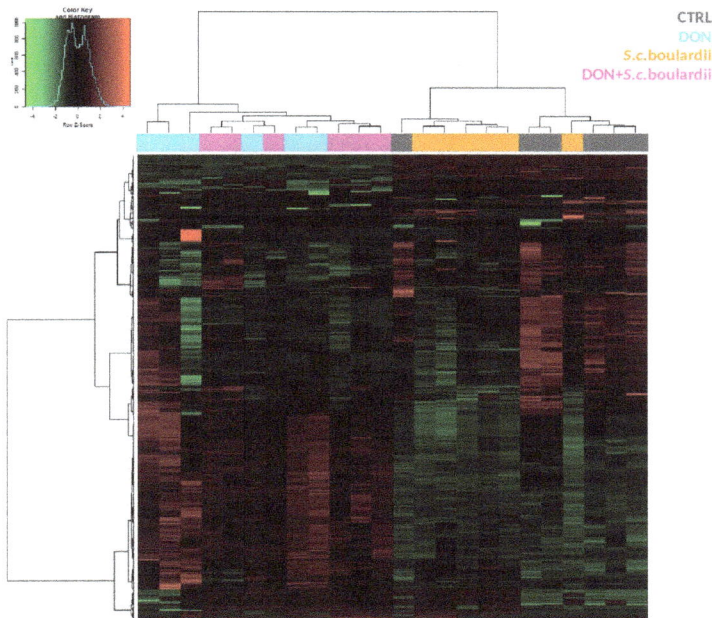

Figure 1. Gene expression profiles of intestinal explants exposed to DON or FX. Heatmap representing differentially expressed probes between the control, DON, *S. cerevisiae* boulardii and DON + *S. cerevisiae* boulardii conditions. Jejunal explants from six different animals were exposed for four hours to DMSO (vehicle), or treated with a *S. cerevisiae* boulardii suspension, or exposed to 10 μM DON. Gene expression was analyzed with a 60 K microarray. Red and green indicate values above and below the mean (average Z-score), respectively. Black indicates values close to the mean.

A.

B.

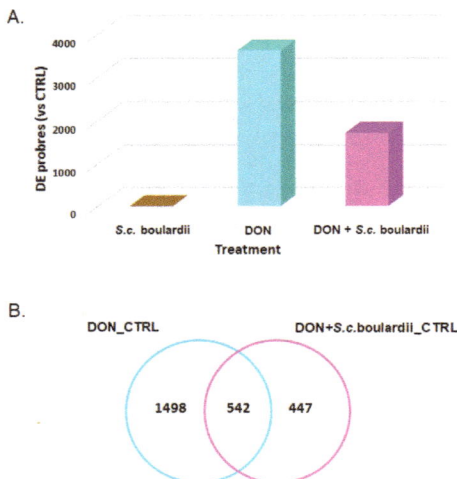

Figure 2. (**A**) Differentially expressed probes on the microarray for the yeast, mycotoxin, and yeast administration followed by mycotoxin exposure conditions; (**B**) Venn diagram of differentially expressed genes in the intestinal tissue after DON exposure or *S. cerevisiae* boulardii administration followed by DON exposure. CTRL represents DMSO control.

Table 1. Top-20 up- and down-regulated genes in the DON and the DON + *S. cerevisiae* boulardii conditions of the microarray experiment.

	DON			DON + *S. cerevisiae* boulardii		
	Gene Symbol	Fold Change *	Adjusted *p* Value	Gene Symbol	Fold Change *	Adjusted *p* Value
	IL-1β	11.37	6.27×10^{-13}	IL-1β	9.56	6.01×10^{-12}
	IL-22	5.62	3.24×10^{-8}	IL-22	5.56	7.73×10^{-8}
	NOR-1	5.09	1.07×10^{-9}	PTGS2	3.96	1.32×10^{-6}
	PTGS2	5.01	3.63×10^{-8}	IL-1α	3.96	2.90×10^{-8}
	CXCL2	4.65	0.00045897	CCL20	3.96	3.85×10^{-7}
	IL-1α	4.17	5.78×10^{-9}	NOR-1	3.88	7.73×10^{-8}
	CCL20	4.17	8.96×10^{-8}	CXCL2	3.22	0.01419023
	CCR7	3.36	1.36×10^{-7}	IL8	2.95	0.0004445
	HAMP	3.34	2.46×10^{-5}	ARX 10G	2.87	7.48×10^{-7}
Up–regulated	PLK2	3.28	1.02×10^{-11}	PRDM1	2.86	8.79×10^{-12}
	AREG	3.26	7.49×10^{-8}	FOSL1	2.82	0.00026329
	PRDM1	3.17	6.27×10^{-13}	GADD45G	2.7	9.54×10^{-6}
	FOSL1	3.11	4.71×10^{-5}	CCR7	2.63	1.35×10^{-5}
	CSF2	2.93	4.60×10^{-5}	PLK2	2.6	2.32×10^{-9}
	ADAMTS1	2.92	9.33×10^{-10}	GADD45A	2.6	2.12×10^{-6}
	CRSP-2	2.9	1.31×10^{-5}	PRDM1	2.59	9.84×10^{-10}
	CD274	2.74	3.47×10^{-7}	ATF3	2.57	4.04×10^{-6}
	RRAD	2.73	0.00150172	PLK2	2.5	3.89×10^{-9}
	IFRD1	2.66	1.47×10^{-8}	RND1	2.48	3.07×10^{-6}
	GADD45G	2.64	7.57×10^{-6}	HAMP	1.31	0.001954

Table 1. *Cont.*

	DON			DON + *S. cerevisiae* boulardii		
	Gene Symbol	Fold Change *	Adjusted *p* Value	Gene Symbol	Fold Change *	Adjusted *p* Value
Down–regulated	CTBS	−3.43	0.0323898	ACTN2	−4.83	0.03632277
	C1QTNF3	−2.38	0.02819327	ACTA1	−4.28	0.03241036
	PDLIM3	−2.2	0.04545171	TPM2	−2.88	0.04875964
	BTC	−2	0.04718046	TPM1	−2.81	0.04897366
	TMEFF2	−1.97	0.02364126	MYL9	−2.66	0.04636262
	HAND1	−1.89	0.04906228	LIMS2	−2.57	0.04897366
	SMPX	−1.82	0.01890697	MYLK	−2.53	0.04955867
	BPI	−1.76	0.03066332	C1QTNF3	−2.49	0.03403947
	LYZ	−1.72	0.02546107	SPOCK3	−2.41	0.02910998
	LECT1	−1.7	0.04314249	BTC	−2.26	0.04788811
	ASPN	−1.67	0.04519455	TPM1	−2.23	0.04179965
	OGN	−1.66	0.03041459	HAND1	−2.2	0.02447994
	RYR2	−1.64	0.03593429	FLNA	−2.1	0.03855459
	DSTN	−1.64	0.00936255	TMX 10FF2	−2.03	0.02907563
	FHL1C	−1.63	0.0438132	CPXM2	−2.02	0.02989774
	CXCL12	−1.63	0.01364805	DNAJA4	−1.94	0.01272008
	CYP4F2	−1.59	0.04673074	PRUNX 102	−1.86	0.0392422
	ITGB1BP2	−1.59	0.0354242	SMARCD3	−1.83	0.04490504
	ACTB	−1.59	0.02928137	FHL1C	−1.81	0.02399939
	MATN2	−1.59	0.0065206	ATP2B4	−1.81	0.04252773

* Fold change compared to DMSO control.

The treatment of the intestinal explants with *S. cerevisiae* boulardii prior to DON exposure decreased the number of DEGs by 50%, as only 1384 genes (1718 probes) were differentially expressed in DON + yeast treated explants (Figure 2A). Nevertheless, the top up-regulated genes in the jejunal tissue treated with either DON alone, or *S. cerevisiae* boulardii prior to DON exposure, were very similar, and inflammation remained the hallmark of the intestinal transcriptome. It is worthy of note that, except for growth arrest and DNA damage-inducible protein gamma gene (*GADD45G*), the 15 other genes expressed in both experimental conditions were slightly less expressed in the DON + yeast condition (Table 1).

Microarray data validation was performed by quantitative real-time polymerase chain reaction (qPCR) on a set of 12 DE genes in DON and DON + yeast conditions. A significant Spearman correlation coefficient (r = 0.896) was observed between the two techniques (Supplementary Figure S1), confirming the reliability of the transcriptome analyses.

2.2. Functional Analysis of the Intestinal Transcriptome Modulation by DON and/or S. cerevisiae boulardii

To further investigate the protective effect of *S. cerevisiae* boulardii, a comparative functional analysis of DEGs in DON and DON + yeast conditions was performed using the core analysis comparative function of Ingenuity Pathway Analysis (IPA) software.

Figure 3 shows that 32 canonical pathways were significantly affected in the jejunal tissue exposed to DON (p-value < 0.05, $-2 >$ IPA Z-score $> +2$). As previously described, the foremost up-regulated signaling pathways in the DON condition, including HMGB1 signaling, IL-6, IL1, TNFR1, p38 MAPK, and TREM1 signaling, were related to immunity/inflammation [21]. The B-cell activating factor, B-cell receptor signaling, and the NF-κB signaling pathway, which not only regulates inflammation and immunity, but also cell survival and cell proliferation, were also up-regulated by DON. Likewise, intestinal exposure to DON resulted in the down regulation of the PPAR and the LXR/RXR activation signaling pathways, which control diverse aspects of cholesterol and fatty acid homeostasis [21,23]. Lastly, a DON-induced oxidative stress in the intestinal tissue was reflected by down-regulation of the antioxidant action of the vitamin C signaling pathway.

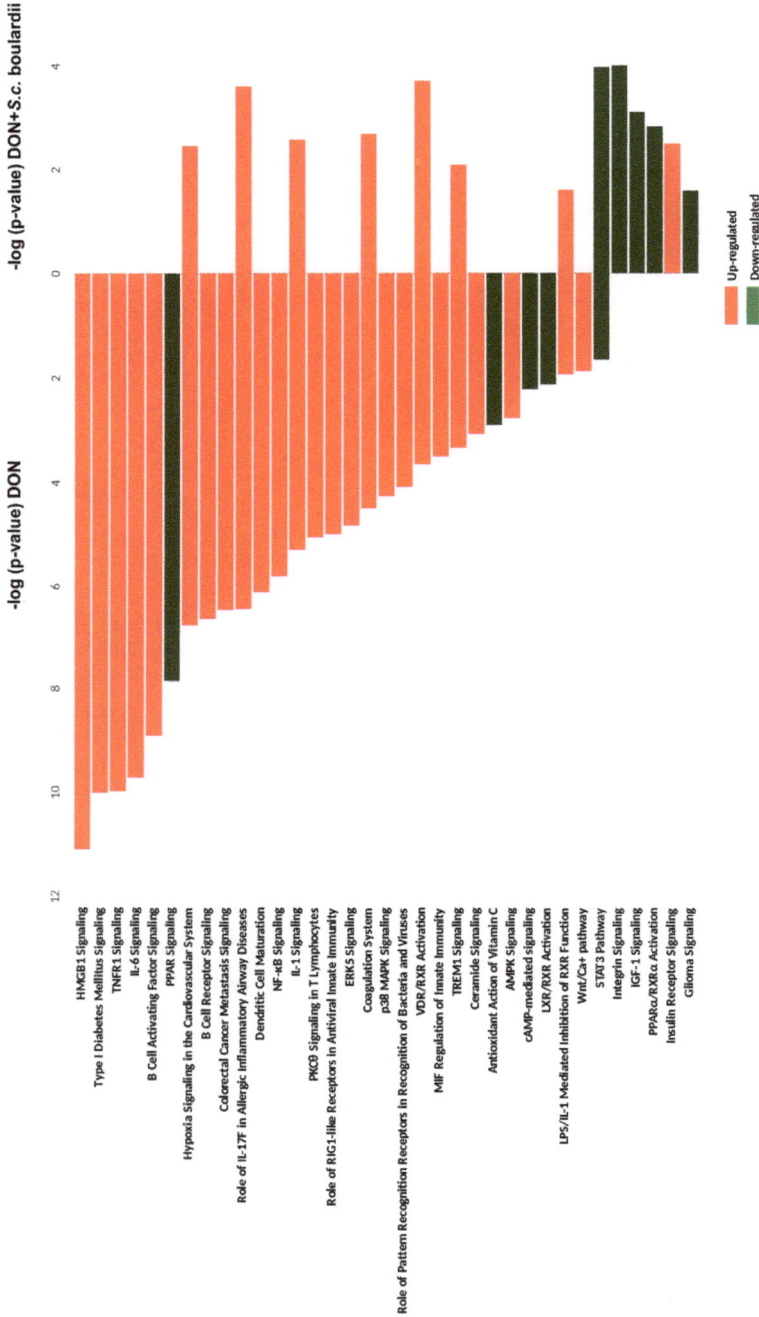

Figure 3. Top canonical pathways significantly modulated in DON and DON + *S. cerevisiae* boulardii conditions. Statistical significance of pathway modulation was calculated via a right-tailed Fisher's exact test in IPA. Only pathways that presented a −log *p*-values exceeding 1.30 and −2 > IPA *Z*-score > +2 were preserved.

Applying *S. cerevisiae* boulardii to the jejunal tissue prior to DON exposure reduced the number of activated canonical pathways from 32 to 13 (Figure 3). In fact, only eight out of the 32 canonical pathways triggered by DON really withstood the protective effects of *S. cerevisiae* boulardii, and five new signaling pathways emerged from a set of DEGs specific to the interaction between DON and yeast on the treated explants (Figures 2B and 3). The pathways expressed in both DON and yeast + DON conditions were the hypoxia signaling, IL-1 signaling, TREM1 signaling, STAT3, the VDR/RXR activation, the LPS/IL-1 mediated inhibition of RXR function, the coagulation system pathway, and the IL-17F pathway in allergic inflammatory diseases. The interaction between DON and *S. cerevisiae* boulardii resulted in the down-regulation of integrin signaling, IGF-1 signaling, glioma signaling, and the PPARa/RXRa activation pathway, as well as the up-regulation of insulin receptor signaling; in contrast, none of these pathways was affected when individually exposed to DON or *S. cerevisiae* boulardii.

Aside from these few cases, the shutdown of the 24 other DON-triggered signaling pathways is evidence that the yeast administration significantly restrained the detrimental effects of this mycotoxin on the intestine. The application of *S. cerevisiae* boulardii was particularly effective on signaling pathways associated with (i) inflammation, (ii) oxidative stress, and (iii) lipid metabolism.

2.3. S. cerevisiae boulardii Reduces the Pro-Inflammatory Effects of DON

Only four out of 19 inflammation/immunity signaling pathways triggered by DON were still observed in explants treated with *S. cerevisiae* boulardii prior to DON exposure. These four signaling pathways were IL-1 and TREM signaling, the LPS/IL-1 mediated inhibition of RXR function, as well as the role of IL-17 in allergic inflammatory disease pathway. Treatment with *S. cerevisiae* boulardii prevented the triggering of other inflammation pathways including HMGB1 signaling, TNFR1 signaling, and the IL-6 signaling pathway, as well as the pivotal NF-kB signaling and p38 MAPK signaling pathways.

HMGB1 belongs to a family of endogenous compounds termed "alarmins", which can be released in the extracellular milieu during states of cellular stress or injury leading to infectious or non-infectious conditions [24]. IL-6 is generated upon activation of the pattern recognition receptors (PRRs) by pathogen-associated molecular patterns (PAMPs) or damage-associated molecular patterns (DAMPs), in the case of infectious lesion or tissue damage [25]. The DON-induced ribotoxic stress has been previously linked with ribosomal RNA cleavage, which could be the starting point of a DAMP-mediated PRR activation of the IL-6 and HMGB1 signaling pathways in the intestine [26]. The hypothesis of cytosolic sensing of cleaved RNA is also supported by the triggering of both a signaling pathway linked with the role of pattern recognition receptors in the recognition of bacteria and viruses, and even more, by another pathway associated with the role of RIG1-like receptors in antiviral innate immunity in presence of DON (Figure 3).

The p38 MAPK pathway is a key regulator of pro-inflammatory cytokines biosynthesis at the transcriptional and translational levels, which makes it critical for normal immune and inflammatory response [27]. In isolated porcine alveolar macrophage cells, *S. cerevisiae* boulardii was shown to attenuate p38 MAPK signaling by alleviating DON-induced phosphorylation and mRNA expression of p38 MAPK protein [17]. A comparison of the activation patterns of the different genes involved in the p38 MAPK in both DON-exposed tissue and *S. cerevisiae* boulardii treated tissue before DON exposure (Figure 4) shows that the remediation action of *S. cerevisiae* boulardii involves many more mechanisms in all the cellular compartments. First, the yeast counteracts the DON-induced upregulation of the transmembrane receptors IL-1R and TNFR/Fas, as well as its adaptor molecule FADD, both of which transduce the triggering signals delivered by IL-1 cytokine and Fas ligand. In the cytosolic compartment, pre-treatment with *S. cerevisiae* boulardii before DON exposure also leads to restoration of the DON-induced downregulation of apoptosis signal-regulating kinase 1 (ASK1) and a member of the cytosolic phospholipase A2 family (cPLA2), and up-regulation of the TNF receptor associated factor 6 (TRAF6). Recent studies revealed the involvement of ASK1 in ROS- or ER stress related diseases, suggesting that ASK1 could be a therapeutic target [28]. The members of the cPLA2 family catalyze the hydrolysis of phospholipids to yield fatty acids and lysophospholipids, and are involved in inflammation by driving arachidonic acid metabolism [29]. Finally, in the intestinal tissue, *S. cerevisiae* boulardii was also seen to downscale the DON-induced activation of the signal transducer and activator of transcription 1 (STAT1), which translocates to the nucleus to promote expression of cytokine response genes [30].

Figure 5 summarizes the effect of DON in the presence, or absence, of *S. cerevisiae* boulardii on the NF-κB signaling pathway. Activation of NF-κB signaling via canonical or alternative pathways regulates various biological processes, including immune response, inflammation, cell growth and survival, and development [31]. We observed that upon intestinal exposure to DON, both canonical and alternative NF-κB signaling pathways were activated. IL-1, TNF-α and bone morphogenetic protein 2 (BMP2) primary signals converged to the nuclear translocation of the heterodimeric NF-κB complex p50/RelA via activation of the catalytic IκB kinase subunits IKKα and IKKβ, while the B-cell activating factor (BAFF) signal led to upregulation and subsequent nuclear translocation of p52/RelB dimer. By contrast, neither p50/RelA, nor p52/RelB complexes showed up-regulation of gene expression when the intestinal explants were treated with *S. cerevisiae* boulardii prior to DON exposure (supplementary Table S1). Interestingly, administration of *S. cerevisiae* boulardii counteracts upstream, the DON-induced upregulation of transmembrane receptors IL-1R/TLR, TNFR and CD40 and adaptor molecules FADD, TRADD and TRAF, on the one hand, and on the other hand, the DON-induced upregulation of BAFF. This suggests that *S. cerevisiae* boulardii may prevent the activation of the canonical pathway of NF-κB signaling by altering the transduction of IL-1 and TNF-α primary signals, and the activation of the alternative pathway by suppressing the initial BAFF signal.

To summarize, the administration of *S. cerevisiae* boulardii prevented the intestinal tissue from the onset of several signaling pathways driving inflammation that is the hallmark of the low-dose exposure to DON and other trichothecene mycotoxins.

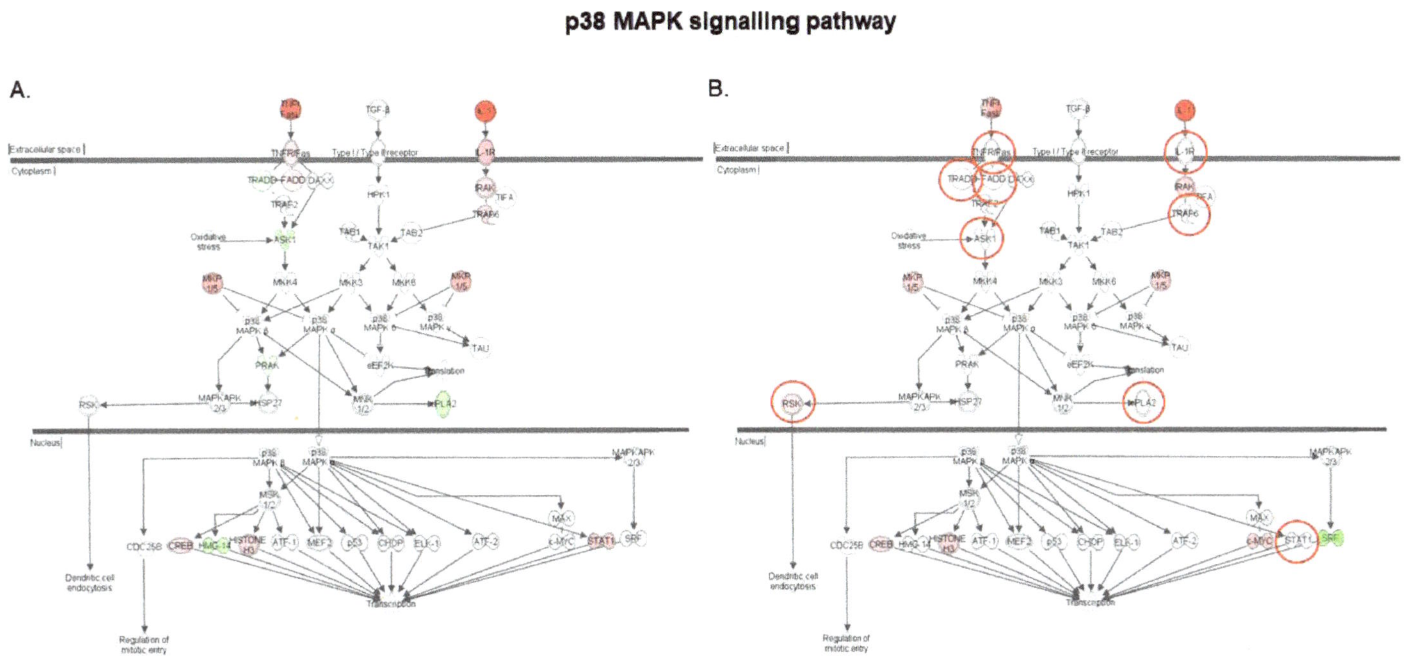

p38 MAPK signalling pathway

Figure 4. Expression patterns of genes of the p38MAPK signaling pathway in the intestinal tissue. (**A**) Intestinal tissue exposed to *S. cerevisiae* boulardii and 10 µM DON; (**B**) Intestinal tissue exposed to 10 µM DON. Red nodes represent up-regulated genes, and green nodes represent down-regulated genes identified in our differential expression analysis. Darker node colors indicate more extreme (high or low) up- or down-regulation of the respective gene. White nodes represent genes that were not identified in the signaling pathway that were not identified in the microarray analysis. The red circles indicate genes showing different expression pattern in both conditions.

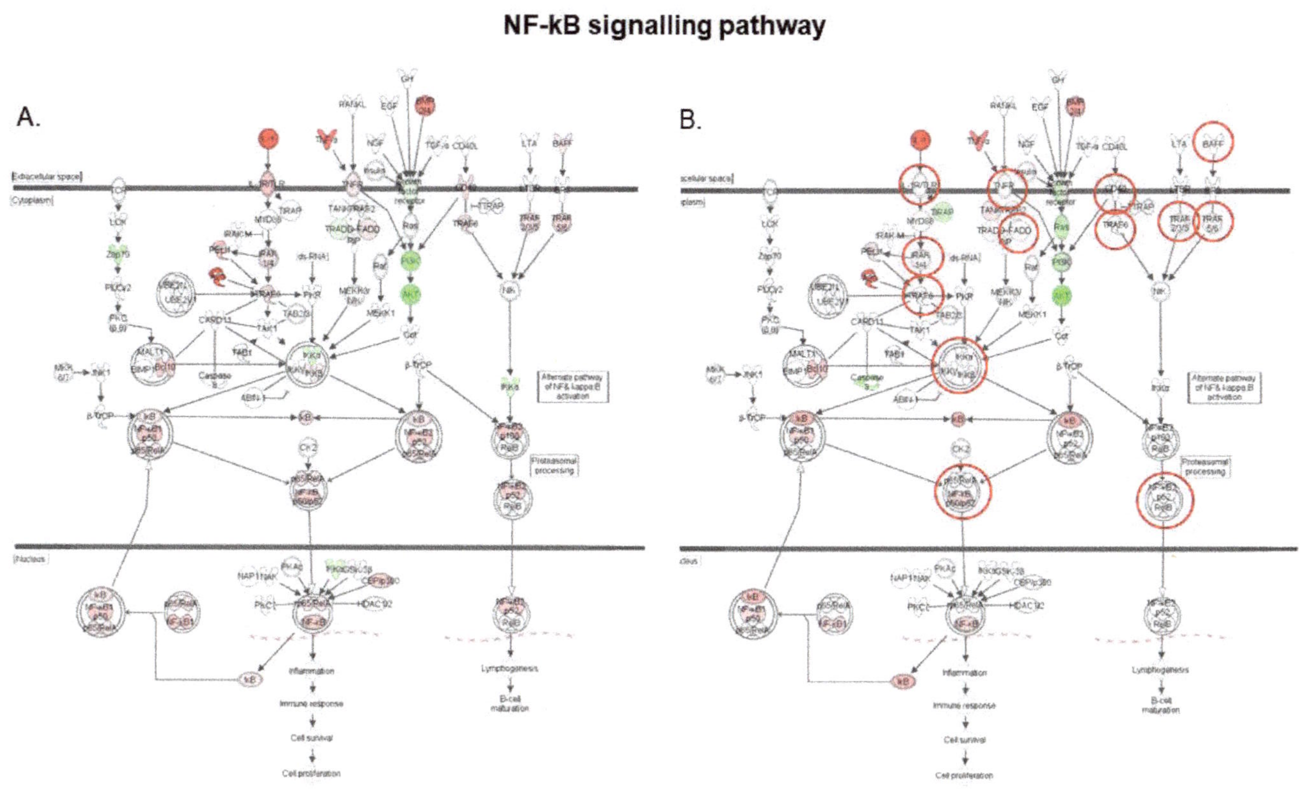

NF-kB signalling pathway

Figure 5. Expression patterns of genes of the NF-κB signaling pathway in the intestinal tissue. (**A**) Intestinal tissue exposed to *S. cerevisiae* boulardii and 10 µM DON; (**B**) Intestinal tissue exposed to 10 µM DON. Red nodes represent up-regulated genes, and green nodes represent down-regulated genes identified in our differential expression analysis. Darker node colors indicate more extreme (high or low) up- or down-regulation of the respective gene. White nodes represent genes involved in the signaling pathway that were not identified in the microarray analysis. The red circles indicate genes showing different expression pattern in both conditions.

2.4. S. cerevisiae boulardii Reverses the Effect of DON on the Antioxidant Action of Vitamin C

The antioxidant action of the vitamin C signaling pathway was down-regulated in the intestinal tissue following exposure to DON (Figure 6). Feeding a DON–contaminated feed to broiler chickens has previously been shown to significantly up-regulate the expression of two sensitive markers of oxidative injury, hypoxia inducible factor 1 subunit alpha (HIF-1α), and heme-oxygenase (HMOX), in intestinal tissue [32]. Oxidative stress is one of the most important underlying mechanisms of the toxicity of DON in eukaryotic cells, and two mechanisms (generation of reactive oxygen species (ROS) and alteration in antioxidant status) have been reported for this mycotoxin [33,34]. Both mechanisms are represented in Figure 6. The DON-induced cytokine signal transduction in the intestinal tissue could generate ROS, while the antioxidant action of vitamin C is repressed. The protective effect of vitamin C as a free radical scavenger warrants its use in the prevention of DON-mediated oxidative stress [35]. Vitamin C can enter the cell directly via sodium-dependent ascorbate co-transporters (SVCT); alternatively, GLUT transporters can carry dehydroascorbic acid that will be reduced to vitamin C by enzymes such as thioredoxin reductase (TXN) and dehydroascorbic acid reductase (DHA), once inside the cell [36]. Hence, by downregulating the TXN gene (Figure 6), DON could impair the conversion of dehydroascorbic acid, and limit intracellular levels of vitamin C, leading to lowered capacity for the inhibition of ROS-mediated events.

As shown by the microarray data in Table 1, and confirmed by the qRT-PCR data in Table 2 and supplementary Table S2, the pre-treatment of the intestinal tissue with *S. cerevisiae* boulardii had a limited effect on the DON induced up-regulation of cytokine expression, which means that the ROS generation was preserved. Nonetheless, comparison of gene activation patterns in the antioxidant action of vitamin C signaling pathway in the DON and DON + *S. cerevisiae* boulardii conditions indicates that the yeast treatment counteracted the DON-induced down-regulation of TXN (Figure 6). This highlights the fact that, although *S. cerevisiae* boulardii could not protect the intestinal tissue from ROS generation, the probiotic helps restore intracellular vitamin C, and could downscale the burden of the DON-induced oxidative stress via ROS generation.

Table 2. Expression of key inflammatory genes in the DON and the DON + *S. cerevisiae* boulardii conditions in microarray and qRT-PCR experiments.

Gene Symbol	DON					DON + S. cerevisiae boulardii			
	FC Microarray *	Adjusted p Value	FC qRT-PCR **	p Value		FC Microarray *	Adjusted p Value	FC qRT-PCR	p Value
IL-1β	11.37	6.27×10^{-13}	6.08	9×10^{-4}		9.56	6.01×10^{-12}	4.96	0.0089
IL-22	5.62	3.24×10^{-8}	5.88	0.0791		5.56	7.73×10^{-8}	3.65	0.0964
IL8	2.22	0.0081	3.13	1.8×10^{-4}		2.95	4.45×10^{-4}	2.91	0.0025
IL17A	2.28	2.4×10^{-4}	7.62	0.0022		1.81	0.0025	1.75	0.018
TNF-α	2.07	1.82×10^{-7}	2.99	0.0085		1.71	6.14×10^{-5}	1.61	0.01

* Fold change compared to DMSO control in the microarray experiment. ** Fold change compared to DMSO control in the qRT-PCR experiment.

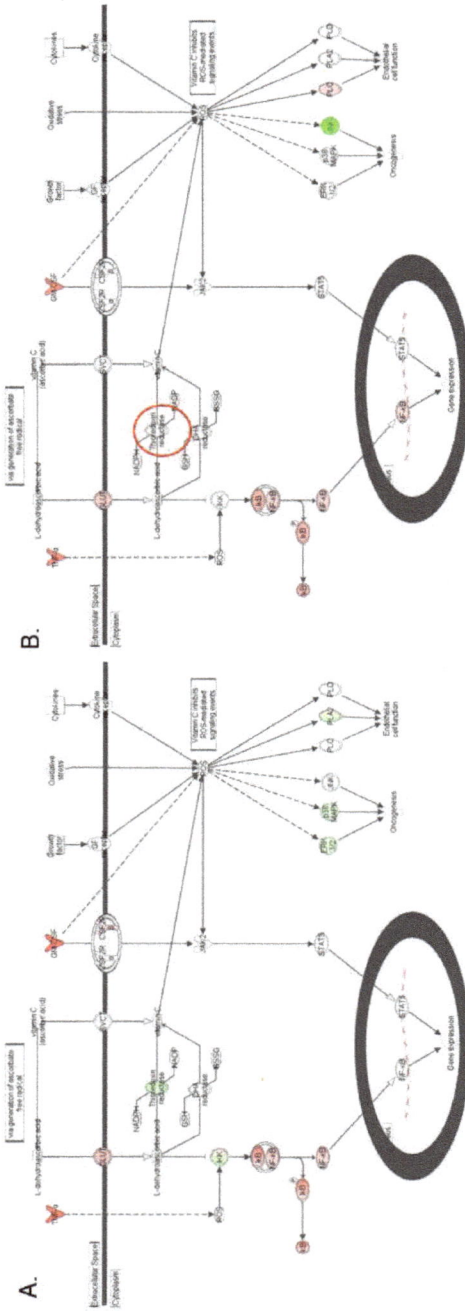

Figure 6. Expression patterns of genes of the antioxidant action of vitamin C signaling pathway in the intestinal tissue. (**A**) Intestinal tissue exposed to 10 μM DON; (**B**) Intestinal tissue exposed to *S. cerevisiae* boulardii and 10 μM DON. Red nodes represent up-regulated genes, and green nodes represent down-regulated genes identified in our differential expression analysis. Darker node colors indicate more extreme (high or low) up- or down-regulation of the respective gene. White nodes represent genes involved in the signaling pathway that were not identified in the microarray analysis. The red circles indicate genes showing different expression pattern in both conditions.

2.5. S. cerevisiae boulardii Restores the Lipid Metabolism Altered by DON

The functional analysis of the intestinal transcriptome upon exposure to DON revealed repression of both PPAR signaling and the LXR/RXR activation which control lipid metabolism (Figure 7). The PPAR/RXR and LXR/RXR heterodimers act as sensors of intracellular lipid metabolism, and thereby, regulate diverse aspects of cholesterol and fatty acid homeostasis [23]. PPARγ is a highly expressed nuclear receptor in macrophages, and its activation increases *LXRα* expression, which in turn transactivates target genes and reduces cell cholesterol levels. As a consequence, deficiency in PPAR signaling is pivotal for the establishment of the foam cells of atherosclerotic lesions [37]. As shown in Figure 7, on the one hand, intestinal exposure to DON repressed *PPARγ* via NF-κB signaling, and on the other hand, down-regulated the expression of *LXRα* gene. By contrast, the DON-induced down regulation of *LXRα* was prevented by the pre-treatment of intestinal tissue with *S. cerevisiae* boulardii along with the canceling of signal transduction at an early-stage of the NF-κB pathway.

Interestingly, expression of the insulin receptor gene and of the platelet-derived growth factor receptor gene (*PDGF*) was also down-regulated. As a phosphoprotein, the transcriptional activity of PPARγ is affected by the extracellular receptor kinase-mitogen activated protein kinase (ERK-MAPK), and thereby its constitutive activators insulin and PDGF [38]. Phosphorylation by ERK has been shown to decrease the transcriptional activity of PPARγ [39,40]. Hence, the down-regulation of the insulin and PDGF receptors observed in tissue treated with yeast prior to exposure to DON could limit the basal inactivation of PPARγ, and function as a potentiating factor for recovery from DON-suppressed PPAR functions.

PPAR signalling pathway

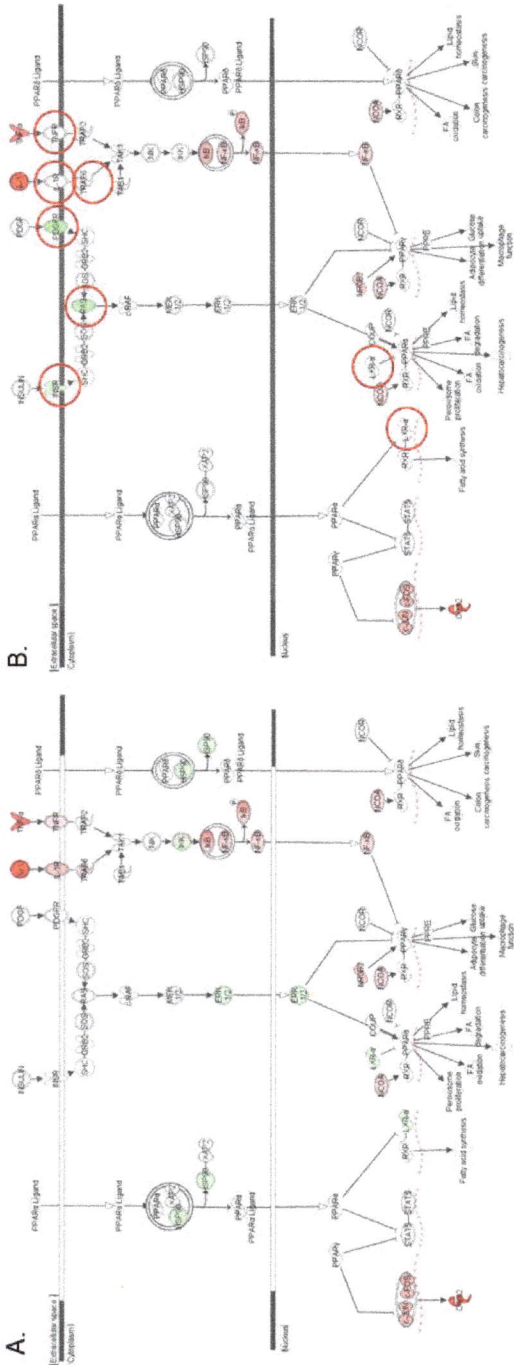

Figure 7. Expression patterns of genes of the PPAR signaling pathway in the intestinal tissue. (**A**) Intestinal tissue exposed to *S. cerevisiae* boulardii and 10 µM DON; (**B**) Intestinal tissue exposed to 10 µM DON. Red nodes represent up-regulated genes, and green nodes represent down-regulated genes identified in our differential expression analysis. Darker node colors indicate more extreme (high or low) up- or down-regulation of the respective gene. White nodes represent genes involved in the signaling pathway that were not identified in the microarray analysis. The red circles indicate genes showing different expression pattern in both conditions.

3. Conclusions

The aim of the present study was to investigate the effects of *S. cerevisiae* boulardii as a strategy to alleviate the effect of DON. To this end, a transcriptional analysis of intestinal explant was performed. On its own, *S. cerevisiae* boulardii induced no differential gene expression in the intestine. However, application of the yeast significantly reduced the global impact of DON on the transcriptome. Prototypical signaling pathways linked to inflammation and immunity, including the NF-κB and the p38 MAPK, triggered by DON were reversed by the *S. cerevisiae* boulardii treatment, although the yeast showed limited efficacy toward some other signaling pathways. Transcriptomic data also suggest that *S. cerevisiae* boulardii reduces the burden of the global DON-induced oxidative stress and restores the PPAR signaling functions which control lipid homeostasis. How these striking observations, made in an oversimplified explant model, apply at a functional level in vivo still remains to be investigated.

4. Materials and Methods

4.1. Toxin

Purified deoxynivalenol (DON) purchased from Sigma (Saint Quentin Fallavier, France) was dissolved to 10 mM in dimethylsulfoxide (DMSO), and stored at −20 °C before dilution in complete culture media.

4.2. Yeast Strain and Culture

Industrial dry yeast Levucell SB20 (*Saccharomyces cerevisiae* boulardii CNCM I-1079) from Lallemand Animal Nutrition (Blagnac, France) was rehydrated (10 g/100 g) in a suspension medium (NaCl, K_2HPO_4, KH_2PO_4, casein peptone and Tween 80) and allowed to rehydrate for 20 min with gentle agitation (120 rpm) in a shaking water bath at 37 °C. Serial dilutions were performed in peptone saline water (NaCl, casein peptone), and a 1/1000 dilution containing 4×10^6 CFU/mL of live cells was used. The yeast solutions were prepared just before use. Whole culture material was used in this experiment, since it is established that the effects of *S. cerevisiae* boulardii on the host result from cell to cell interactions, as well as from interactions between yeast secreted molecules and epithelial cells [41,42].

4.3. Culture of Jejunum Explants

Jejunal explants were obtained from 5-week old crossbred castrated male piglets, as described previously [7,43,44]. Briefly, 5 cm middle jejunum segments were collected in complete William's Medium E (Sigma, Saint Quentin Fallavier, France). Four to six washes were performed with William's Medium E. After removing external *tunica muscularis*, each jejunum segment was opened longitudinally, and pieces of 6 mm diameter were obtained with biopsy punches (Kruuse, Centravet, Dinan, France). Two explants/wells were deposited villi upward on 1-cm^2 biopsy sponges (Medtronic, Minneapolis, MN, USA) in six well plates (Cellstar, Greiner Bio-One, Frickenhausen, Germany) containing the control medium, supplemented or not with *S. cerevisiae* boulardii containing medium. The culture medium contained 100 U/mL penicillin, 100 µg/mL streptomycin, and 50 µg/mL gentamycin (Eurobio, Courtaboeuf, France). All these operations were achieved in less than one hour after the piglets were euthanized.

The experiment was conducted according to the guidelines of the French Ministry of Agriculture for animal research. All animal experimentation procedures were approved by the Ethics committee of Pharmacology-Toxicology of Toulouse-Midi-Pyrénées in animal experimentation (Toxcométhique), N° TOXCOM/0017/IO PP, in accordance with the European Directive on the protection of animals used for scientific purposes (Directive 2010/63/EU). The date of approval is 1 September 2017. The three authors (I.A.K, I.P.O. and P.P) have an official agreement with the French Veterinary Services allowing animal experimentation. The explants were pre-treated, or not, with 75 µL of the *S. cerevisiae* boulardii. I-1079 (which corresponds to 3×10^5 colony forming units) for 30 min, and then challenged with

10 μM DON for 4 h at 39 °C. The dose of DON and *S. cerevisiae* boulardii I-1079 were chosen to reflect doses in feed equivalent to 3 ppm of DON and 2×10^9 CFU/kg of feed of *S. cerevisiae* boulardii I-1079, respectively. A toxin vehicle (DMSO) condition, and an *S. cerevisiae* boulardii I-1079 condition, were used as controls. After incubation, treated explants were stored at −80 °C before RNA extraction.

4.4. RNA Extraction

Jejunal explants were lysed in 1 mL of Extract All reagent (Eurobio, Les Ulis, France) with ceramic beads (Bertin Technologies, Saint Quentin en Yvelines, France). Total RNA was extracted according to the manufacturer's recommendations, as previously described [45,46]. The RNA concentration was determined by measuring the optical density at 260 nm, and the RNA integrity was assessed using both NanoDrop spectrophotometric analysis (Labtech International, Paris, France) and Agilent capillary electrophoresis (Agilent 2100 Bioanalyzer, Agilent Technologies Inc., Santa Clara, CA, USA). The mean (±SD) RNA integrity number (RIN) of these mRNA preparations was 6.85 (±0.8).

4.5. Microarray Processing and Functional Analysis of Expressed Genes

The microarray GPL16524 (Agilent technology, Santa Clara, CA, USA, 8 × 60 K) used in this experiment consisted of 43,603 spots derived from the 44 K (V2:026440 design) Agilent porcine-specific microarray [21]. This microarray was enhanced with 9532 genes from adipose tissue, 3776 genes from the immune system, and 3768 genes from skeletal muscle. A total of 24 samples (6 replicates per treatment group) were processed. For each sample, cyanine-3 (Cy3)-labeled cRNA was prepared from 200 ng of total RNA using the One-Color Quick Amp Labeling kit (Agilent, Santa Clara, CA, USA), according to the manufacturer's instructions, followed by the Agencourt RNAClean XP (Agencourt Bioscience Corporation, Beverly, MA, USA). Approximately 600 ng of Cy3-labeled cRNA was hybridized onto the SurePrint G3 Porcine GE microarray (8 × 60 K), following the manufacturer's instructions. Immediately after washing, the slides were scanned on an Agilent G2505C Microarray Scanner using Agilent Scan Control A.8.5.1 software, and the fluorescence signals were extracted using the Agilent Feature Extraction software v10.10.1.1 with the default parameters. The microarray data were analyzed using R (www.r-project.org, R v. 3.1.2) and the Bioconductor packages (www.bioconductor.org, v 3.0), as described in GEO entry GSE97821, which also contains all the details of the experiments.

Network analysis and functional analysis of the DE genes were performed using the Ingenuity Pathway Analysis tool (IPA, http://www.ingenuity.com) to identify gene networks and signaling pathways affected by each treatment. The IPA output included statistical assessment of the significance of gene networks and signaling pathways based on Fisher's exact test; only networks and pathways that presented a p value < 0.05 or a $-\log p$ value exceeding 1.30 (FDR q-values < 0.05) and a Z-score with an absolute value ≥ 2 were retained.

4.6. Quantitative Real-Time Polymerase Chain Reaction (qRT-PCR) Analysis

The reverse transcription and real-time qPCR steps were performed on total RNA samples ($n = 6$ per treatment group), as previously described [47]. The primers for selected differentially expressed genes on the microarray (Supplementary Table S3) were designed using Primer Express Software, and purchased from Invitrogen (Invitrogen, Life Technologies Corporation, Paisley, UK). Non-reverse transcribed RNA was used as the non-template control for verification of the genomic DNA amplification signal. The specificity of the qPCR products was assessed at the end of the reactions by analyzing the dissociation curves. The expression stability of five candidate reference genes, (Cyclophylin A (*CycloA*), β-actin, β2-microglobulin, Ribosomal Protein L32 (*RPL32*), and Hypoxanthine Phosphoribosyl transferase 1 (*HPRT-1*)) across different experimental samples has been investigated; it was demonstrated that *RPL32* showed the highest stability (SD = 0.82; r = 0.971) [21]. *RPL32* and *CycloA* were chosen as housekeeping genes, and the 2-ΔΔCt method was used to calculate the fold change in gene expression. For comparison with microarray data, the Spearman correlation between the microarray Log2 (FC) and qPCR Log2 (2-ΔΔCt) values was calculated.

4.7. Statistical Analysis

The microarray data were analyzed using the R Bioconductor packages and the limma lmFit function, as previously described [21]. Probes with adjusted p values ≤ 0.05 (FDR correction using the Benjamini Hochberg procedure) were differentially expressed between the treated and control conditions. Hierarchical clustering was applied to the samples and the probes, using the 1-Pearson correlation coefficient as the distance and Ward's criterion for agglomeration, and was then illustrated as a heatmap presenting gene expression profiles of selected regulated genes.

For gene expression quantification by qRT-PCR, the mRNA expression of the target genes was normalized to the expressed housekeeping genes using REST© 2009 software (Qiagen, Valencia, CA, USA), which uses the pair-wise fixed reallocation randomization test as the statistical model [10].

Supplementary Materials: The following are available online at http://www.mdpi.com/2072-6651/10/5/199/s1, Table S1: Expression of the genes involved in the NF-κB signalling pathway, Table S2: List of probes with a fold change >2 in the DON and DON+*S.c.* boulardii conditions, Table S3: Primer sequences used for qRT-PCR analysis (F: Forward; R: Reverse), Figure S1: Comparison between microarray-based Log2 (FC) and qRT-PCR-based results Log2 (2-ΔΔCt) by Spearman correlation scattered plots.

Author Contributions: I.A.-K., P.P., S.C., M.C. and I.P.O. conceived and designed the experiments. I.A.-K., P.P., and J.-F.H. performed the ex-vivo experiments. Y.L. and M.N. performed microarray analysis. I.A.-K. performed IPA analysis of the microarray data. I.A.-K. and M.N. performed the qPCR analysis. I.A.-K., J.-F.H. and I.P.O. wrote the paper.

Funding: This study was supported by projects from the Agence Nationale de la Recherche ANR ExpoMycoPig (ANR-17-Carn012) and by project from region Occitanie CLE2014 (funded by the Occitanie Region and Lallemand).

Acknowledgments: The authors are grateful to the Bioinformatics platform from Toulouse Midi-Pyrenees Génopole (GenoToul) for providing resources for the microarray analysis and to A.M. Cossalter for technical assistance with the animal experiments. The authors thank D. Goodfellow for English editing.

Conflicts of Interest: The authors declare no conflict of interest.

References

1. Robert, H.; Payros, D.; Pinton, P.; Theodorou, V.; Mercier-Bonin, M.; Oswald, I.P. Impact of mycotoxins on the intestine: Are mucus and microbiota new targets? *J. Toxicol. Environ. Health Part B Crit. Rev.* **2017**, *20*, 249–275. [CrossRef] [PubMed]

2. Pinton, P.; Oswald, I.P. Effect of deoxynivalenol and other type B trichothecenes on the intestine: A review. *Toxins* **2014**, *6*, 1615–1643. [CrossRef] [PubMed]

3. Cano, P.M.; Seeboth, J.; Meurens, F.; Cognie, J.; Abrami, R.; Oswald, I.P.; Guzylack-Piriou, L. Deoxynivalenol as a new factor in the persistence of intestinal inflammatory diseases: An emerging hypothesis through possible modulation of TH17-mediated response. *PLoS ONE* **2013**, *8*, e53647. [CrossRef] [PubMed]

4. Maresca, M. From the gut to the brain: Journey and pathophysiological effects of the food-associated trichothecene mycotoxin deoxynivalenol. *Toxins* **2013**, *5*, 784–820. [CrossRef] [PubMed]

5. Payros, D.; Alassane-Kpembi, I.; Pierron, A.; Loiseau, N.; Pinton, P.; Oswald, I.P. Toxicology of deoxynivalenol and its acetylated and modified forms. *Arch. Toxicol.* **2016**, *90*, 2931–2957. [CrossRef] [PubMed]

6. Pestka, J.J. Deoxynivalenol: Mechanisms of action, human exposure, and toxicological relevance. *Arch. Toxicol.* **2010**, *84*, 663–679. [CrossRef] [PubMed]

7. Pierron, A.; Mimoun, S.; Murate, L.S.; Loiseau, N.; Lippi, Y.; Bracarense, A.P.; Liaubet, L.; Schatzmayr, G.; Berthiller, F.; Moll, W.D.; et al. Intestinal toxicity of the masked mycotoxin deoxynivalenol-3-beta-D-glucoside. *Arch. Toxicol.* **2016**, *90*, 2037–2046. [CrossRef] [PubMed]

8. Alassane-Kpembi, I.; Kolf-Clauw, M.; Gauthier, T.; Abrami, R.; Abiola, F.A.; Oswald, I.P.; Puel, O. New insights into mycotoxin mixtures: The toxicity of low doses of type B trichothecenes on intestinal epithelial cells is synergistic. *Toxicol. Appl. Pharmacol.* **2013**, *272*, 191–198. [CrossRef] [PubMed]

9. Alassane-Kpembi, I.; Puel, O.; Pinton, P.; Cossalter, A.M.; Chou, T.C.; Oswald, I.P. Co-exposure to low doses of the food contaminants deoxynivalenol and nivalenol has a synergistic inflammatory effect on intestinal explants. *Arch. Toxicol.* **2017**, *91*, 2677–2687. [CrossRef] [PubMed]

10. Alassane-Kpembi, I.; Puel, O.; Oswald, I.P. Toxicological interactions between the mycotoxins deoxynivalenol, nivalenol and their acetylated derivatives in intestinal epithelial cells. *Arch. Toxicol.* **2015**, *89*, 1337–1346. [CrossRef] [PubMed]

11. Garcia, G.R.; Payros, D.; Pinton, P.; Dogi, C.A.; Laffitte, J.; Neves, M.; Gonzalez Pereyra, M.L.; Cavaglieri, L.R.; Oswald, I.P. Intestinal toxicity of deoxynivalenol is limited by lactobacillus rhamnosus RC007 in pig jejunum explants. *Arch. Toxicol.* **2018**, *92*, 983–993. [CrossRef] [PubMed]

12. Hemarajata, P.; Versalovic, J. Effects of probiotics on gut microbiota: Mechanisms of intestinal immunomodulation and neuromodulation. *Ther. Adv. Gastroenter.* **2013**, *6*, 39–51. [CrossRef] [PubMed]

13. Pontier-Bres, R.; Rampal, P.; Peyron, J.F.; Munro, P.; Lemichez, E.; Czerucka, D. The *Saccharomyces boulardii* CNCM I-745 strain shows protective effects against the B. Anthracis lt toxin. *Toxins* **2015**, *7*, 4455–4467. [CrossRef] [PubMed]

14. Trevisi, P.; Latorre, R.; Priori, D.; Luise, D.; Archetti, I.; Mazzoni, M.; D'Inca, R.; Bosi, P. Effect of feed supplementation with live yeast on the intestinal transcriptome profile of weaning pigs orally challenged with *Escherichia coli* f4. *Animal* **2017**, *11*, 33–44. [CrossRef] [PubMed]

15. Weaver, A.C.; See, M.T.; Hansen, J.A.; Kim, Y.B.; De Souza, A.L.; Middleton, T.F.; Kim, S.W. The use of feed additives to reduce the effects of aflatoxin and deoxynivalenol on pig growth, organ health and immune status during chronic exposure. *Toxins* **2013**, *5*, 1261–1281. [CrossRef] [PubMed]

16. Sougioultzis, S.; Simeonidis, S.; Bhaskar, K.R.; Chen, X.; Anton, P.M.; Keates, S.; Pothoulakis, C.; Kelly, C.P. *Saccharomyces boulardii* produces a soluble anti-inflammatory factor that inhibits NF-kappab-mediated IL-8 gene expression. *Biochem. Biophys. Res. Commun.* **2006**, *343*, 69–76. [CrossRef] [PubMed]

17. Chang, C.; Wang, K.; Zhou, S.N.; Wang, X.D.; Wu, J.E. Protective effect of *Saccharomyces boulardii* on deoxynivalenol-induced injury of porcine macrophage via attenuating p38 MAPK signal pathway. *Appl. Biochem. Biotechnol.* **2017**, *182*, 411–427. [CrossRef] [PubMed]

18. Pinton, P.; Nougayrede, J.P.; Del Rio, J.C.; Moreno, C.; Marin, D.E.; Ferrier, L.; Bracarense, A.P.; Kolf-Clauw, M.; Oswald, I.P. The food contaminant deoxynivalenol, decreases intestinal barrier permeability and reduces claudin expression. *Toxicol. Appl. Pharmacol.* **2009**, *237*, 41–48. [CrossRef] [PubMed]

19. Knutsen, H.K.; Alexander, J.; Barregard, L.; Bignami, M.; Bruschweiler, B.; Ceccatelli, S.; Cottrill, B.; Dinovi, M.; Grasl-Kraupp, B.; Hogstrand, C.; et al. Risks to human and animal health related to the presence of deoxynivalenol and its acetylated and modified forms in food and feed. *EFSA J.* **2017**, *15*. [CrossRef]

20. Aquilina, G.; Azimonti, G.; Bampidis, V.; Bastos, M.D.; Bories, G.; Chesson, A.; Cocconcelli, P.S.; Flachowsky, G.; Gropp, J.; Kolar, B.; et al. Safety and efficacy of Levucell® SB (*Saccharomyces cerevisiae* CNCM I-1079) as a feed additive for weaned piglets and sows. *EFSA J.* **2016**, *14*, e04478.

21. Alassane-Kpembi, I.; Gerez, J.R.; Cossalter, A.M.; Neves, M.; Laffitte, J.; Naylies, C.; Lippi, Y.; Kolf-Clauw, M.; Bracarense, A.P.L.; Pinton, P.; et al. Intestinal toxicity of the type B trichothecene mycotoxin fusarenon-x: Whole transcriptome profiling reveals new signaling pathways. *Sci. Rep.* **2017**, *7*, 7530. [CrossRef] [PubMed]

22. Pierron, A.; Mimoun, S.; Murate, L.S.; Loiseau, N.; Lippi, Y.; Bracarense, A.P.; Schatzmayr, G.; He, J.W.; Zhou, T.; Moll, W.D.; et al. Microbial biotransformation of DON: Molecular basis for reduced toxicity. *Sci. Rep.* **2016**, *6*, 29105. [CrossRef] [PubMed]

23. Ricote, M.; Valledor, A.F.; Glass, C.K. Decoding transcriptional programs regulated by ppars and LXRS in the macrophage: Effects on lipid homeostasis, inflammation, and atherosclerosis. *Arterioscler. Thromb. Vasc. Biol.* **2004**, *24*, 230–239. [CrossRef] [PubMed]

24. Klune, J.R.; Dhupar, R.; Cardinal, J.; Billiar, T.R.; Tsung, A. Hmgb1: Endogenous danger signaling. *Mol. Med.* **2008**, *14*, 476–484. [CrossRef] [PubMed]

25. Tanaka, T.; Narazaki, M.; Kishimoto, T. IL-6 in inflammation, immunity, and disease. *Csh Perspect. Biol.* **2014**, *6*, a016295. [CrossRef] [PubMed]

26. Li, M.; Pestka, J.J. Comparative induction of 28S ribosomal RNA cleavage by ricin and the trichothecenes deoxynivalenol and T-2 toxin in the macrophage. *Toxicol. Sci.* **2008**, *105*, 67–78. [CrossRef] [PubMed]

27. Cuenda, A.; Rousseau, S. P38 map-kinases pathway regulation, function and role in human diseases. *Biochim. Biophys. Acta* **2007**, *1773*, 1358–1375. [CrossRef] [PubMed]

28. Nagai, H.; Noguchi, T.; Takeda, K.; Ichijo, H. Pathophysiological roles of ASK1-map kinase signaling pathways. *J. Biochem. Mol. Biol.* **2007**, *40*, 1–6. [CrossRef] [PubMed]

29. Murakami, M.; Yamamoto, K.; Miki, Y.; Murase, R.; Sato, H.; Taketomi, Y. The roles of the secreted phospholipase A$_2$ gene family in immunology. *Adv. Immunol.* **2016**, *132*, 91–134. [PubMed]

30. Majoros, A.; Platanitis, E.; Kernbauer-Holzl, E.; Rosebrock, F.; Muller, M.; Decker, T. Canonical and non-canonical aspects of JAK-STAT signaling: Lessons from interferons for cytokine responses. *Front. Immunol.* **2017**, *8*, 29. [CrossRef] [PubMed]

31. Sun, S.C. The noncanonical NF-kappab pathway. *Immunol. Rev.* **2012**, *246*, 125–140. [CrossRef] [PubMed]

32. Osselaere, A.; Santos, R.; Hautekiet, V.; De Backer, P.; Chiers, K.; Ducatelle, R.; Croubels, S. Deoxynivalenol impairs hepatic and intestinal gene expression of selected oxidative stress, tight junction and inflammation proteins in broiler chickens, but addition of an adsorbing agent shifts the effects to the distal parts of the small intestine. *PLoS ONE* **2013**, *8*, e69014. [CrossRef] [PubMed]

33. Mishra, S.; Dwivedi, P.D.; Pandey, H.P.; Das, M. Role of oxidative stress in deoxynivalenol induced toxicity. *Food Chem. Toxicol.* **2014**, *72*, 20–29. [CrossRef] [PubMed]

34. Wu, Q.H.; Wang, X.; Yang, W.; Nussler, A.K.; Xiong, L.Y.; Kuca, K.; Dohnal, V.; Zhang, X.J.; Yuan, Z.H. Oxidative stress-mediated cytotoxicity and metabolism of T-2 toxin and deoxynivalenol in animals and humans: An update. *Arch. Toxicol.* **2014**, *88*, 1309–1326. [CrossRef] [PubMed]

35. Rizzo, A.F.; Atroshi, F.; Ahotupa, M.; Sankari, S.; Elovaara, E. Protective effect of antioxidants against free radical-mediated lipid peroxidation induced by don or T-2 toxin. *Zentralb Vet. Reihe A* **1994**, *41*, 81–90. [CrossRef]

36. Nimse, S.B.; Pal, D. Free radicals, natural antioxidants, and their reaction mechanisms. *Rsc Adv.* **2015**, *5*, 27986–28006. [CrossRef]

37. Chinetti, G.; Lestavel, S.; Bocher, V.; Remaley, A.T.; Neve, B.; Torra, I.P.; Teissier, E.; Minnich, A.; Jaye, M.; Duverger, N.; et al. PPAR-alpha and PPAR-gamma activators induce cholesterol removal from human macrophage foam cells through stimulation of the abca1 pathway. *Nat. Med.* **2001**, *7*, 53–58. [CrossRef] [PubMed]

38. Burns, K.A.; Vanden Heuvel, J.P. Modulation of ppar activity via phosphorylation. *Biochim. Biophys. Acta* **2007**, *1771*, 952–960. [CrossRef] [PubMed]

39. Adams, M.; Reginato, M.J.; Shao, D.; Lazar, M.A.; Chatterjee, V.K. Transcriptional activation by peroxisome proliferator-activated receptor gamma is inhibited by phosphorylation at a consensus mitogen-activated protein kinase site. *J. Biol. Chem.* **1997**, *272*, 5128–5132. [CrossRef] [PubMed]

40. Hu, E.; Kim, J.B.; Sarraf, P.; Spiegelman, B.M. Inhibition of adipogenesis through map kinase-mediated phosphorylation of ppargamma. *Science* **1996**, *274*, 2100–2103. [CrossRef] [PubMed]

41. Canonici, A.; Pellegrino, E.; Siret, C.; Terciolo, C.; Czerucka, D.; Bastonero, S.; Marvaldi, J.; Lombardo, D.; Rigot, V.; Andre, F. *Saccharomyces boulardii* improves intestinal epithelial cell restitution by inhibiting alphaVSeta5 integrin activation state. *PLoS ONE* **2012**, *7*, e45047. [CrossRef] [PubMed]

42. Czerucka, D.; Piche, T.; Rampal, P. Review article: Yeast as probiotics—*Saccharomyces boulardii*. *Aliment. Pharmacol. Ther.* **2007**, *26*, 767–778. [CrossRef] [PubMed]

43. Kolf-Clauw, M.; Castellote, J.; Joly, B.; Bourges-Abella, N.; Raymond-Letron, I.; Pinton, P.; Oswald, I.P. Development of a pig jejunal explant culture for studying the gastrointestinal toxicity of the mycotoxin deoxynivalenol: Histopathological analysis. *Toxicol. In Vitro* **2009**, *23*, 1580–1584. [CrossRef] [PubMed]

44. Lucioli, J.; Pinton, P.; Callu, P.; Laffitte, J.; Grosjean, F.; Kolf-Clauw, M.; Oswald, I.P.; Bracarense, A.P. The food contaminant deoxynivalenol activates the mitogen activated protein kinases in the intestine: Interest of ex vivo models as an alternative to in vivo experiments. *Toxicon* **2013**, *66*, 31–36. [CrossRef] [PubMed]

45. Devriendt, B.; Gallois, M.; Verdonck, F.; Wache, Y.; Bimczok, D.; Oswald, I.P.; Goddeeris, B.M.; Cox, E. The food contaminant fumonisin B_1 reduces the maturation of porcine CD11R1$^+$ intestinal antigen presenting cells and antigen-specific immune responses, leading to a prolonged intestinal ETEC infection. *Vet. Res.* **2009**, *40*, 1–4. [CrossRef] [PubMed]

46. Pinton, P.; Graziani, F.; Pujol, A.; Nicoletti, C.; Paris, O.; Ernouf, P.; Di Pasquale, E.; Perrier, J.; Oswald, I.P.; Maresca, M. Deoxynivalenol inhibits the expression by goblet cells of intestinal mucins through a PKR and MAP kinase dependent repression of the resistin-like molecule beta. *Mol. Nutr. Food Res.* **2015**, *59*, 1076–1087. [CrossRef] [PubMed]

47. Grenier, B.; Bracarense, A.P.; Schwartz, H.E.; Trumel, C.; Cossalter, A.M.; Schatzmayr, G.; Kolf-Clauw, M.; Moll, W.D.; Oswald, I.P. The low intestinal and hepatic toxicity of hydrolyzed fumonisin B_1 correlates with its inability to alter the metabolism of sphingolipids. *Biochem. Pharmacol.* **2012**, *83*, 1465–1473. [CrossRef] [PubMed]

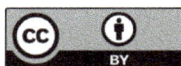

toxins

MDPI

Article

Protective Effect of N-Acetylcysteine against Oxidative Stress Induced by Zearalenone via Mitochondrial Apoptosis Pathway in SIEC02 Cells

Jingjing Wang †, Mengmeng Li †, Wei Zhang, Aixin Gu, Jiawen Dong, Jianping Li * **and Anshan Shan ***

Institute of Animal Nutrition, Northeast Agricultural University, Harbin 150030, China;
JF_JING@hotmail.com (J.W.); limengmeng@outlook.com (M.L.); zhangwei910315@hotmail.com (W.Z.);
aixingu@hotmail.com (A.G.); dongjiawen2018@outlook.com (J.D.)
* Correspondence: ljpneau@gmail.com (J.L.); asshan@neau.edu.cn (A.S.); Tel.: +86-0451-5519-1439 (J.L.)
† These authors contributed equally to the paper.

Received: 5 August 2018; Accepted: 2 October 2018; Published: 9 October 2018

Abstract: Zearalenone (ZEN), a nonsteroidal estrogen mycotoxin, is widely found in feed and foodstuffs. Intestinal cells may become the primary target of toxin attack after ingesting food containing ZEN. Porcine small intestinal epithelial (SIEC02) cells were selected to assess the effect of ZEN exposure on the intestine. Cells were exposed to ZEN (20 μg/mL) or pretreated with (81, 162, and 324 μg/mL) N-acetylcysteine (NAC) prior to ZEN treatment. Results indicated that the activities of glutathione peroxidase (Gpx) and glutathione reductase (GR) were reduced by ZEN, which induced reactive oxygen species (ROS) and malondialdehyde (MDA) production. Moreover, these activities increased apoptosis and mitochondrial membrane potential ($\Delta\Psi$m), and regulated the messenger RNA (mRNA) expression of Bax, Bcl-2, caspase-3, caspase-9, and cytochrome c (cyto c). Additionally, NAC pretreatment reduced the oxidative damage and inhibited the apoptosis induced by ZEN. It can be concluded that ZEN-induced oxidative stress and damage may further induce mitochondrial apoptosis, and pretreatment of NAC can degrade this damage to some extent.

Keywords: Zearalenone; N-acetylcysteine; SIEC02 cells; Mitochondrial apoptosis

Key contribution: The gastrointestinal tract is the primary target of mycotoxin attack, and ZEN produced cytotoxic effects on SIEC02 cells. Oxidative stress and mitochondrial apoptosis of SIEC02 cells, produced after exposure to ZEN and NAC pretreatment, can alleviate the negative effect of ZEN on SIEC02 cells.

---

1. Introduction

Zearalenone (ZEN), a secondary metabolite produced by fungi of the genus *Fusarium*, can seriously affect animal growth, reproduction, and immune function [1–3]. Studies estimate that one-fourth of the global food and feed output is contaminated by mycotoxins, and the number is likely to be closer to 50% if new fungal toxins are considered for limited data [4,5]. ZEN is being increasingly recognized as a frequent contaminant in animal feeding, which has a significant effect on human and animal health [6,7]. According to a recent report, the United States Department of Agriculture (USDA), the European Food Safety Authority (EFSA), and China are concerned about mycotoxin contamination in cereals, and they have renewed the maximum residue limits (MRLs) in food and feeds [8]. The MRLs in food is 350 μg/kg, 350 μg/kg, and 60 μg/kg, respectively. EFSA and China also reiterated that the MRLs in feed is 2000 μg/kg and 500 μg/kg [8].

It is shown that most animals have a certain sensitivity to ZEN, and the pig is the most sensitive animal [9]. The primary attack target of toxins from ingested food or feed is the gastrointestinal tract, and thus it affects intestinal function [10,11]. The main metabolites of ZEN are α-zearalenol (α-ZOL) and β-zearalenol (β-ZOL) [12]. Establishing a barrier model (IPEC-1) in vitro, study has shown that ZEN and its metabolites damage barrier function by reducing the immune response [13]. It has been reported that ZEN affects the villous structures and reduces the expression of junction proteins in a dose-dependent manner in pregnant rats [14]. The estrogen-like effects of ZEN and its derivatives have been determined in vivo and in vitro [13,15]. A further experiment has demonstrated that oxidative damage is likely to be evoked as one of the main pathways of ZEN toxicity [16]. Moreover, data suggested that ZEN induced apoptosis in a dose-dependent manner in many cell lines (HepG2, porcine granulosa, and SHSY-5Y cells) [6,17,18]. Therefore, it is necessary to analyze the effect of ZEN on the intestinal tract.

N-acetylcysteine (NAC), the precursor of glutathione, is a water-soluble molecule that has antioxidant, anti-inflammatory, and tumor-inhibitory properties [19,20]. A previous study has shown that NAC can exert antioxidant effects both in vitro and in vivo [21]. It is generally assumed that the action of NAC is to scavenge free radicals by increasing the intracellular glutathione (GSH) level [22]. More recently, studies have found that NAC can directly inhibit the production of reactive oxygen species (ROS), and thus inhibit apoptosis [23,24]. Similarly, NAC pretreatment can reduce lipid peroxidation and inhibit apoptosis [25]. In addition, NAC also plays an important role in protecting renal function by reducing oxidative stress [26,27].

Cells were poisoned by ZEN, cells may undergo complex and different pathways of damage, including apoptosis [16,18]. The SIEC02 cells retained the morphological and functional characteristics that were typical of primary swine intestinal epithelial cells by introducing the human telomerase reverse transcriptase, and thus they provide a cell model in vitro [28]. However, the mechanism underlying the apoptosis of intestinal cells after exposure to ZEN is still not totally understood. Therefore, the purpose of this study was to evaluate whether ZEN-induced oxidative damage could further lead to apoptosis, and whether the addition of NAC could alleviate this negative effect on SIEC02 cells.

2. Results

2.1. Effects of ZEN and NAC on Cell Viability

To examine the cytotoxic effects of ZEN, SIEC02 cells were incubated with ZEN (5, 10, 15, 20, 25 and 30 μg/mL) for 24 h. After incubation, ZEN treatment inhibited the cell viability markedly in a dose-dependent manner (Figure 1A). Cell viability was only 36.30% at a ZEN concentration of 30 μg/mL, and the inhibitory concentration of IC_{50} (50% inhibitory concentration) was 22.68 ± 0.80 μg/mL. Hence, a cytotoxic concentration of ZEN (20 μg/mL) was selected for subsequent experiments. In addition, NAC alone did not show any cytotoxicity at concentrations (81, 162, and 324 μg/mL) of incubation for 6 h. However, compared with the control group, cell viability was significantly reduced when cells were treated by NAC (162 and 324 μg/mL) for 12 h ($P < 0.05$). All three concentrations of NAC significantly reduced cell viability for 24 h ($P < 0.01$) (Figure 1B). Based on the additions shown in Figure 1B, NAC concentrations (81, 162 and 324 μg/mL) were selected for pretreating the cells for 6 h prior to the ZEN treatment.

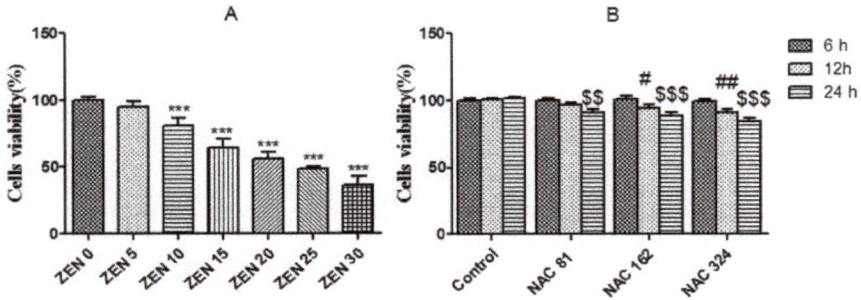

Figure 1. Effects of zearalenone (ZEN) and N-acetylcysteine (NAC) on SIEC02 cells viability. Cells were treated without or with different concentrations of ZEN (0, 5, 10, 15, 20, 25 and 30 μg/mL) for 24 h (**A**). Cells were pretreated without or with different concentrations of NAC (81, 162 and 324 μg/mL) for 6 h, 12 h, and 24 h (**B**). Cells survival was measured by Cell Counting Kit-8 (CCK-8) assay. The values are mean ± SD of three independent experiments. *** indicates a significant difference between ZEN and control at $P < 0.001$. #, ## indicates a significant difference of 12 h between NAC and control, with significant differences at $P < 0.05$ and $P < 0.01$. $$, $$$ indicates a significant difference of 24 h between NAC and the control at $P < 0.01$ and $P < 0.001$.

2.2. Effects of ZEN and NAC on Oxidative Stress

2.2.1. Glutathione peroxidase (Gpx) Activity

Data on the activity of antioxidative enzymes and related products in SIEC02 cells is summarized in Figure 2. As shown in Figure 2A, Gpx activity was significantly reduced after ZEN treatment on 0.227 μmol/mg of protein, compared with the control group (0.325 μmol/mg) ($P < 0.001$). The Gpx activity was restored to a certain extend by the pretreatment of cells with NAC (81, 162 and 324 μg/mL) ($P < 0.001$) and increased to 0.247, 0.248 and 0.254 μmol/mg of protein, respectively. Based on these data, NAC pretreatment could significantly increase the reduction in Gpx activity induced by ZEN, and the optimal concentration of NAC was 324 μg/mL ($P < 0.05$).

2.2.2. Glutathione reductase (GR) Activity

According to Figure 2B, compared with the control group (11.307 U/mg), the GR activity of ZEN treatment was significantly reduced to 0.857 U/mg of protein ($P < 0.001$). The reduction in GR activity induced by ZEN was restored to a certain extend by the treatment of cells with NAC (81, 162 and 324 μg/mL) ($P < 0.05$) and increased to 3.859, 3.537 and 3.269 U/mg of protein, respectively. Based on these data, NAC pretreatment could significantly increase the activity of GR. Three concentrations of NAC did not reach a significant level.

2.2.3. Malondialdehyde (MDA) Level

As shown in Figure 2C, the MDA level of ZEN treatment was significantly higher (151.9 nmol/mg of protein) than the control group (32.2 nmol/mg) ($P < 0.001$). Pretreatment with NAC (81, 162 and 324 μg/mL) significantly reduced the increase in the MDA level as induced by ZEN ($P < 0.001$), and decreased to 132.2, 130.2 and 132.5 nmol/mg of protein, respectively. Three concentrations of NAC did not reach a significant level.

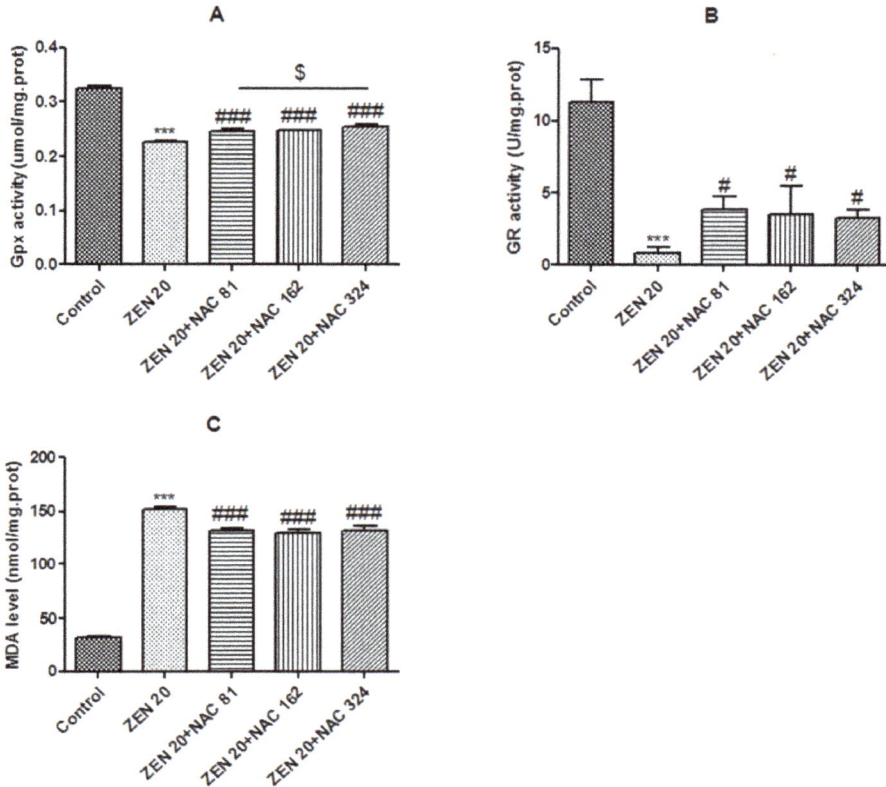

Figure 2. Effect of ZEN (20 µg/mL) and NAC (81, 162 and 324 µg/mL) on intracellular glutathione peroxidase (Gpx), glutathione reductase (GR) activity, and malondialdehyde (MDA) levels. Cells were exposed to ZEN for 24 h, including NAC pretreatment for 6 h. The results of Gpx, GR, and MDA were µmol/mg, U/mg, nmol/mg of protein, respectively. Each set of data shows the mean ± SD of three independent experiments. *** indicates a significant difference between ZEN and control $P < 0.001$. #, ###, indicates a significant difference between ZEN and NAC in mutual treatment at $P < 0.05$ and $P < 0.001$. $ indicates a significant difference between three concentrations of NAC at $P < 0.05$ (**A**–**C**).

2.3. Effects of ZEN and NAC on Intracellular ROS Generation

ROS was generated as by-products of cellular metabolism, which could trigger oxidative stress at high concentrations [29] . ROS production was monitored by measuring the fluorescence intensity of DCFH-DA (2',7'-dichlorodihydrofluorescein diacetate dye). DCFH-DA is a fluorescent probe of ROS. The non-fluorescent fluorescin DCFH-DA derivatives will emit fluorescence after being oxidized by the radicals generated by the toxins. In the presence of ROS, H_2-DCF is rapidly oxidized to become highly fluorescent DCF [30,31]. The result indicated that ZEN could significantly induce ROS accumulation in SIEC02 cells ($P < 0.001$) (Figure 3) and the ROS content in the ZEN group was significantly higher than that in control group. As observed in Figure 3, NAC pretreatment significantly reduced ZEN-induced ROS production ($P < 0.01$), and the optimal concentration of NAC was 162 µg/mL ($P < 0.05$).

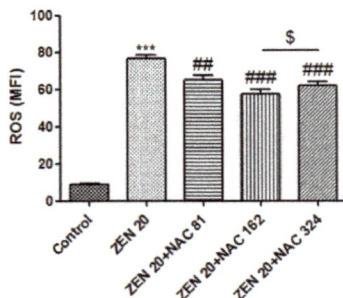

Figure 3. Effect of ZEN (20 µg/mL) and NAC (81, 162 and 324 µg/mL) on intracellular reactive oxygen species (ROS) production. Cells were exposed to ZEN for 24 h, including NAC pretreatment for 6 h. The results are expressed as mean fluorescent intensity (MFI). Each set of data shows the mean ± SD of the three independent experiments. *** indicates a significant difference between ZEN and control at $P < 0.001$. ##, ### indicates a significant difference between ZEN and NAC in mutual treatment at $P < 0.01$ and $P < 0.001$. $ indicates a significant difference between three concentrations of NAC at $P < 0.05$.

2.4. Effects of ZEN and NAC on Apoptosis

Cells were stained with Annexin V-FITC/PI to determine whether ZEN induced cell apoptosis and its consequences following alleviation with NAC were evaluated. Compared with the control group (Figure 4A), the number of living cells were decreased and the early apoptosis of ZEN treatment, and the late apoptotic cells were significantly increased ($P < 0.05$) (Figure 4B and 4F). As seen in Figure 4C,D,E and F, the apoptotic cells of Q2 and Q4 were reduced compared with Figure 4B, and the apoptotic rate was also significantly reduced ($P < 0.01$) by NAC pretreatment. The optimal concentration of NAC was 324 µg/mL ($P < 0.05$) (Figure 4F).

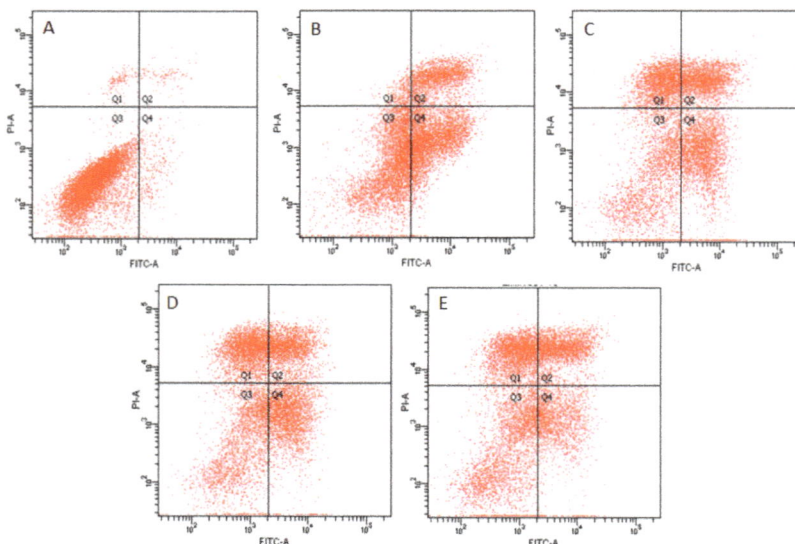

Figure 4. *Cont.*

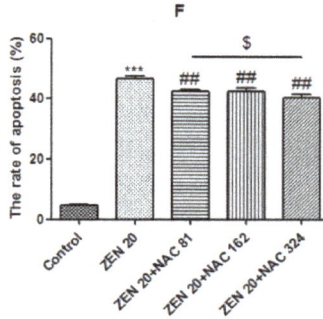

Figure 4. Annexin V-FITC/PI flow cytometry was used to detect SIEC02 cells treated with ZEN (20 µg/mL) and NAC (81, 162 and 324 µg/mL). The Q1, Q2, Q3, and Q4 gates, respectively, represented dead cells, the late stage of cell apoptosis, normal cells, and the early stage of cell apoptosis (**A, B, C, D** and **E** are control, ZEN 20 µg/mL, ZEN 20 µg/mL + NAC 81 µg/mL, ZEN 20 µg/mL + NAC 162 µg/mL, and ZEN 20 µg/mL + NAC 324 µg/mL, respectively). Apoptosis results are expressed as the rate of apoptosis. Each set of data shows the mean ± SD of the three independent experiments. *** indicates a significant difference between ZEN and control at $P < 0.001$. ## indicates a significant difference between ZEN and NAC in mutual treatment at $P < 0.01$. \$ indicates a significant difference between three concentrations of NAC at $P < 0.05$ (**F**).

2.5. Effects of ZEN and NAC on the Change of ΔΨm

JC-1 (mitochondrial probe) formed J-aggregates in the mitochondrial matrix (red) at high ΔΨm in nonapoptotic cells, and formed monomeric (green) at low ΔΨm in apoptotic cells (Figure 5). Therefore, the change of ΔΨm was reflected by decreasing the red and green fluorescence ratio. The effects of different treatments on mitochondrial membrane potential in SIEC02 cells are shown in Figure 5A–E. As shown in Figure 5B, the green aggregates were increased compared with the control group (Figure 5A), indicating that the ΔΨm was decreased, the cell membrane was severely damaged, and the apoptosis rate was significantly increased ($P < 0.001$) (Figure 5F). After NAC pretreatment, green aggregates showed signs of weakening (Figure 5C,D and E) compared with the ZEN group (Figure 5B). The apoptosis rate of the cells was significantly decreased by NAC pretreatment ($P < 0.01$) and it did not reach a significant level in the three concentrations of NAC (Figure 5F).

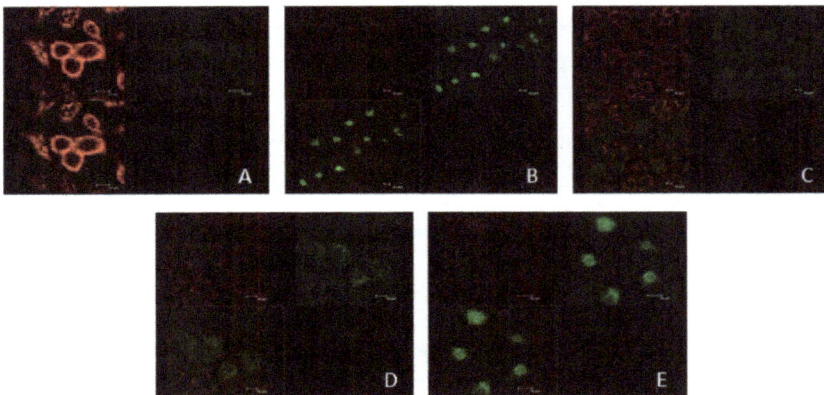

Figure 5. *Cont.*

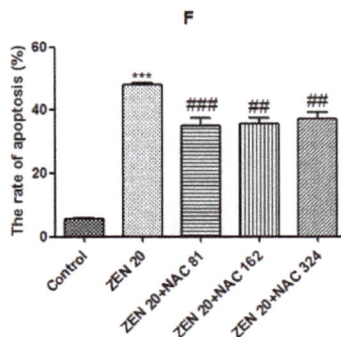

Figure 5. A laser scanning confocal microscope was used to observe the changes of mitochondrial membrane potential ($\Delta\Psi$m) in SIEC02 cells treated with ZEN and NAC. The scanning pictures were as shown in the figure (**A–E** are control, ZEN 20 µg/mL, ZEN 20 µg/mL + NAC 81 µg/mL, ZEN 20 µg/mL + NAC 162 µg/mL and ZEN 20 µg/mL + NAC 324 µg/mL, respectively). Scale bar: 10 µm. The results are expressed as apoptosis rate (**F**); each set of data shows the mean ± SD of the three independent experiments. *** indicates a significant difference between ZEN and control at $P < 0.001$. ##, ### indicates a significant difference between ZEN and NAC in mutual treatment at $P < 0.01$ and $P < 0.001$ (**F**).

2.6. Effects of ZEN and NAC on Apoptosis-Related mRNA Expression

2.6.1. Bax

The effects of ZEN and NAC protection apoptosis-related mRNA levels via caspase pathways are shown in Figure 6. As shown in Figure 6A, the mRNA expression levels of Bax were significantly increased by ZEN, compared with the control group ($P < 0.001$). Compared with the ZEN treatment, the NAC-pretreated significantly reduced the mRNA expression of Bax ($P < 0.001$). Three concentrations of NAC did not reach a significant level.

2.6.2. Bcl-2

The expression of Bcl-2 mRNA was opposite to that of Bax. As shown in Figure 6B, the mRNA expression levels of Bax were significantly decreased in the ZEN group ($P < 0.01$). Compared with ZEN treatment, the production of Bcl-2 could not be significantly decreased at a NAC concentration of 324 µg/mL. When the concentration of NAC were 81 and 162 µg/mL, the mRNA expression of Bcl-2 significantly increased ($P < 0.001$), and the optimal concentration of NAC was 162 µg/mL ($P < 0.01$).

2.6.3. Cytochrome c (Cyto c)

As shown in Figure 6C, the mRNA expression levels of cyto c were significantly increased by ZEN ($P < 0.01$). Compared with ZEN treatment, the production of cyto c could not be significantly decreased at a NAC concentration of 81 µg/mL. When the NAC concentration of NAC were 162 and 324 µg/mL, cyto-c production was significantly decreased ($P < 0.01$).

2.6.4. Caspase-9 and Caspase-3

Similar to cyto c mRNA expression, caspase-9 and caspase-3 mRNA levels were significantly increased by ZEN ($P < 0.05$) (Figure 6D,E). Compared with ZEN treatment, the mRNA expression of caspase-9 was significantly reduced at the NAC concentrations of 81 and 162 µg/mL ($P < 0.05$). At the same time, when the NAC concentration of NAC were 162 and 324 µg/mL, the mRNA expression of caspase-3 was significantly increased ($P < 0.001$).

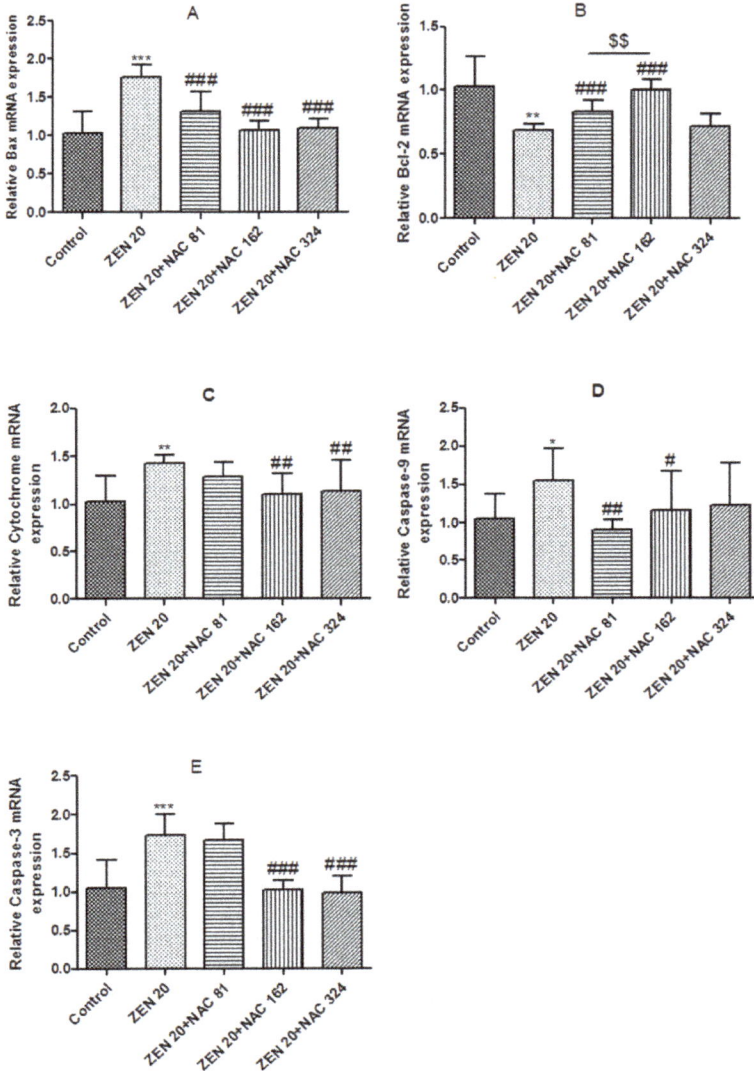

Figure 6. The results of the ZEN (20 µg/mL) and NAC (81, 162 and 324 µg/mL) expression levels of each apoptotic gene (Bcl-2, Bax, cytochrome c, caspase-9, caspase-3) in the SIEC02 cells. Cells were exposed to ZEN for 24 h, including NAC pretreatment for 6 h. The results are expressed relative to the expression of actin; each set of data shows the mean ± SD of the three independent experiments. *, **, *** indicates a significant difference between ZEN and control at $P < 0.05$, $P < 0.01$, and $P < 0.001$. #, ##, ### indicates a significant difference between ZEN and NAC in mutual treatment at $P < 0.05$, $P < 0.01$, and $P < 0.001$. $$ indicates a significant difference between three concentrations of NAC at $P < 0.01$ (**A–E**).

3. Discussion

ZEN and its major metabolites are secondary metabolites of *Fusarium* fungi that produce cell damage [12,32]. A number of studies have found that ZEN has an inhibitory effect on cell proliferation [15,16]. The most direct indicator is the number of living cells due to toxic changes. The IC_{50} is an important indicator of the cellular response to chemical effects. In human hepatoma cells (HepG2) and colorectal cancer cells (HCT116), the IC_{50} is 100 μM and 60 μM, respectively, and cell proliferation undergoes a dose-dependent reduction after ZEN treatment [18,33]. In this experiment, Cell Counting Kit-8 (CCK-8) method was used to detect the effect of ZEN on the activity of SIEC02 cells cultured in vitro. The results showed that after treatment with ZEN for 24 h, the IC_{50} range was 22.68 ± 0.80 μg/mL (62.89 μM). This value might differ slightly from that just mentioned, because of differences in cell lines. With the increase in ZEN concentration, the cell activity gradually decreased and showed a dose-response relationship.

The gastrointestinal tract is the primary site of toxin interaction, and intestinal epithelial cells are an important first target site for mycotoxin [34,35]. Most studies of toxicity have shown that the cytotoxicity of ZEN is determined by the production of ROS, DNA damage, and an increased formation of lipid peroxidation [36,37]. In normal physiological processes, small amounts of ROS are generated as by-products of cellular metabolism, primarily in the mitochondria [29,32]. ROS are highly reactive molecules, among which oxygen-free radicals can destroy cell structures, and increase lipid peroxidation of biofilms [38,39]. MDA, as the final product of lipid peroxidation, which can cause cell serious injuries in membrane structure, changes the permeability of cell membranes, leading to cell apoptosis, and necrosis [40]. Therefore, the measurement of MDA content can indirectly reflect the degree of lipid peroxidation. In this experiment, our results showed that 20 μg/mL of ZEN significantly increased ROS and MDA contents in SIEC02 cells. Previous studies have found similar effects in different cell types that are exposed to ZEN. These results were consistent with the findings that ZEN can significantly increase ROS in CHO-K1 and IPEC-J2 cells and MDA in Caco-2 cells [36,41,42].

NAC, a precursor of GSH that is a free radical scavenger, which plays an important role as an antagonistic foreign chemical to the oxidative damage caused by biological organisms [22,43]. The antioxidant activity of NAC is evaluated by the enzymatic system. The antioxidant enzymes and other regulatory enzymes can be used as the first line of defense, and they play a role in scavenging free radical damage intracellularly and extracellularly [38]. GR and Gpx are the intrinsic anti-oxidative enzymes of cells [44]. Gpx catalyzes GSH to decompose H_2O_2 into water, and to form Glutathione oxidized (GSSG), and the GR enzyme can reduce GSSG to GSH, to scavenge excess H_2O_2 [45,46]. NAC could increase intracellular glutathione and produce sulfhydryl groups that directly eliminate ROS, such as hypochlorous acid, hydrogen peroxide, superoxide, and hydroxyl radicals [47,48]. Consequently, NAC increases the activity of the antioxidant enzymes Gpx and GR by restoring intracellular GSH content, thereby eliminating ROS. In this experiment, our data clearly demonstrated that the activities of Gpx and GR were significantly increased after NAC pretreatment, and that ROS was significantly reduced. Our study showed that NAC preconditioning could alleviate the activity of antioxidant enzymes in SIEC02 cells, and this result is also consistent with another team's results on the pig kidney PK15 cells [49]. In addition, pretreatment with NAC positively reduced ROS generation, suggesting a potential antioxidant for NAC, which is conformed to reduce cellular ROS by adding NAC in Jurkat T cells [50].

Apoptosis, a form of programmed cell death, is an essential process in cell growth, reproduction, and self-adjustment and it is characterized by morphological changes such as nucleosome fracture and the formation of apoptotic bodies [51,52]. In apoptosis caused by exposure to mycotoxins, mitochondrial-mediated apoptosis is the main pathway, which is activated programmed cell death by ROS via mediated by mycotoxins [53]. The mitochondria are an important source of ROS within most mammalian cells [54]. In response to apoptotic stimuli, DNA damage and oxidative stress occur, and eventually the mitochondrial pathway is triggered [30]. The mitochondrial outer membrane is highly permeability in mitochondria [31,55]. Indeed, a previous study reported that when cells are poisoned or subjected to other stimuli, the ΔΨm decreases [56]. The ΔΨm disruption is an important trigger in managing apoptosis [57]. Studies have found that ZEN may cause mitochondrial membrane hyperpolarization over a short period of time, followed by loss of the ΔΨm [58,59]. Previous in vitro experiments demonstrate that ZEN directly causes apoptosis through the mitochondrial pathway at low concentrations. Subsequently, numerous studies show that ZEN causes intracellular ROS and MDA levels to rise and $\Delta\Psi m$ decreases, leading to cell apoptosis [32,60,61]. Based on these findings, to reveal whether ZEN-induced apoptosis involves $\Delta\Psi m$, our study focused on detecting $\Delta\Psi m$ in SIEC02 cells by JC-1 fluorescence to detect changes in membrane potential. Green fluorescence is indicative of the $\Delta\Psi m$ decline by JC-1 staining [62,63]. Our results showed that treatment with ZEN caused an increase in ROS and loss of $\Delta\Psi m$, suggesting that ZEN passed the mitochondrial-mediated pathway. In this study, the percentage of ZEN cells with green fluorescence increased by NAC. This may be because NAC is deacetylated to cysteine, rapidly oxidized, and then transported to cells, which is reduced to GSH, thereby restoring the cell state [6]. The results showed that after addition of NAC pretreatment, $\Delta\Psi m$ increased, inhibiting apoptosis in SIEC02 cells. This result is consistent with recent studies that have promoted apoptosis of the mitochondria-mediated pathway through ZEN [64].

When mitochondrial membrane permeability changes, cyto c is first released from the mitochondrial membrane space into the cytoplasm, resulting in subsequent activation of capase-9 [65,66]. Next, activation of caspase-9 activates the downstream performer (caspase-3), thereby triggering apoptosis in the cascade [67]. In the mitochondrial apoptosis pathway, caspase-9 is a key activator of the caspase cascade; caspase-3 is located downstream of the apoptotic ordered cascade reaction and it is the key executor of the transfer, and its activation marks the process of apoptosis [68,69]. Previous studies have found that the production of ROS can proceed from the release of cyto c [70]. Furthermore, a study has shown that ROS can further release cyto c from the mitochondria into the cytoplasm [64]. In this experiment, after ZEN exposure, both intracellular ROS and cyto c increased significantly consistent with previous studies. The Bcl-2 protein family may regulate mitochondrial permeability through both permeabilization of the mitochondrial membrane or translocation of cyto c [28]. Bax is the representative of apoptosis-promoting proteins, and Bcl-2 is a gene that inhibits apoptosis [71]. When the cell damage is serious, Bcl-2 protein expression decreases and Bax protein expression increases [72]. The current study showed that ZEN downregulated Bcl-2 and upregulated Bax mRNA expression, which triggered apoptosis in SIEC02 cells. In the current study, our results showed that after treatment with ZEN toxins, a significant increase in apoptosis was observed. ZEN treatment upregulated mRNA expression of cyto c, caspase-3, and caspase-9. According to the results of this experiment, pretreatment with NAC could inhibit the expression of proapoptotic genes in cells, increase the expression of antiapoptotic genes, and reduce the cell damage induced by ZEN.

4. Conclusions

In conclusion, the results of this study suggested that ZEN induced oxidative stress in SIEC02 cells and sequentially promoted apoptosis through the mitochondrial pathway. ZEN produced substantial cytotoxicity to SIEC02 cells because of elevated ROS levels, which in turn led to increased caspase-3 activation and apoptosis. In addition, NAC pretreatment increased antioxidant enzyme activity, elevated $\Delta\Psi m$, and inhibited ZEN-induced apoptosis through the mitochondrial pathway. Based on these results, this study provides new insights into the mechanism of action of ZEN on intestinal cells in vitro, and the mitigation of this effect by pretreatment with NAC. However, all of the effects of ZEN and its protective mechanisms for the intestine are still not fully understood, and further research is needed.

5. Materials and Methods

5.1. Chemicals and Reagents

ZEN and NAC were supplied by Sigma-Aldrich (St. Louis, MO, USA). Dulbecco modified Eagle medium (DMEM)-F:12 cell culture medium was purchased from Thermo Fisher (Hyclone, Shanghai, China). Fetal bovine serum (FBS) was supplied by Gibco (Invitrogen Corporation, Grand Island, NY, USA). CCK-8 was supplied by Dojindo (Kumamoto, Japan). ROS assay kit, MDA, Gpx, and GR antioxidant kits, and ΔΨm assay kit with JC-1 were supplied by Beyotime Biotechnology (Nantong, China). Phosphate buffered saline (PBS) was purchased from Biotopped (Beijing, China). Ethanol at a concentration of 0.25% was chosen as an organic solvent for the dilution of ZEN pure product for subsequent testing.

5.2. Cell Culture and Conditions

SIEC02 cells were donated by Northwest A&F University. The SIEC02 cell line was derived from the mid-jejunum of neonatal, un-suckled, and 1-day-old Landrace piglets [73]. Cells (passages 15–30) were grown in DMEM-F:12 supplemented with 10% fetal calf serum, and 1% penicillin and streptomycin, and cultured at 37 °C in an atmosphere of 5% CO_2 in a cell incubator. The cells were inoculated in a 25 cm^2 cell culture flask (Nest, Eimer Biotechnology Company, Wuxi, China), and the culture medium was changed after 24 h. When the cells were confluent to approximately 80%–90%, the cell monolayer was washed with PBS and digested with 1× trypsin/EDTA (Beyotime Institute of Biotechnology, Nantong, China) for subsequent testing.

5.3. Cell Viability Assay

The cytotoxicity of ZEN on SIEC02 cells was measured by CCK-8. Cells (0.5–0.8×10^6/mL) were seeded in 96-well culture plates for 24 h (Nest, Eimer Biotechnology Company, Wuxi, China) and then treated with ZEN (0, 5, 10, 15, 20, 25 and 30 μg/mL). Similarly, cells were seeded in the same culture plates (6, 12, and 24 h) and then treated with NAC (81, 162, and 324 μg/mL). After all treatments were completed, cells were washed twice with PBS. CCK-8 was then added to a final concentration of 10% in a serum-free medium and cultured at 37 °C for 3 h. The viability rate was measured by measuring the absorbance on a microplate reader with an emission wavelength of 450 nm (SpectraMax M5, Molecular Devices, Sunnyvale, CA, USA).

5.4. Experiment Design

For all experiments, cells were used at 80%–90% confluence and assigned into five treatment groups: control group (cells were incubated with FBS-DMEM-F:12 culture medium for 24 h); ZEN group (cells were incubated with 20 μg/mL ZEN for 24 h); NAC+ZEN group after cells were pretreated with NAC (81, 162 and 324 μg/mL) for 6 h, then placed with fresh culture medium containing 20 μg/mL ZEN for 24 h. The cells of the subsequent experiments (0.5–0.8×10^6/mL) were seeded in 6-well culture plates (Nest, Eimer Biotechnology Company, Wuxi, China) and treated with drugs as described in this section.

5.5. Determination of Antioxidant Enzyme Activity and Oxidative Products

SIEC02 cells were used for the analysis of antioxidative enzyme and related products. Briefly, cells were washed with 4 °C precooled PBS and resuspended, then lysed on ice. Antioxidant enzyme activities such as Gpx and GR were measured using the assay kit according to the manufacturer's instructions. The results were expressed as μmol/mg or U/mg of protein, respectively. The level of MDA was measured according to the kit instructions, and the results were expressed as nmol/mg of protein. The density of each protein was detected by Enhanced BCA Protein Assay Kit (Beyotime Institute of Biotechnology, Nantong, China).

5.6. Detection of ROS Generation

The balance between the generation and clearance of ROS is important to maintain intracellular redox states. A flow cytometry technique was used to assess the intracellular amounts of ROS with dichlorofluorescein diacetate (DCFH-DA). Briefly, cells were washed with PBS and incubated with 10 μM DCFH-DA at 37 °C for 20 min. After incubated, cells were washed thrice with serum-free cell culture medium. Intracellular production of ROS was measured by a FACS flow cytometry

(Becton-Dickinson, San Jose, CA, USA) with an excitation wavelength of 488 nm and an emission wavelength of 525 nm. The DCF fluorescence intensity indicates the amount of intracellular ROS and the results were analyzed by mean fluorescent intensity (MFI).

5.7. Apoptosis Detection

5.7.1. Annexin V-FITC/PI Double Staining

The apoptosis of SIEC02 cells was measured by the Annexin V-FITC/PI apoptosis detection kit (Biosea Biochemicals, Shanghai, China). Briefly, cells were trypsinized and harvested via centrifugation at 2000×g and 4 °C for 5 min, then re-suspended in 500 μL binding buffer. Annexin-FITC (10 μL) was injected into the solutions and incubated for 40 min at 37 °C in the dark. Finally, 5 μL PI (10 μg/mL) was added. Scattering signals were detected by FACS flow cytometry as described in the previous section.

5.7.2. ΔΨm Assay

In this experiment, ΔΨm was monitored by the cationic dye JC-1. Briefly, after treatment and washing three times with PBS, culture medium (1 mL) and JC-1 staining solution (1 mL) are added; after being fully mixed, the cells are incubated at 37 °C for 20 minutes. During incubation, according to 1 mL JC-1 staining buffer (5×) with 4 mL distilled water, JC-1 staining is mixed with JC-1 staining buffer (1×). An increase in the green/red fluorescence intensity ratio indicates mitochondrial membrane depolarization. To each well, 0.5 mL culture medium was added, and the results were detected using a laser scanning confocal microscope (LEICA, Hesse, Germany).

5.7.3. RNA Extraction and Quantitative real time polymerase chain reaction (qRT-PCR)

Total RNA was extracted using RNA fast 200 (Fastagen, Shanghai, China), according to the manufacturer's instruction. The A_{260}/A_{280} ratio was measured by using a using a Nano Photometer P-Class (Implen GmbH, Munich, Germany) to ensure the purity of the RNA sample, and agarose gel electrophoresis was used to ensure the integrity of the total RNA sample. The complementary DNA (cDNA) was amplified by qRT-PCR using a SYBR Premix Ex Taq RT-PCR kit (Takara, Dalian, China) and used for RT-PCR. SYBR Green I RT-PCR kit (Takara, Dalian, China) was used to measure the mRNA expression of apoptosis-related genes (Bcl-2, Bax, cyto c, caspase-9, caspase-3), and β-actin was used as the internal control gene to correct for differences. The sequences of the specific primers used were as follows in Table 1 [49]. The sequences of the specific primers in this study used were designed from published GenBank sequences, and they were synthesized by Sangon (Shanghai, China).

Table 1. Primers used for qRT-PCR.

Genes	Accession Number	Orientation	Sequences (5′→3′)	Fragments Size (bp)	Tm (°C)
β-actin	AY550069	Forward	ATGCTTCTAGGCGGACTGT	211	58.2
		Reverse	CCATCCAACCGACTGCT		
Bcl-2	AB271960.1	Forward	GCGACTTTGCCGAGATGT	116	55.9
		Reverse	CACAATCCTCCCCCAGTTC		
Bax	XM_003127290.3	Forward	TTTGCTTCAGGGTTTCATCC	113	54.4
		Reverse	GACACTCGCTCAACTTCTTGG		
Cyto c	NM_001129970.1	Forward	CTCTTACACAGATGCCAACAA	139	56.1
		Reverse	TTCCCTTTCTCCCTTCTTCT		
Caspase-9	XM_013998997.1	Forward	GGACATTGGTTCTGGAGGATT	116	52.3
		Reverse	TGTTGATGATGAGGCAGTGG		
Caspase-3	NM_214131.1	Forward	GACACTCGCTCAACTTCTTGG	121	54.5
		Reverse	TTGGACTGTGGGATTGAGAC		

RT-PCR was performed by an ABI PRISM 7500 SDS thermal cycler (Applied Biosystems, Foster City, CA, USA). The reaction was carried out using a 10 µL system of PCR, including 1.0 µL of cDNA and 0.2 µL of each primer. The cycle numbers and annealing temperature were optimized for each primer pair. The PCR cycling conditions were as follows: a denaturation step at 95 °C for 30 s, followed by 40 cycles of denaturing at 95 °C for 5 s and annealing at 60 °C for 34 s. The relative expression of the apoptosis cytokine mRNA was measured by the $2^{-\Delta\Delta Ct}$ method [74].

5.8. Statistical Analysis

Data were analyzed using SPSS 17.0 software (SPSS Inc., Chicago, IL, USA, 2008), and the data of three independent experiments were expressed as mean ± standard deviation (SD). All the experimental data were analyzed for variance uniformity. When the variance was uniform, data were analyzed by a one-way ANOVA followed by Least-Significant Difference (LSD). When the variance was uneven, data were converted into logarithms, and then analyzed by one-way ANOVA followed by LSD. The significance was considered to be at the probability level of $P < 0.05$.

Author Contributions: Conceptualization, J.L.; Data curation, J.W., W.Z., and A.G.; Formal analysis, J.W. and M.L.; Funding acquisition, J.L. and A.S.; Investigation, J.L.; Methodology, J.W. and M.L.; Project administration, J.L.; Software, W.Z. and J.D.; Supervision, J.L. and A.S.; Writing—original draft, J.W. and M.L.; Writing—review & editing, J.L.

Funding: This research was funded by the National Key R&D Program (2016YFD0501207), the Natural Science Foundation of Heilongjiang Province of China (LC2018007), and the China Agriculture Research System (CARS-35).

Conflicts of Interest: The authors declare no conflict of interest.

References

1. Rui, G.; Meng, Q.; Li, J.; Min, L.; Zhang, Y.; Bi, C.; Shan, A. Modified halloysite nanotubes reduce the toxic effects of zearalenone in gestating sows on growth and muscle development of their offsprings. *J. Anim. Sci. Biotechno.* **2016**, *7*, 570–578.
2. Gao, X.; Sun, L.; Zhang, N.; Li, C.; Zhang, J.; Xiao, Z.; Qi, D. Gestational zearalenone exposure causes reproductive and developmental toxicity in pregnant rats and female offspring. *Toxins* **2017**, *9*, 21. [CrossRef] [PubMed]
3. Wu, L.; Li, J.; Li, Y.; Li, T.; He, Q.; Tang, Y.; Liu, H.; Su, Y.; Yin, Y.; Liao, P. Aflatoxin b1, zearalenone and deoxynivalenol in feed ingredients and complete feed from different province in china. *J. Anim. Sci. Biotechno.* **2016**, *7*, 63. [CrossRef] [PubMed]
4. Moretti, A.; Logrieco, A.F.; Susca, A. Mycotoxins: An underhand food problem. In *Mycotoxigenic Fungi*; Moretti, A., Susca, A., Eds.; Humana Press: New York, NY, USA, 2017; Volume 1542, pp. 3–12.
5. Stanciu, O.; Banc, R.; Cozma, A.; Filip, L.; Miere, D.; Mañes, J.; Loghin, F. Occurence of fusarium mycotoxins in wheat from europe—a review. *Acta. Universitatis. Cibiniensis.* **2015**, *19*, 35–60. [CrossRef]
6. Venkataramana, M.; Nayaka, S.C.; Anand, T.; Rajesh, R.; Aiyaz, M.; Divakara, S.T.; Murali, H.S.; Prakash, H.S.; Rao, P.V.L. Zearalenone induced toxicity in shsy-5y cells: The role of oxidative stress evidenced by n-acetyl cysteine. *Food Chem. Toxicol.* **2014**, *65*, 335–342. [CrossRef] [PubMed]
7. Pietsch, C.; Noser, J.; Wettstein, F.E.; Burkhardt-Holm, P. Unraveling the mechanisms involved in zearalenone-mediated toxicity in permanent fish cell cultures. *Toxicon* **2014**, *88*, 44–61. [CrossRef] [PubMed]
8. Sun, X.D.; Su, P.; Shan, H. Mycotoxin contamination of maize in china. *Compr. Rev. Food Sci. F.* **2017**, *16*, 835–849. [CrossRef]
9. Knutsen, H.K.; Alexander, J.; Barregård, L.; Bignami, M.; Brüschweiler, B.; Ceccatelli, S.; Cottrill, B.; Dinovi, M.; Edler, L.; Grasl-Kraupp, B. Risks for animal health related to the presence of zearalenone and its modified forms in feed. *EFSA J.* **2017**, *15*, e04851.
10. Pinton, P.; Nougayrede, J.P.; Del Rio, J.C. The food contaminant deoxynivalenol, decreases intestinal barrier permeability and reduces claudin expression. *Toxicol. Appl. Pharm.* **2009**, *237*, 41–48. [CrossRef] [PubMed]
11. Goossens, J.; Pasmans, F.; Verbrugghe, E.; Vandenbroucke, V.; De Baere, S.; Meyer, E.; Haesebrouck, F.; De Backer, P.; Croubels, S. Porcine intestinal epithelial barrier disruption by the fusarium mycotoxins deoxynivalenol

and T-2 toxin promotes transepithelial passage of doxycycline and paromomycin. *BMC Vet. Res.* **2012**, *8*, 245. [CrossRef] [PubMed]

12. Tatay, E.; Font, G.; Ruiz, M.J. Cytotoxic effects of zearalenone and its metabolites and antioxidant cell defense in cho-k1 cells. *Food Chem. Toxicol.* **2016**, *96*, 43–49. [CrossRef] [PubMed]

13. Marin, D.E.; Taranu, I.; Pistol, G.; Stancu, M. Effects of zearalenone and its metabolites on the swine epithelial intestinal cell line: Ipec 1. *Proc. Nutr. Soc.* **2013**, *72*, 85–89. [CrossRef]

14. Liu, M.; Gao, R.; Meng, Q.; Zhang, Y.; Bi, C.; Shan, A. Toxic effects of maternal zearalenone exposure on intestinal oxidative stress, barrier function, immunological and morphological changes in rats. *PLoS ONE* **2014**, *9*, e106412. [CrossRef] [PubMed]

15. Cortinovis, C.; Caloni, F.; Schreiber, N.B.; Spicer, L.J. Effects of fumonisin b1 alone and combined with deoxynivalenol or zearalenone on porcine granulosa cell proliferation and steroid production. *Theriogenology.* **2014**, *81*, 1042–1049. [CrossRef] [PubMed]

16. Hassen, W.; Ayedboussema, I.; Oscoz, A.A.; Lopez, A.C.; Bacha, H. The role of oxidative stress in zearalenone-mediated toxicity in hep g2 cells: Oxidative DNA damage, gluthatione depletion and stress proteins induction. *Toxicology* **2007**, *232*, 294–302. [CrossRef] [PubMed]

17. Zhu, L.; Yuan, H.; Guo, C.; Lu, Y.; Deng, S.; Yang, Y.; Wei, Q.; Wen, L.; He, Z. Zearalenone induces apoptosis and necrosis in porcine granulosa cells via a caspase-3- and caspase-9-dependent mitochondrial signaling pathway. *J. Cell. Physiol.* **2012**, *227*, 1814–1820. [CrossRef] [PubMed]

18. Ayed-Boussema, I.; Bouaziz, C.; Rjiba, K.; Valenti, K.; Laporte, F.; Bacha, H.; Hassen, W. The mycotoxin zearalenone induces apoptosis in human hepatocytes (hepg2) via p53-dependent mitochondrial signaling pathway. *Toxicol. in Vitro* **2008**, *22*, 1671–1680. [CrossRef] [PubMed]

19. Schneider, R., Jr.; Santos, C.F.; Clarimundo, V.; Dalmaz, C.; Elisabetsky, E.; Gomez, R. N-acetylcysteine prevents behavioral and biochemical changes induced by alcohol cessation in rats. *Alcohol* **2015**, *49*, 259–263.

20. Wang, W.; Dan, L.; Ding, X.; Zhao, Q.; Chen, J.; Tian, K.; Yang, Q.; Lu, L. N-acetylcysteine protects inner ear hair cells and spiral ganglion neurons from manganese exposure by regulating ros levels. *Toxicol. Lett.* **2017**, *279*, 77–86. [CrossRef] [PubMed]

21. Aruoma, O.I.; Halliwell, B.; Hoey, B.M.; Butler, J. The antioxidant action of n-acetylcysteine: Its reaction with hydrogen peroxide, hydroxyl radical, superoxide, and hypochlorous acid. *Free Radical Biol. Med.* **1989**, *6*, 593–597. [CrossRef]

22. Moreira, M.A.; Irigoyen, M.C.; Saad, K.R.; Saad, P.F.; Koike, M.K.; Montero, E.F.; Martins, J.L. N-acetylcysteine reduces the renal oxidative stress and apoptosis induced by hemorrhagic shock. *J. Surg. Res.* **2016**, *203*, 113–120. [CrossRef] [PubMed]

23. Halasi, M.; Wang, M.; Chavan, T.S.; Gaponenko, V.; Hay, N.; Gartel, A.L. Ros inhibitor n-acetyl-l-cysteine antagonizes the activity of proteasome inhibitors. *Biochem. J.* **2013**, *454*, 201–208. [CrossRef] [PubMed]

24. Cazzola, M.; Calzetta, L.; Facciolo, F.; Rogliani, P.; Matera, M.G. Pharmacological investigation on the anti-oxidant and anti-inflammatory activity of n-acetylcysteine in an ex vivo model of copd exacerbation. *Resp. Res.* **2017**, *18*, 26. [CrossRef] [PubMed]

25. Xue, C.; Liu, W.; Wu, J.; Yang, X.; Xu, H. Chemoprotective effect of n-acetylcysteine (nac) on cellular oxidative damages and apoptosis induced by nano titanium dioxide under uva irradiation. *Toxicol. in Vitro* **2011**, *25*, 110. [CrossRef] [PubMed]

26. Sharma, M.; Kaur, T.; Singla, S.K. Role of mitochondria and nadph oxidase derived reactive oxygen species in hyperoxaluria induced nephrolithiasis: Therapeutic intervention with combinatorial therapy of n-acetyl cysteine and apocynin. *Mitochondrion* **2016**, *27*, 15–24. [CrossRef] [PubMed]

27. Kondakçı, G.; Aydın, A.F.; Doğru-Abbasoğlu, S.; Uysal, M. The effect of n-acetylcysteine supplementation on serum homocysteine levels and hepatic and renal oxidative stress in homocysteine thiolactone-treated rats. *Arch. Physiol. Biochem.* **2017**, *123*, 128–133. [CrossRef] [PubMed]

28. Wang, Y.; Zheng, W.; Bian, X.; Yuan, Y.; Gu, J.; Liu, X.; Liu, Z.; Bian, J. Zearalenone induces apoptosis and cytoprotective autophagy in primary leydig cells. *Toxicol. Lett.* **2014**, *226*, 182–191. [CrossRef] [PubMed]

29. Thannickal, V.J.; Fanburg, B.L. Reactive oxygen species in cell signaling. *Am. J. Physiol. Lung Cell. Mol. Physiol.* **2000**, *279*, L1005. [CrossRef] [PubMed]

30. Prosperini, A.; Juan-García, A.; Font, G.; Ruiz, M.J. Beauvericin-induced cytotoxicity via ros production and mitochondrial damage in caco-2 cells. *Toxicol. Lett.* **2013**, *222*, 204–211. [CrossRef] [PubMed]

31. Wu, J.; Jing, L.; Yuan, H.; Peng, S.-q. T-2 toxin induces apoptosis in ovarian granulosa cells of rats through reactive oxygen species-mediated mitochondrial pathway. *Toxicol. Lett.* **2011**, *202*, 168–177. [CrossRef] [PubMed]

32. Tatay, E.; Espín, S.; Garcíafernández, A.J.; Ruiz, M.J. Oxidative damage and disturbance of antioxidant capacity by zearalenone and its metabolites in human cells. *Toxicol. in Vitro* **2017**, *45*, 334. [CrossRef] [PubMed]

33. Bensassi, F.; Gallerne, C.; Sharaf el Dein, O.; Hajlaoui, M.R.; Lemaire, C.; Bacha, H. In vitro investigation of toxicological interactions between the fusariotoxins deoxynivalenol and zearalenone. *Toxicon* **2014**, *84*, 1–6. [CrossRef] [PubMed]

34. Cornelia, B.; Sonia, S.; Roxana, C.P.; Raduly, L.; Ovidiu, B.; Ionelia, T.; Eliza, M.D.; Monica, M.; Ancuta, J.; Patriciu, A.C. Evaluation of cellular and molecular impact of zearalenone andescherichia colico-exposure on ipec-1 cells using microarray technology. *BMC Genomics* **2016**, *17*, 576.

35. Wan, L.Y.; Turner, P.C.; Elnezami, H. Individual and combined cytotoxic effects of fusarium toxins (deoxynivalenol, nivalenol, zearalenone and fumonisins b1) on swine jejunal epithelial cells. *Food Chem. Toxicol.* **2013**, *57*, 276–283. [CrossRef] [PubMed]

36. Ferrer, E.; Juangarcía, A.; Font, G.; Ruiz, M.J. Reactive oxygen species induced by beauvericin, patulin and zearalenone in cho-k1 cells. *Toxicol. in Vitro* **2009**, *23*, 1504–1509. [CrossRef] [PubMed]

37. Kang, C.; Lee, H.; Yoo, Y.S.; Hah, D.Y.; Kim, C.H.; Kim, E.; Kim, J.S. Evaluation of oxidative DNA damage using an alkaline single cell gel electrophoresis (scge) comet assay, and the protective effects of n-acetylcysteine amide on zearalenone-induced cytotoxicity in chang liver cells. *Toxicol. Res.* **2013**, *29*, 43–52. [CrossRef] [PubMed]

38. Birben, E.; Sahiner, U.M.; Sackesen, C.; Erzurum, S.; Kalayci, O. Oxidative stress and antioxidant defense. *World Allergy Organ. J.* **2012**, *5*, 9–19. [CrossRef] [PubMed]

39. Pundir, M.; Arora, S.; Kaur, T.; Singh, R.; Singh, A.P. Effect of modulating the allosteric sites of n-methyl-d-aspartate receptors in ischemia-reperfusion induced acute kidney injury. *J. Surg. Res.* **2013**, *183*, 668–677. [CrossRef] [PubMed]

40. Yan, S.H.; Wang, J.H.; Zhu, L.S.; Chen, A.M.; Wang, J. Thiamethoxam induces oxidative stress and antioxidant response in zebrafish (danio rerio) livers. *Environ. Toxicol.* **2016**, *31*, 2006–2015. [CrossRef] [PubMed]

41. Abid, E.S.; Ee, B.C.B. Comparative study of toxic effects of zearalenone and its two major metabolites alpha-zearalenol and beta-zearalenol on cultured human caco-2 cells. *J. Biochem. Mol. Toxicol.* **2009**, *23*, 233–243. [CrossRef] [PubMed]

42. Fan, W.; Shen, T.; Ding, Q.; Lv, Y.; Li, L.; Huang, K.; Yan, L.; Song, S. Zearalenone induces ros-mediated mitochondrial damage in porcine ipec-j2 cells. *J. Biochem. Mol. Toxicol.* **2017**, *31*, e21944. [CrossRef] [PubMed]

43. Dennog, C.; Radermacher, P.; Barnett, Y.A.; Speit, G. Antioxidant status in humans after exposure to hyperbaric oxygen. *Mutat. Res.* **1999**, *428*, 83–89. [CrossRef]

44. Phamhuy, L.A.; He, H.; Phamhuy, C. Free radicals, antioxidants in disease and health. *Int. J. Biomed. Sci.* **2008**, *4*, 89–96.

45. Assady, M.; Farahnak, A.; Golestani, A.; Esharghian, M. Superoxide dismutase (sod) enzyme activity assay in fasciola spp. Parasites and liver tissue extract. *Iran. J. Parasitol.* **2011**, *6*, 17. [PubMed]

46. Wu, G.; Fang, Y.Z.; Yang, S.; Lupton, J.R.; Turner, N.D. Glutathione metabolism and its implications for health. *J. Nutr.* **2004**, *134*, 489. [CrossRef] [PubMed]

47. Ashrafzadeh, T.H.; Saeed, H.; Foad, R.; Ashrafzadeh, T.M.; Hadi, H. Effects of n-acetylcysteine and pentoxifylline on remote lung injury in a rat model of hind-limb ischemia/reperfusion injury. *J. Bras. Pneumol.* **2016**, *42*, 9.

48. Nazıroğlu, M.; Şenol, N.; Ghazizadeh, V.; Yürüker, V. Neuroprotection induced by n-acetylcysteine and selenium against traumatic brain injury-induced apoptosis and calcium entry in hippocampus of rat. *Cell Mol. Neurobiol.* **2014**, *34*, 895. [CrossRef] [PubMed]

49. Wei, Z.; Zhang, S.; Zhang, M.; Yang, L.; Cheng, B.; Li, J.; Shan, A. Individual and combined effects of fusarium toxins on apoptosis in pk15 cells and the protective role of n-acetylcysteine. *Food Chem. Toxicol.* **2017**, *111*, 27–43.

50. Yeo, E.H.; Goh, W.L.; Chow, S.C. The aminopeptidase inhibitor, z-l-cmk is toxic and induced cell death in jurkat t cells through oxidative stress. *Toxicol. Mech. Methods.* **2017**, *28*, 157–166. [CrossRef] [PubMed]

51. Zhao, J.; Kyotani, Y.; Itoh, S.; Nakayama, H.; Isosaki, M.; Yoshizumi, M. Big mitogen-activated protein kinase 1 protects cultured rat aortic smooth muscle cells from oxidative damage. *J. Pharmacol. Sci.* **2011**, *116*, 173–180. [CrossRef] [PubMed]

52. Hotchkiss, R.S.; Strasser, A.; McDunn, J.E.; Swanson, P.E. Cell death. *N. Engl. J. Med.* **2009**, *361*, 1570–1583. [CrossRef] [PubMed]

53. Borys, S.; Khozmi, R.; Kranc, W.; Bryja, A.; Dyszkiewiczkonwińska, M.; Jeseta, M.; Kempisty, B. Recent findings of the types of programmed cell death. *Adv. Cell Biol.* **2017**, *5*, 43–49. [CrossRef]

54. Murphy, M.P. How mitochondria produce reactive oxygen species. *Biochem. J.* **2009**, *417*, 1–13. [CrossRef] [PubMed]

55. Guo, Z.Y.; Xu, M.H.; He, W.; Wang, S.T.; Guo, Z.Y.; Xu, M.H.; He, W.; Wang, S.T. Effect of mitochondria permeability transition pore on h9c2 myocardial cell apoptosis induced by lipopolysaccharide. *J. Shanghai Jiaotong Univ.* **2017**, *37*, 942–949.

56. Vaca, C.E.; Wilhelm, J.; Harms-Ringdahl, M. Interaction of lipid peroxidation products with DNA. A review. *Mutat. Res.* **1988**, *195*, 137–149. [CrossRef]

57. Hüttemann, M.; Pecina, P.; Rainbolt, M.; Sanderson, T.H.; Kagan, V.E.; Samavati, L.; Doan, J.W.; Lee, I. The multiple functions of cytochrome c and their regulation in life and death decisions of the mammalian cell: From respiration to apoptosis. *Mitochondrion* **2011**, *11*, 369–381. [CrossRef] [PubMed]

58. Bras, M.; Queenan, B.; Susin, S.A. Programmed cell death via mitochondria: Different modes of dying. *Biochemistry (Moscow)* **2005**, *70*, 231–239. [CrossRef]

59. Leal, A.M.D.S.; Queiroz, J.D.F.D.; Lima, T.K.D.S.; Agnezlima, L.F. Violacein induces cell death by triggering mitochondrial membrane hyperpolarization in vitro. *BMC Microbiol.* **2015**, *15*, 1–8. [CrossRef] [PubMed]

60. Abbès, S.; Salahabbès, J.B.; Ouanes, Z.; Houas, Z.; Othman, O.; Bacha, H.; Abdelwahhab, M.A.; Oueslati, R. Preventive role of phyllosilicate clay on the immunological and biochemical toxicity of zearalenone in balb/c mice. *Int. Immunopharmacol.* **2006**, *6*, 1251–1258. [CrossRef] [PubMed]

61. Eraslan, G.; Kanbur, M.; Aslan, Ö.; Karabacak, M. The antioxidant effects of pumpkin seed oil on subacute aflatoxin poisoning in mice. *Environ. Toxicol.* **2013**, *28*, 681–688. [CrossRef] [PubMed]

62. Wu, L.L.; Dunning, K.R.; Yang, X.; Russell, D.L.; Norman, R.J.; Robker, R.L. In Oocytes exhibit lipid accumulation, endoplasmic reticulum stress, mitochondrial dysfunction, and apoptosis in response to high fat diet. *Biol. Reprod.* **2010**, *83*, 185. [CrossRef]

63. Ly, J.D.; Grubb, D.R.; Lawen, A. The mitochondrial membrane potential ($\delta\psi$ m) in apoptosis; an update. *Apoptosis* **2003**, *8*, 115–128. [CrossRef] [PubMed]

64. Yun, Y.; Zong, M.; Xu, W.; Yang, Z.; Bo, W.; Yang, M.; Tao, L. Natural pyrethrins induces apoptosis in human hepatocyte cells via bax- and bcl-2-mediated mitochondrial pathway. *Chem. Biol. Interact.* **2017**, *262*, 38–45.

65. Guo, L.; Peng, Y.; Yao, J.; Sui, L.; Gu, A.; Wang, J. Anticancer activity and molecular mechanism of resveratrol-bovine serum albumin nanoparticles on subcutaneously implanted human primary ovarian carcinoma cells in nude mice. *Cancer Biother. Radiopharm.* **2010**, *25*, 471. [CrossRef] [PubMed]

66. Tsai, C.H.; Yang, S.H.; Chien, C.M.; Lu, M.C.; Lo, C.S.; Lin, Y.H.; Hu, X.W.; Lin, S.R. Mechanisms of cardiotoxin iii-induced apoptosis in human colorectal cancer colo205 cells. *Clin. Exp. Pharmacol. Physiol.* **2006**, *33*, 177–182. [CrossRef] [PubMed]

67. Deng, L.; Ding, D.; Su, J.; Manohar, S.; Salvi, R. Salicylate selectively kills cochlear spiral ganglion neurons by paradoxically up-regulating superoxide. *Neurotox. Res.* **2013**, *24*, 307–319. [CrossRef] [PubMed]

68. Hua, P.; Liu, J.; Tao, J.; Liu, J.; Yang, S. Influence of caspase-3 silencing on the proliferation and apoptosis of rat bone marrow mesenchymal stem cells under hypoxia. *Int. J. Clin. Exp. Med.* **2015**, *8*, 1624–1633. [PubMed]

69. Wang, X.; Diao, Y.; Liu, Y.; Gao, N.; Gao, D.; Wan, Y.; Zhong, J.; Jin, G. Synergistic apoptosis-inducing effect of aspirin and isosorbide mononitrate on human colon cancer cells. *Mol. Med. Rep.* **2015**, *12*, 4750. [CrossRef] [PubMed]

70. Vacca, R.A.; Valenti, D.; Bobba, A.; Merafina, R.S.; Passarella, S.; Marra, E. Cytochrome c is released in a reactive oxygen species-dependent manner and is degraded via caspase-like proteases in tobacco bright-yellow 2 cells en route to heat shock-induced cell death. *Plant Physiol.* **2006**, *141*, 208–219. [CrossRef] [PubMed]

71. Czabotar, P.E.; Lessene, G.; Strasser, A.; Adams, J.M. Control of apoptosis by the bcl-2 protein family: Implications for physiology and therapy. *Nat. Rev. Mol. Cell. Biol.* **2014**, *15*, 49–63. [CrossRef] [PubMed]

72. Sun, L.H.; Lei, M.Y.; Zhang, N.Y.; Gao, X.; Li, C.; Krumm, C.S.; Qi, D.S. Individual and combined cytotoxic effects of aflatoxin b1, zearalenone, deoxynivalenol and fumonisin b1 on brl 3a rat liver cells. *Toxicon* **2015**, *95*, 6. [CrossRef] [PubMed]

73. Wang, J.; Hu, G.; Lin, Z.; He, L.; Xu, L.; Zhang, Y. Characteristic and functional analysis of a newly established porcine small intestinal epithelial cell line. *PLoS ONE* **2014**, *9*, e110916. [CrossRef] [PubMed]

74. Bousquet, L.; Pruvost, A.; Guyot, A.; Farinotti, R.; Mabondzo, A. Combination of tenofovir and emtricitabine plus efavirenz: In vitro modulation of abc transporter and intracellular drug accumulation. *Antimicrob. Agents Chemother.* **2009**, *53*, 896. [CrossRef] [PubMed]

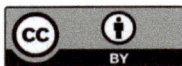

toxins

MDPI

Article

Effects of Adding *Clostridium* sp. WJ06 on Intestinal Morphology and Microbial Diversity of Growing Pigs Fed with Natural Deoxynivalenol Contaminated Wheat

FuChang Li [1], JinQuan Wang [2], LiBo Huang [1], HongJu Chen [1] and ChunYang Wang [1],*

[1] Shandong Provincial Key Laboratory of Animal Biotechnology and Disease Control and Prevention, Shandong Agricultural University, 61 Daizong Street, Taian City 271018, China; chlf@sdau.edu.cn (F.L.); huanglibo123@126.com (L.H.); hjchen72@sdau.edu.cn (H.C.)

[2] Feed Research Institute, Chinese Academy of Agricultural Sciences, Beijing 100081, China; wangjinquan@caas.net.cn

* Correspondence: wcy@sdau.edu.cn; Tel.: +86-135-0548-0263

Academic Editors: Isabelle P. Oswald, Philippe Pinton and Imourana Alassane-Kpembi
Received: 3 October 2017; Accepted: 22 November 2017; Published: 27 November 2017

Abstract: Deoxynivalenol (DON) is commonly detected in cereals, and is a threat to human and animal health. The effects of microbiological detoxification are now being widely studied. A total of 24 pigs (over four months) were randomly divided into three treatments. Treatment A was fed with a basal diet as the control group. Treatment B was fed with naturally DON-contaminated wheat as a negative control group. Treatment C was fed with a contaminated diet that also had *Clostridium* sp. WJ06, which was used as a detoxicant. Growth performance, relative organ weight, intestinal morphology, and the intestinal flora of bacteria and fungi were examined. The results showed that after consuming a DON-contaminated diet, the growth performance of the pigs decreased significantly ($p < 0.05$), the relative organ weight of the liver and kidney increased significantly ($p < 0.05$), and the integrity of the intestinal barrier was also impaired, though the toxic effects of the contaminated diets on growing pigs were relieved after adding *Clostridium* sp. WJ06. The data from MiSeq sequencing of the 16S ribosomal ribonucleic acid (rRNA) gene and internal transcribed spacer 1 (ITS1) gene suggested that the abundance of intestinal flora was significantly different across the three treatments. In conclusion, the application of *Clostridium* sp. WJ06 can reduce the toxic effects of DON and adjust the intestinal microecosystem of growing pigs.

Keywords: *Clostridium* sp. WJ06; deoxynivalenol; pig; intestinal morphology; microbial diversity

---

1. Introduction

Deoxynivalenol (DON), also known as vomitoxin, is synthesized mainly by the toxigenic fungi of the *Fusarium* genus, which is commonly detected in cereals, particularly wheat, barley, maize, and their by-products all over the world [1]. This mycotoxin remains stable for many years when stored at room temperature, or even when heated at 135 °C. Its deactivation occurs through the destruction of the epoxide ring under drastic acid or alkaline conditions, reactions with aluminum and lithium hydrates or peroxides, and hydration in autoclave [2]. Therefore, DON readily enters the human and animal food chains [3–5]. DON causes toxic effects in humans as well as in all animal species investigated to date. Among animal species, pigs show a relatively high sensitivity to DON because of the high percentage of cereals in their diet and the lack of microorganisms in the front of their small intestine, which are able to degrade mycotoxins before DON is absorbed by the small intestine [6,7].

The intestinal tract is the first target for mycotoxins following ingestion of contaminated feed. Consumption of DON-contaminated feed in pigs impacts the gastrointestinal tract, causing epithelial injuries of the stomach and the intestine, and leading to intestinal inflammatory response [8,9]. In vitro and in vivo studies have also demonstrated that DON inhibits intestinal nutrient absorption, alters intestinal cell functions, and compromises the intestinal barrier [10]. Additionally, stability of the intestinal flora appeared to be an important factor in animal health. Surprisingly, the effect of DON on intestinal microflora has been poorly investigated [11]. Direct impact of DON on intestinal microflora composition has never been reported, and only few data are available for other members of the trichothecene toxin group [12,13].

Due to the detrimental effects of mycotoxins, some strategies have been developed to prevent the growth of mycotoxigenic fungi and also to decontaminate and detoxify foods and feeds [14]. These strategies include: (1) the prevention of mycotoxin contamination; (2) the detoxification of mycotoxins present in foods and feeds; and (3) the inhibition of mycotoxin absorption in the gastrointestinal tract. Although numerous physical and chemical detoxification methods have been tested, none really provide the necessary efficacy and safety [15]. Since cost-effective methods to detoxify mycotoxin-contaminated grains and foods are urgently needed to minimize potential losses to the farmer and toxicological hazards to the consumer, it is a necessity to find new suitable methods for the decontamination of mycotoxins. Therefore, the development of microbiological detoxification measures is essential for improving the safety of these foods for human consumption. Microbes or their enzymes could be used for mycotoxin detoxification, and such biological approaches are now being widely studied [16,17]. DON, as well as other trichothecenes, may have its chemical structure altered by bacteria or fungi, which utilize their enzymatic systems as a carbon source.

Therefore, the present study aims to: (i) investigate the influence of naturally DON-contaminated wheat on the intestinal morphology and intestinal microflora of growing pigs; and (ii) evaluate the effect of *Clostridium* sp. WJ06 on the intestinal morphology and intestinal microflora of growing pigs as a detoxicant.

2. Results

2.1. Effect of Clostridium sp. WJ06 on Growth Performance and Relative Organ Weight of Growing Pigs

The effect of *Clostridium* sp. WJ06 and DON-contaminated wheat on the growth performance of growing pigs is shown in Table 1. In this study, average daily body weight gain (ADG) and average daily feed issue (ADFI) decreased significantly more than in the control group after feeding DON-contaminated wheat ($p < 0.05$), while the ratio of feed intake to body weight gain (F/G) increased significantly ($p < 0.05$). There were no significant differences ($p \geq 0.05$) from the control group after adding *Clostridium* sp. WJ06.

Table 1. Effect of *Clostridium* sp. WJ06 on the growth performance of pigs.

Treatment *	Initial Weight (kg)	Final Weight (kg)	ADG (g) [#]	ADFI (kg) [#]	F/G [#]
A	54.38 ± 1.21	78.3 ± 1.78	885.93±72	2.14±0.38	2.41 ± 0.32
B	56.44 ± 1.63	71.33 ± 2.98 [a]	551.48±46 [a]	1.66±0.33 [a]	3.01 ± 0.41 [a]
C	56.06 ± 1.78	76.07 ± 3.15	741.16 ± 62	1.98 ± 0.27	2.68 ± 0.36

Values are presented as Mean ± SD, $n = 8$. The values with different small letters [(a)] in the same column differ significantly ($p < 0.05$). [#] ADG, average daily body weight gain; ADFI, average daily feed intake; F/G, the ratio of feed intake to body weight gain, indicating feeding efficiency. Feed was calculated based on dry weight. * Treatment A refers to the control diet; Treatment B refers to the contaminated diet; Treatment C refers to the contaminated diet with *Clostridium* sp. WJ06 added.

The effect of *Clostridium* sp. WJ06 on the relative organ weight of growing pigs is shown in Figure 1. The results showed that the relative weights of the liver, kidney, and spleen of growing pigs increased significantly more than in the control group after feeding DON-contaminated wheat

($p < 0.05$), while there were no significant differences ($p \geq 0.05$) for the relative weights of the heart and lungs. After adding *Clostridium* sp. WJ06, the relative weight of the liver and kidney were not significantly different ($p \geq 0.05$) to the control group, while the spleen increased significantly ($p < 0.05$).

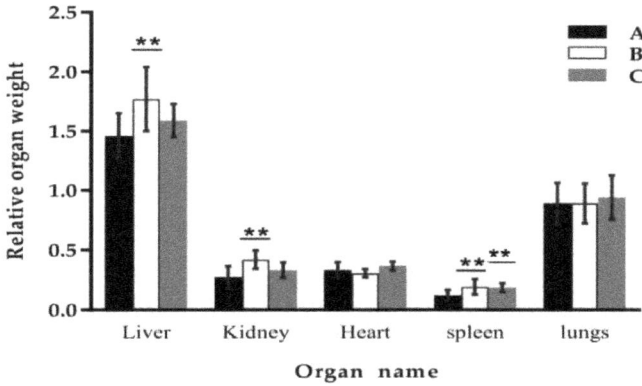

Figure 1. Effect of *Clostridium* sp. WJ06 on relative organ weight [1] of growing pigs. [1] Relative organ weight (kg/kg) = organ weight (kg)/live weight (kg). A, B, and C represent the samples of different treatments. Bars are presented as mean ± SD, $n = 3$. ** Indicates that results differ significantly between treatments ($p < 0.05$).

2.2. Effects of Clostridium sp. WJ06 on Intestinal Morphology of Growing Pigs

Representative morphologies of the ileum, caecum and colon are illustrated in Figure 2. Scanning electron microscope observations revealed that the mucosa of ileum, caecum and colon were severely damaged after pigs were fed with DON-contaminated wheat compared with the control group, especially for ileum. Additionally, epithelial cells on the surface of the intestinal villus were not integrated and exhibited histological lesions. In contrast, the damage to the villus barriers of the intestine from contaminated diets were relieved significantly after adding *Clostridium* sp. WJ06 to the diets of pigs.

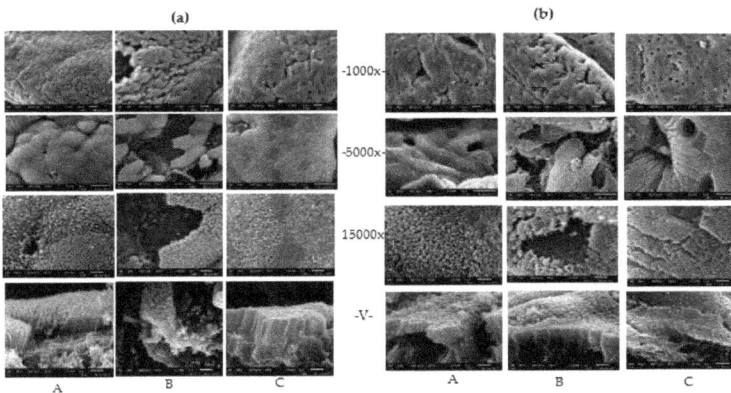

Figure 2. *Cont.*

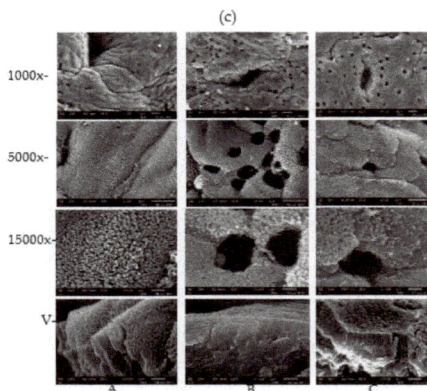

Figure 2. The effect of *Clostridium* sp. WJ06 on the morphology of different intestine regions of growing pigs via scanning electron microscopy (*n* = 3). (**a–c**) refer to samples of the ileum, caecum, and colon, respectively. A, B, and C refer to the samples of different treatments. 1000×, 5000×, and 15,000× represent the magnification of electron microscopy at transverse sections. V represents the photo of a vertical section magnified 15,000×.

2.3. Analysis of Operational Taxonomic Units (OTUs) and the Alpha Diversity of Bacteria Flora and Fungal Flora in all Samples

Alpha diversity was applied in analyzing the complexity of species diversity for one sample, and two indices (rarefaction curves and rank-abundance curves) were selected to identify community richness and diversity (Figure 3). Rarefaction curves reflect the reasonability of the number of sequencing reads used for analysis, and can be used to infer species richness in the sample. A flat curve means that the number of sequencing reads is reasonable, and less new species can be detected with increasing sequencing reads. Rank abundance curves directly reflect the richness and evenness of species in the sample. Species richness can be viewed as the range of the curve in the horizontal direction. The results demonstrated that the curves of all of the samples have almost approached the saturation plateau, which indicates that the 16s ribosomal ribonucleic acid (rRNA) gene and the internal transcribed spacer 1 (ITS1) gene sequence database was very abundant, and the current analysis had adequate depth to capture most microbial diversity information.

In the present study, a total number of 253,708 qualified sequence reads were obtained from nine samples via V3–V4 16S rRNA sequencing, with an average of 43,177 effective sequence reads for each sample (the minimum sample was 34,392, and the maximum was 47,673), and the average length of the effective bacterial sequence reads was 389 bp (Table 2). At the same time, the data of the operational taxonomic units (OTUs) and the richness estimator by ITS1 sequencing are listed in Table 3. A total number of 605,933 qualified sequence reads were obtained from nine samples, with an average of 67,326 effective sequence reads for each sample (the minimum sample was 46,157, and the maximum was 102,600), and the average length of the effective fungal sequence reads was 227 bp (Table 3).

In order to analyze the species diversity within samples, we clustered all of the effective tags to operational taxonomic units (OTUs) at 97% similarity. Then, we performed species annotation based on the OTUs' representative tags. According to the results of species annotation, the statistics of the sequence numbers in different classification levels (kingdom, phylum, class, order, family, genus, and species) are calculated and displayed in Figure 4. The composition of each sample and differences among samples can be understood through Figure 4. The results in our study showed that the sequence number of fungi flora varied significantly in the three treatments at several classification levels, while that of bacteria flora were not shifted significantly; that is, the structure of intestinal bacteria flora were relatively simple and stable.

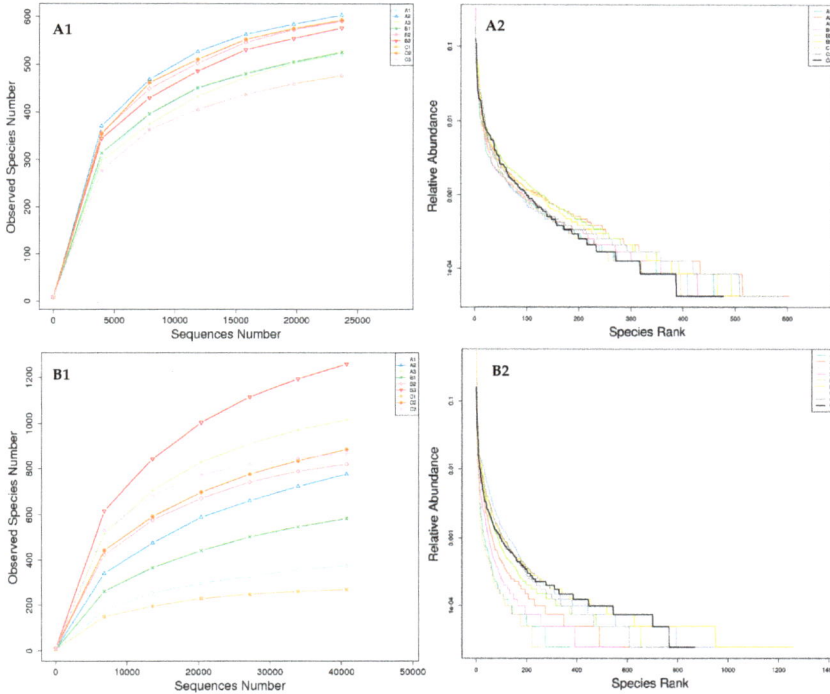

Figure 3. Rarefaction curve and rank abundance curve in nine libraries. (**A1,A2**) represented the data from 16S ribosomal ribonucleic acid (rRNA) gene sequencing. (**B1,B2**) represented the data from internal transcribed spacer 1 (ITS1) gene sequencing. In the rarefaction curves plot (**A1 & B1**), the x-axis is number sequencing reads randomly chosen from a certain sample to obtain operational taxonomic units (OTUs). The y-axis is corresponding OTUs. In the rank-abundance curves plot (**A2 & B2**), the x-axis is the abundance rank, and the y-axis is the relative abundance. The higher the abundance, the smaller the rank. Curves for different samples are represented by different colors.

Table 2. OTUs [1] data and richness estimator of nine libraries via 16S rRNA gene sequencing.

Sample Name *	Raw PE [#]	Qualified [#]	Base (nt) [#]	AvgLen (nt) [#]	Effective% [#]	Chao Ave [2]	Observed Species	Shannon Ave [2]
A1	64,782	34,392	10,231,113	390	40.5	564.27	426	4.93
B1	69,691	41,156	14,360,310	388	53.05	496.63	380	4.66
C1	68,531	40,201	13,531,583	384	51.41	538.44	443	5.44
A2	72,117	47,250	15,233,409	389	54.37	434.19	365	5.21
B2	64,769	45,377	14,399,002	389	57.1	436.26	389	5.90
C2	69,357	45,332	14,537,019	385	54.4	379.02	329	5.53
A3	75,203	47,673	14,834,644	392	50.28	489.40	406	4.85
B3	68,288	41,553	14,224,802	396	52.59	468.35	382	5.05
C3	70,715	45,665	14,628,909	386	53.59	586.57	485	6.00
Total	409,247	253,708	82,292,436	2325	311	4393	3605	48
Average	69,272	43,177	13,997,865	389	51.92	488.13	401	5.29

* A1, B1, and C1 represent the sequences of ileum from different treatments. A2, B2, and C2 represent the sequences of caecum from different treatments. A3, B3, and C3 represent the sequences of colon from different treatments. [1] The operational taxonomic units (OTUs) were defined at 3% dissimilarity level. [2] The richness estimators (Chao) and diversity indices (Shannon) were calculated using the program QIIME. [#] Raw PE means original PE reads tested by the Illumina MiSeq platform. Qualified means the raw reads with chimeric sequences and low quality sequences removed. Base refers to the final effective data of the basic group. AveLen refers to the average length of effective tags. Effective means Effective Tags/Raw PE × 100%.

Table 3. OTUs [1] data and richness estimator of nine libraries via ITS1 gene sequencing.

Sample Name *	Raw PE [#]	Qualified [#]	Base (nt) [#]	AvgLen (nt)[#]	Effective% [#]	Chao Ave [2]	Observed Species	Shannon Ave [2]
A1	123,899	72,335	18,813,512	267	56.92	798.77	611	5.18
B1	70,194	54,056	12,893,920	246	74.80	389.73	287	2.92
C1	121,183	102,600	22,150,221	218	83.97	656.80	447	3.46
A2	103,737	79,891	17,630,954	221	76.95	843.35	570	5.07
B2	72,542	46,157	10,630,776	234	62.49	992.45	667	5.71
C2	95,418	78,657	16,739,208	213	82.33	656.80	665	3.46
A3	78,988	64,817	12,797,508	198	81.95	959.79	748	6.87
B3	83,591	62,692	13,180,068	211	74.72	1195.65	918	6.52
C3	72,307	44,728	10,577,687	238	61.34	886.02	769	5.96
Total	821,859	605,933	135,413,854	2046	655.47	7379.36	5681	45.14
Average	91,318	67,326	15,045,984	227	72.83	819.93	631	5.02

* A1, B1, and C1 represent the sequences of ileum from different treatments. A2, B2, and C2 represent the sequences of caecum from different treatments. A3, B3, and C3 represent the sequences of colon from different treatments. [1] The operational taxonomic units (OTUs) were defined at 3% dissimilarity level. [2] The richness estimators (Chao) and diversity indices (Shannon) were calculated using the program QIIME. [#] Raw PE means original PE reads tested by the Illumina MiSeq platform. Qualified means the raw reads with chimeric sequences and low quality sequences removed. Base refers to the final effective data of the basic group. AveLen refers to the average length of effective tags. Effective means Effective Tags/Raw PE × 100%.

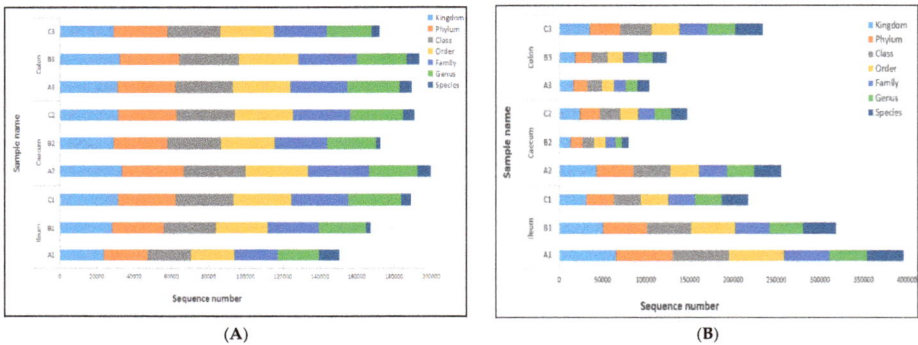

(A)   (B)

Figure 4. Tag abundance of each sample at different classification levels. Sequence number indicates the number of sequences annotated to that level, which are expressed in different colors. Bars are presented as means, *n* = 3. (**A**) The sequence number of bacteria flora in different treatments. (**B**) The sequence number of fungi flora.

2.4. Effects of Clostridium sp. WJ06 on Intestinal Bacterial Flora of Pigs via 16S rRNA Gene Sequencing

In this paper, the top 10 species of bacteria flora with the highest relative abundance at the phylum and genus levels are shown in Figures 5 and 6, respectively. Based on relative abundance, *Firmicutes*, *Spirochaetes*, *Bacteroidetes*, and *Proteobacteria* were identified as the major bacterial taxa of the pig bacterial community in all of the samples. For *Firmicutes* in particular, the average relative abundance was over 86% in different treatments. As shown in Figure 5, the abundance of *Firmicutes* in the ileum and colon decreased significantly after being fed with contaminated diets, while that of *Spirochaetes* and *Bacteroidetes* in the ileum and colon were significantly increased. However, the abundance of these bacteria was not affected after adding *Clostridium* sp. WJ06. The result also showed that the dominant bacteria of caecum were not significantly affected by contaminated diets.

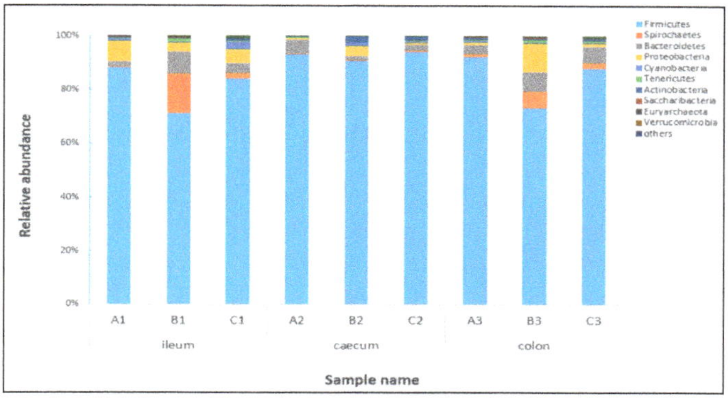

Figure 5. Relative abundance of the dominant bacterial phyla level in nine libraries. Each bar represents the relative abundance of each sample. Each color represents a particular bacterial family. Sequences that could not be classified into the top 10 were classified as 'others'. A, B, and C represent the samples from three treatments, and 1, 2, and 3 represent the samples of the ileum, caecum and colon, respectively.

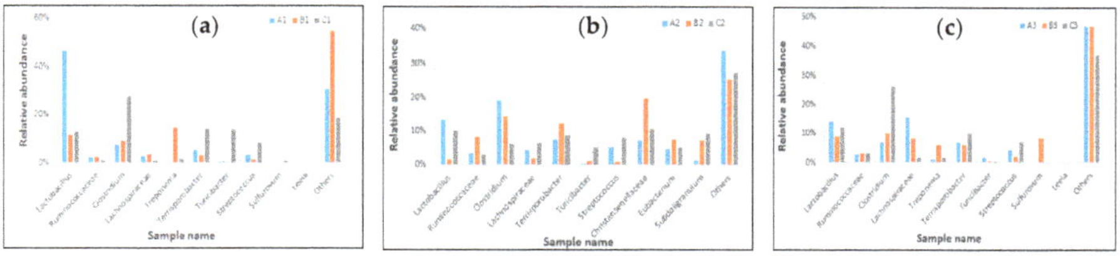

Figure 6. Relative abundance of the dominant bacteria at the same gut region at the genus level. Each bar represents the relative abundance of each sample. Each color represents a particular bacterial family. (**a**) A1, B1, and C1 represent the samples of the ileum in different treatments. (**b**) A2, B2, and C2 represent the samples of the caecum in different treatments. (**c**) A3, B3, and C3 represent the samples of the colon in different treatments.

Lactobacillus represented the largest number of bacteria in the ileum (47%), ceacum (13%), and colon (14%) at the genus level, especially for ileum. The abundance of *Lactobacillus* was significantly decreased in the ileum (11%), ceacum (2%) and colon (9%) after being fed with contaminated diets, while that of *Lactobacillus* was higher than the control group in the ceacum (10%) and colon (12%), but not in the ileum (13%) after adding *Clostridium* sp. WJ06 (Figure 6). Meanwhile, the abundance of *Clostridium* increased significantly after the use of *Clostridium* sp. WJ06. The abundance of *Clostridium* in the ileum and colon of the control treatment were all 7%, while that of *Clostridium* in the ileum and colon increased to 28% and 27%, respectively, after adding *Clostridium* sp. WJ06. The abundance of *Clostridium* in the ceacum of the control treatment was 19%, but fell to 6% after adding *Clostridium* sp. WJ06. However, the abundance of *Clostridium* was not affected by contaminated diets, which may be connected with the reproductive ability of *Clostridium* sp. WJ06 and was different in the ileum, caecum, and colon, respectively.

In our study, the result showed that the structure of porcine cecal flora was quite different from that of the flora of the ileum and colon. *Christensenellaceae*, *Eubacterium*, and *Subdoligranulum* belong to the dominant flora in the ceacum, but not in the colon and ileum. At the same time, *Sulfurovum*, *Leeia*, and *Treponema* formed dominant populations in the ileum and colon, but not in the ceacum. The shifts of the bacterial community compositions were further corroborated by a clear clustering of the dominant bacterial genus corresponding to different treatment in the heat map, as shown in Figure 7. The result revealed that the bacterial composition in the ileum, ceacum, and colon of growing pigs varied significantly in different diets, but the structure of bacteria was relatively stable and simple.

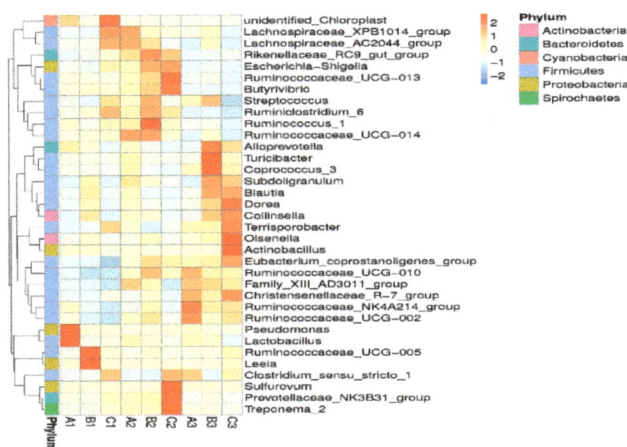

Figure 7. Hierarchically clustered heat map of the highly represented fungal taxa (at the genus level) in nine libraries. The relative percentages (%) of the bacterial families are indicated by varying color intensities, according to the legend at the top of the figure. The darker the color of samples, the higher the relative abundance shown in the picture.

2.5. Effects of Clostridium sp. WJ06 on Intestinal Bacterial Flora of Pigs via ITS1 Gene Sequence

In this paper, the top 10 species of fungal flora with the highest relative abundance at the phylum and genus levels are shown in Figures 8 and 9, respectively. It can be seen from Figure 8 that the number of dominant fungi species varied significantly in the ileum, caecum, and colon in different diets, especially in regard to the abundance of *Basidiomycota* and *Ascomycota*.

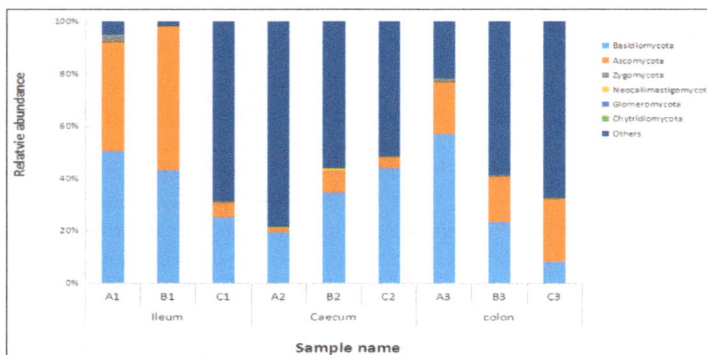

Figure 8. Dominant fungi composition of the different communities at the phyla level. Each bar represents the relative abundance of each sample. Each color represents a particular bacterial family. Sequences that could not be classified into top 10 were assigned as 'others'. A, B, and C represent the samples from three treatments, and 1, 2, and 3 represent the samples of the ileum, caecum, and colon, respectively.

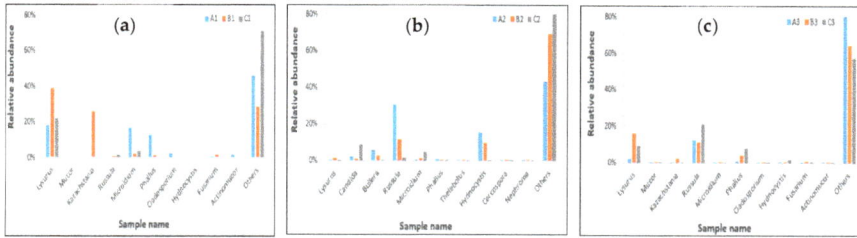

Figure 9. Relative abundance of the dominant fungi at the same gut region at the genus level. Each bar represents the relative abundance of each sample. Each color represents a particular bacterial family. (**a**) A1, B1, and C1 represent the samples of ileum in different treatments. (**b**) A2, B2, and C2 represent the samples of caecum in different treatments. (**c**) A3, B3, and C3 represent the samples of the colon in different treatments.

As shown in Figure 9, the results revealed that the abundance of *Lysurus, Kazachstania,* and *Fusarium* were significantly increased in the ileum and colon at the genus level after being fed with contaminated diets, and that these bacteria had not significantly increased after adding *Clostridium* sp. WJ06. The result indicated that the species structure of the caecum was significantly different from that of the ileum and colon.

The shifts of the fungal community compositions were further corroborated by clear clustering of the dominant bacterial genus corresponding to different treatments in the heat map, as shown in Figure 10. The results suggested that the number of fungi in the treatment groups varied greatly.

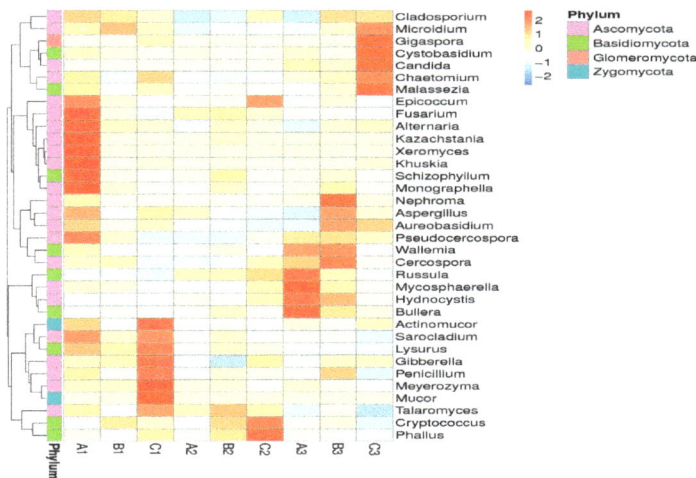

Figure 10. Hierarchically clustered heat map of the highly represented fungal taxa (at the genus level) in nine samples. The relative percentages (%) of the bacterial families are indicated by varying color intensities according to the legend at the top of the figure. The more brunette the samples' color, the higher relative abundance shown in the picture.

2.6. Analysis of Beta Diversity of all Samples

Beta diversity analysis was used to evaluate the differences of samples in species complexity, and principal component analysis (PCA) was carried out for this paper [18]. The PCA plot based on the relative abundance of bacterial OTUs revealed a separation between the different treatments and different intestinal regions on the basis of the first two PC scores, which accounted for 11.72% and 18.16% of the total variation, respectively (Figure 11A). The more similar the composition of samples, the closer the distance shown in the PCA picture. Our data showed that the bacterial flora diversity varied significantly in the different intestinal regions, but there was no significant difference in the different treatments.

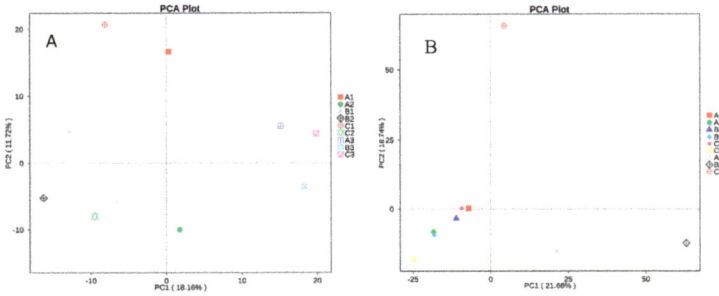

Figure 11. Principal component analysis (PCA) in nine libraries. Scatterplot of PCA score depicting the variance in fingerprints derived from different bacterial communities. The more similar the composition of samples, the closer the distance shown in the PCA picture. (**A**) The sequence number of bacteria flora. (**B**) The sequence number of fungi flora.

At the same time, the fungal diversity was analyzed by PCA, and the two PC scores accounted for 18.74% and 21.68% of the total variation, respectively (Figure 11B). Our data showed that the fungal flora diversity varied significantly more in the colon than in the ileum and caecum in different diets.

2.7. Analysis of the Concentration of DON and De-Epoxy-DON (DOM-1) in Urine and Feces

De-epoxydeoxynivalenol (DOM-1) had not been found in porcine urine in any experimental group. The concentration of DON in urine at different trail periods is displayed in Figure 12. The result indicated that on the 14th, 21st, and 35th day of the experiment, the DON value in group B was significantly higher ($p < 0.05$) when compared with the other groups. Meanwhile, the DON value in group C was significantly lower when compared to group B ($p < 0.05$), but significantly higher than the control group ($p < 0.05$). No significant differences were found in each group on different exposure days.

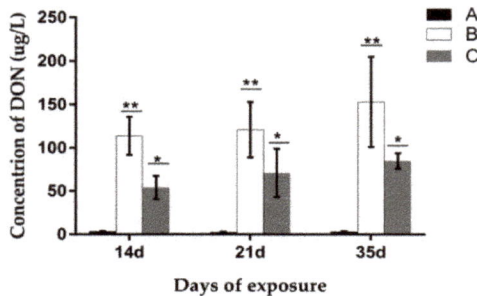

Figure 12. Concentration of deoxynivalenol (DON) in porcine urine at different exposure days. A, B, and C represent the samples of different treatments. Bars are presented as mean ± SD, $n = 5$. The values with different asterisks (* or **) differed significantly on the same exposure day ($p < 0.05$).

The concentration of DON and DOM-1 in porcine feces is displayed in Figure 13. The result showed that the DON value in group B increased significantly compared with the other groups ($p < 0.05$), and a gradual increasing trend of the DON value from day 14 to day 35 appeared in groups B and C. The concentration of DOM-1 had not been found in group A in our study. The DOM-1 value of group B decreased significantly more than that of group C ($p < 0.05$), while the values at days 21 and 35 were significantly higher than the value at day 14 ($p < 0.05$). This result indicated that DOM-1 was mainly converted in the intestinal tract by *Clostridium* sp. WJ06.

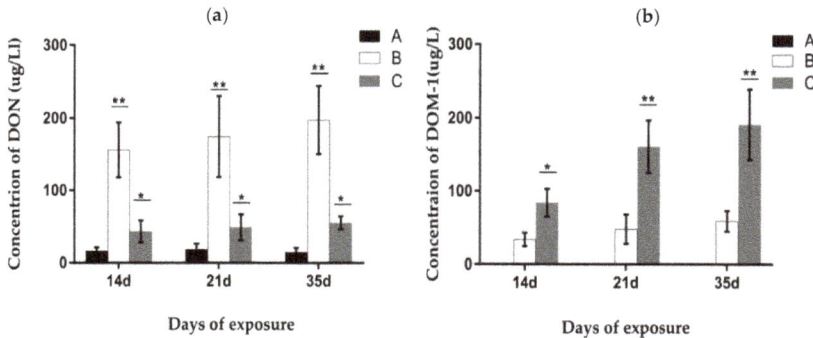

Figure 13. Concentration of DON and de-epoxy-DON (DOM-1) in porcine feces at different exposure days. (**a**) The concentration of DON. (**b**) The concentration of DOM-1. A, B, and C represent the samples of different treatments. Bars are presented as mean ± SD, $n = 5$. The values with different asterisks (* or **) in the same exposure day differ significantly ($p < 0.05$).

3. Discussion

3.1. DON Metabolism and the Toxic Effects of DON

Since the discrepancy existed in the absorption, metabolism and clearance procedures, the tolerance for the toxicity and pathogenic dose of DON were different for different animal species in vivo [19,20]. DON was degraded by microorganisms into a variety of products (such as de-epoxy-DON) in the digestive tract or in the intestinal mucosa, liver, kidney, and other organs. Chemical structure of DON and DOM-1 was listed in Figure 14. Residual DON and DOM-1 were the highest in the pig kidney, followed by the liver, and the high DON residue in the kidney may be associated with urine enrichment [21–23].

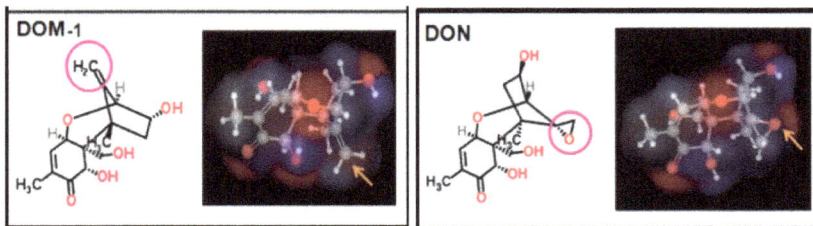

Figure 14. Chemical structure of DON and DOM-1 was cited by Maresca [24]. DON and DOM-1 were drawn using Marvin software. Images on the right show an electrostatic map of the molecules, with the blue color indicating a positive region, the red color indicating a negative region, and the gray color indicating a neutral region. The purple circles on the left images and the yellow arrows on the right images indicate the position of the epoxide or de-epoxide functions in DON and DOM-1, respectively.

In this study, the relative weight of the liver and kidney of growing pigs increased significantly after being fed with DON-contaminated wheat, indicating that the toxicity of DON was related to its metabolism and residual presence in the liver and kidney, which was consistent with the result reported before [21–23]. Meanwhile, the toxin effects on the liver and kidney of growing pigs were relieved after adding *Clostridium* sp. WJ06. These results come from the analysis of DON and DOM-1 in porcine feces and urine, and revealed that DOM-1 was mainly converted in the intestinal tract by *Clostridium* sp. WJ06. This indicated that the detoxified effect of *Clostridium* sp. WJ06 may be because it can convert DON to DOM-1 in the intestinal tract, and then reduce the absorption of DON in the intestine.

The results of this study also showed that DON-contaminated wheat can also cause a significant increase in the relative weight of the spleen, which was inconsistent with previous results [21,22]. *Clostridium* sp. WJ06 had no protective effect on the spleen of pigs, which may be due to the coexistence of other mycotoxins in the naturally contaminated wheat. The special metabolic pathways may exist in the spleen, so that *Clostridium* sp. WJ06 cannot decompose the toxicity of a variety of mycotoxins on the spleen of pigs.

3.2. Intestinal Morphological Structural Integrity and Toxic Effects of DON

The integrity of the intestinal barrier can effectively prevent intestinal bacteria, toxins, inflammatory mediators, and other harmful substances from passing through the intestinal mucosa into the blood [12,25]. DON is mainly absorbed in the small intestine, and it can pass through the intestinal barrier, enter the blood circulation and distribution system, and travel to the peripheral organs, thereby affecting the activity and function of the cells [26–28]. The absorption rate of DON exhibited the great difference between animal species; for example, the absorption rates of pigs, chickens, sheep, and cows were 82%, 19%, 9.9%, and 1%, respectively [29,30]. These differences are mainly related to the distribution of parasitic flora before or after the small intestine [31]. Before entering the small intestine of ruminants and poultry, DON is exposed to higher concentrations of microorganisms, which can convert DON to DOM-1 [32]. For humans and monogastric animals, there are a lack of microorganisms in the front of the small intestine, so humans and pigs are more sensitive to DON than poultry and ruminants [33,34].

In this study, the results suggested the microstructure of the ileum, caecum, and colon were destroyed by DON, especially ileum, which may be due to fewer microorganisms in the ileum of pigs than the caecum and colon. After adding *Clostridium* sp. WJ06, the damage to the intestinal barrier were alleviated significantly. The results indicated that DON may induce intestinal lesions by disrupting the integrity of the intestinal barrier, which is consistent with previous findings [35]. *Clostridium* sp. WJ06's protection of the intestine is probably because it can convert DON to DOM-1 in the intestine, thereby reducing its absorption and protecting the intestinal barrier of growing pigs. In the future, a study concerning the mechanism of *Clostridium* sp. WJ06 on degrading DON needs to be carried out.

3.3. Effects of Clostridium sp. WJ06 on Intestinal Microflora Diversity

The animal digestive tract, especially that of mammals, is very suitable for microbial mass reproduction. The complex microbial communities that survive in the intestine are called microbial flora [36]. Intestinal microflora planted in the small intestine and large intestine play an important role in maintaining the host's functions, including the energy intake of food, generation of the host's key metabolites, development of the immune system, response to gastrointestinal diseases, and so on [37]. In this research, the effects of *Clostridium* sp. and DON on the diversity of bacteria and fungi in the pig intestine were studied by MiSeq sequencing of the 16S rRNA gene and the ITS1 gene.

At the phylum level, *Firmicutes* is the predominant group of bacteria in the intestinal tract of mammals, with a proportion of more than 80%. *Bacteroidetes* is in the intestinal tract of second heterotic groups, which are connected with fermentation of carbohydrates, glucose metabolism, and bile acid metabolism. In the analysis of the genus level, *Lactobacillus* was the largest number of bacteria in the ileum, caecum and colon, especially in the ileum. The abundance of *Lactobacillus* was significantly decreased in all of the intestinal regions. A number of physiological influences of *Lactobacillus* on their hosts have been examined, including antimicrobial effects, microbial interference, supplementary effects on nutrition, antitumor effects, the reduction of cholesterol in serum, and immunomodulatory effects, and so on [38,39]. The analysis concerning the diversity of fungal flora of growing pigs in different diets was listed in this paper.

In conclusion, the results indicated that the bacterial and fungal composition in the ileum, caecum and colon of growing pigs varied significantly in different diets, but the structure of bacteria was relatively stable and simple. The effect of detoxification of *Clostridium* sp. WJ06 may be connected with the adjustment effect on the composition and diversity of intestinal microflora. Meanwhile, our results suggested that the composition and structure of the caecum of pigs was different significantly compared with that of the ileum and colon.

4. Materials and Methods

4.1. Ethics Statement

All procedures were carried out in accordance with the Guidelines for Experimental Animals of the Ministry of Science and Technology (Beijing, China) for the ethical use of experimental animals. The protocol were reviewed and approved by the Animal Care and Use Committee in the Shandong Agricultural University of China. (Permit Number ACSA-2016-036, 15 September 2016).

4.2. Bacteria Culture

Clostridium sp. WJ06 (Patent No: CN102485883.B) was separated from the intestinal tract of adult chickens, provided by Dr. Wang Jinquan of the Chinese Academy of Agricultural Sciences. L10 broth or agar was used to culture *Clostridium* sp. WJ06 at 37 °C for 48–72 h in an anaerobic chamber with an atmosphere of 85% N_2, 10% CO_2, and 5% H_2. At the same time, the conversion of DON was determined by high performance liquid chromatography (HPLC), and the results showed that the DON can be converted into DOM-1 with a degradation rate of over 90% by *Clostridium* sp. WJ06 (Figure 15) and has good stability.

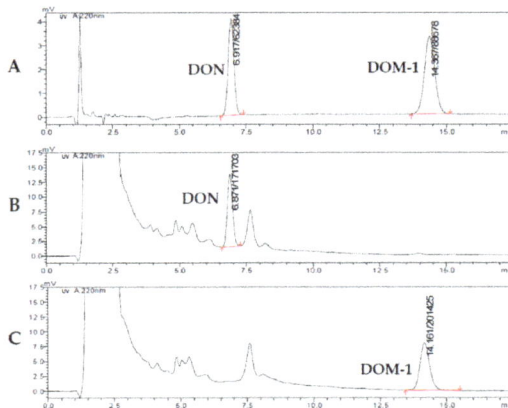

Figure 15. The effect of *Clostridium* sp. WJ06 culture on degrading DON in vitro via high performance liquid chromatography (HPLC). (**A**) The chromatogram of standard DON and DOM-1. (**B**) The chromatogram of the co-culture of DON (20 ppm) and L10. (**C**) The chromatogram of the co-culture of DON (20 ppm), L10, and *Clostridium* sp. WJ06.

4.3. Diets, Animals, and Experimental Design

The basal diet on the basis of de Blas and Wiseman (1998) and the addition of DON-contaminated wheat diets (33.3%) were completed before the trial of the seventh day, and the diet composition and nutrition level are shown in Table 4. DON, Aflatoxin B1 (AFB1), Fumonisin B1 (FB1) and Zearalenone (ZEA) were all examined by LC-MS/MS in the Institute of Quality Standards and Detection Technology, Chinese Academy of Agricultural Sciences (Beijing, China).

Table 4. Composition of the experimental diets.

	Basal Diet	Contaminated Diet
Ingredients (%)		
Corn	60.0	32.7
Soybean Meal	23.0	18.0
Extruded soybean	2.0	1.0
Contaminated wheat	0	33.3
Concentrate feed [#]	15	15
Total	100	100
Calculated composition (%)		
Dry matter	85.4	86.62
Crude ash	4.79	4.88
Calcium	0.63	0.58
Available phosphorus	0.57	0.62
Crude fibre	53.75	52.55
Crude protein	16.67	16.70
Crude fat	3.78	2.72
Digestible energy (MJ/kg)	17.17	16.69
Content of mycotoxin (ug/kg) [2]		
DON	371.2	1904.44
Aflatoxin B1 (AFB1)	1.56	1.59
Fumonisin B1 (FB1)	256.3	325.7
Zearalenone (ZEA)	145.16	96.08

[#] Concentrate feed provided per kg diet: Ca 2.1 g; P 1.2 g; Mn 6 mg; Fe 150 mg; Zn 150 mg; Cu 9 mg; I 0.21 mg; Se 0.45 mg; vitamin A 3300 IU; vitamin D 290 IU; vitamin E 24 IU; vitamin K 30.75 mg; vitamin B1 1.50 mg; vitamin B2 5.25 mg; vitamin B6 2.25 mg; vitamin B 120.026 mg; pantothenic acid 15 mg; nicotinic acid 22.50 mg.
[2] Measured by HPLC methods.

Twenty-four commodity generation PIC pigs (quinary crossbred Pig improve Co. England, four months of age) of both sexes (equal male to female ratio per treatment and 55.58 ± 1.83 kg in mass) were used for experiments after an adaptation period of seven days. The pigs were divided into eight healthy pigs per treatment group and assigned to the three experimental diets by average liver mass, which was monitored every day. Treatment A was only fed with basal diet as a control group. Treatment B was fed with the basal diet with the addition of DON-contaminated wheat as the negative control group. Treatment C was fed with the basal diet with the addition of DON-contaminated wheat, but using *Clostridium* sp. WJ06 as a detoxicant every day. The addition amount of *Clostridium* sp. was 30 mL per pig every day, and the culture solution of *Clostridium* sp. WJ06 was poured into the feed and mixed completely before feeding in the morning. The feeding experiment was carried out at a Kongjiazhuang farm in Shandong province.

The experiment lasted for 35 days, including a seven-day adaptation period and a 28-day experimental period. Feeds and water were provided ad libitum and offered at 8:30 am and 5:30 pm daily. The residual feed was collected daily. Pigs were weighed individually at the beginning and the end of the experiment, and the average daily weight gain (ADG) was calculated. The average daily feed intake (ADFI) was recorded, and the feed intake to body weight gain (F/G) ratio was calculated.

On days 14, 21, and 35 of the experiment, the urine and feces of 20 pigs (five pigs per treatment) were collected and stored at −20 °C for further analysis. On the 35th day of the experiment, three healthy pigs randomly selected from each treatment group were euthanized by electric shock at the same time (8:00 am). The liver, kidney, heart, and other organs were separated and weighed. The relative weight of the organ (kg/kg) = organ weight (kg)/live weight (kg) was calculated. Meanwhile, their digestive tracts had been removed within less than 15 min. The content of the intestines (including the ileum, caecum, and colon) were collected and frozen immediately in liquid nitrogen, and subsequently stored at −70 °C until analyzed. Then, the approximately two-centimeter segment of the middle portion of the ileum, caecum, and colon was fixed in 2.5% glutaraldehyde at room temperature for observation under a scanning electron microscope.

4.4. DNA Extraction

Twenty-seven samples (200 mg of the intestinal content of the ileum, caecum, and colon) were suspended in 1.4 mL of ASL buffer (stool lysis buffer, Qiagen, Hilden, Germany), and DNA was extracted using a QIAamp DNA Stool Mini kit (Qiagen, Hilden, Germany), following the manufacturer's instructions. The bacterial cells were disrupted by a bead beater with sterile zirconia beads added to the samples, which improved extraction yield and the quality of the community DNA [40]. For each sample, DNA was extracted in duplicate to avoid bias [41], and the extracts from the same sample were pooled for 16S rRNA sequencing. To assess the DNA quality, A 260/280 measurements were performed using a DU640 Nucleic Acids and Protein Analyzer (Beckman Coulter, Brea, CA, USA). The DNA samples were diluted to 20 ng/uL using sterile ultrapure water. After the extracted DNA was detected and quantified strictly, equal moles of three DNA samples of the same treatment and the intestinal regions were mixed [42]. Therefore, the total number of mixed DNA samples was nine, and then nine libraries were coded as A1, A2, A3, B1, B2, B3, C1, C2, and C3; that is, A, B, and C represented the samples from three treatments, and 1, 2, and 3 represented the samples of the ileum, caecum, and colon, respectively. Then, all of the samples were stored at −20 °C until use.

4.5. MiSeq Sequencing of 16S rRNA Gene and ITS1 Gene

For all of the samples collected, we used a barcoded high-throughput sequencing approach similar to that described in Jia et al. [43] and McGuire et al. [44] to survey the diversity and composition of the bacterial and fungal species in each of these samples. PCR amplifications were conducted with the barcoded primer pair 341F/806R set that amplifies the V3–V4 fragments of the 16S rRNA gene (341F: CCTAYGGGRBGCASCAG, 806: GGACTACNNGGGTATCTAAT). Meanwhile, the first internal transcribed spacer region (ITS1) of the fungal rRNA gene was amplified using the ITS5-1737F (GGAAGTAAAAGTCGTAACAAGG) and ITS2-2043R (GCTGCGTTCTTCATCGATGC) as the primer pair. All of the amplicon sequencing samples were accomplished using the Illumina MiSeq platform at the Novogene Bioinformatics Technology Co., Ltd., Beijing, China.

At first, all of the initial template DNA concentrations were normalized between samples. PCR reactions were performed according to protocols described by Caporaso et al. [45]. All of the PCR reactions were carried out with Phusion® High-Fidelity PCR Master Mix (NEB, Beijing, China).

We mixed the same volume of 1× loading buffer (contained SYB green) with PCR products and operate electrophoresis on 2% agarose gel for detection. Samples with a bright main strip between 400–450 bp were chosen for further experiments. PCR products were mixed in equidensity ratios. Then, the mixture of PCR products was purified with a Qiagen Gel Extraction Kit (Qiagen, Hilden, Germany). Sequencing libraries were generated using a TruSeq® DNA PCR-Free Sample Preparation Kit (Illumina, San Diego, CA, USA) following the manufacturer's recommendations, and index codes were added. The library quality was assessed on the Qubit® 2.0 Fluorometer (Thermo Scientific, Waltham, MA, USA) and Agilent Bioanalyzer 2100 system (Agilent, Waldbronn, Germany). At last, the library was sequenced on an IlluminaHiSeq2500 platform and 250 bp paired-end reads were generated.

4.6. Bioinformatics Analysis

Paired-end reads were assigned to each sample based on their unique barcode and truncated by cutting off the barcode and primer sequence. The high-quality clean tags were obtained, which complied with the method reported by Jia et al. [43]. These sequences were classified into the same OTUs (operational taxonomic units) at an identity threshold of 97% similarity using UPARSE software (UPARSE v7.0.1001, Edgar, Tiburon, California, USA, http://drive5.com/uparse/) [46]. For each representative sequence, the GreenGene Database (http://greengenes.lbl.gov/cgi-bin/nph-index.cgi) was used based on the Ribosomal Database Project (RDP) classifier (Version 2.2, http://sourceforge.net/projects/rdp-classifier/) algorithm to annotate taxonomic information. The taxon abundance of each sample was generated into phylum, class, order, family, and genera levels. In order to study the phylogenetic relationship of different OTUs, and the difference of the dominant species in different samples (groups), multiple sequence alignments were conducted using the MUSCLE software (Version 3.8.31, http://www.drive5.com/muscle/) [47].

We processed the ITS1 fungal amplicon data following methods outlined in McGuire et al. [47]. We used the QIIME pipeline in a similar way as for the 16S rRNA data, except the Unite Database (https://unite.ut.ee/) was used based on the Blast algorithm, which was calculated by QIIME software (Version 1.9.1, http://qiime.org/scripts/assign_taxonomy.html) to annotate taxonomic information.

All of the analyses from clustering to alpha diversity (within each sample) and beta diversity (between samples) were performed with QIIME (Version 1.9.10,) and displayed with R software (Version 2.15.3) [48].

4.7. Analysis of the Concentration of DON and DOM-1 in Urine and Feces

The concentrations of DON and de-epoxy-DON (DOM-1) in urine and feces were analyzed by LC-MS/MS (liquid chromatography-tandem mass spectrometry). The sample preparation methods were described in detail earlier [49]. LC-MS/MS analysis was performed using an Agilent 1200 liquid chromatograph (Agilent Technologies, Palo Alto, CA, USA) coupled to a 3200 QTrap® mass spectrometry system (Applied Biosystems, Foster City, CA, USA) equipped with a Turbo electrospray ionization (ESI) interface. All investigations concerning the concentration of DON and DOM-1 were carried out in the Institute of Quality Standards and Detection Technology, Chinese Academy of Agricultural Sciences.

4.8. Statistical Analysis

The data analyses for growth performance and the relative weight of organs were performed using one-way analysis with SPSS for Windows, version 14.0, and differences between means were compared by Duncan's least significant difference. p value < 0.05 was considered a significant difference, and the analysis result was noted with mean ± standard deviation (mean ± SD).

Acknowledgments: We would like to thank our anonymous reviewers and our colleagues from the Animal Nutrition Laboratory for their valuable critiques and suggestions. This work was supported by grants from key Research and Development Program of China (S2016G4513) and form the Funds of Shandong "Double Tops" Program. All authors report no conflicts of interest relevant to this paper.

Author Contributions: For this research, FuChang Li performed the experiments and wrote a draft of the paper. JinQuan Wang contributed reagents/materials/analysis tools. LiBo Huang and HongJu Chen performed a part of experiments and analyzed the data. ChunYang Wang conceived and designed the experiments and revised the paper.

Conflicts of Interest: The authors declare no conflict of interest.

References

1. Rohweder, D.; Kersten, S.; Valenta, H.; Sondermann, S.; Schollenberger, M.; Drochner, W.; Dänicke, S. Bioavailability of the *Fusarium* toxin deoxynivalenol (DON) from wheat straw and chaff in pigs. *Arch. Anim. Nutr.* **2013**, *67*, 37–47. [CrossRef] [PubMed]
2. Garda-Buffon, J.; Kupsk, L.; Badiale-Furlong, E. Deoxynivalenol (DON) degradation and peroxidase enzyme activity in submerged fermentation. *Ciênc. Tecnol. Aliment.* **2011**, *31*, 198–203. [CrossRef]
3. Fodor, J.S. Individual and Combined Effects of Subchronic Exposure of Three Fusarium Toxins (Fumonisin B, Deoxynivalenol and Zearalenone) in Rabbit Bucks. *J. Toxicol. Clin. Toxicol.* **2015**, *5*, 2–11. [CrossRef]
4. Kachlek, M.J.; Szabó-Fodor, A.; Szabó, I.; Bors, C.; Celia, Z.; Gerencsér, Z.; Matics, Z.; Szendrő, T.; Tuboly, E.; Balogh-Zándoki, R.; et al. Subchronic exposure to deoxynivalenol exerts slight effect on the immune system and liver morphology of growing rabbits. *Acta Vet. Brno* **2017**, *86*, 37–44. [CrossRef]
5. Pestka, J.J. Mechanisms of Deoxynivalenol-Induced Gene Expression and Apoptosis. *Food Addit. Contam.* **2008**, *25*, 1128–1140. [CrossRef]
6. Ghareeb, K.; Awad, W.A.; Böhm, J.Q.; Zebeli, K.G. Impacts of the feed contaminant deoxynivalenol on the intestine of monogastric animals: Poultry and swine. *J. Appl. Toxicol.* **2015**, *35*, 327–340. [CrossRef] [PubMed]
7. Lewczuk, B.B.; Przybylska-Gornowicz, M.; Gajecka, K.; Targonska, N.; Ziolkowska, M.; Gajecki, M. Histological structure of duodenum in gilts receiving low doses of zearalenone and deoxynivalenol in feed. *Exp. Toxicol. Pathol.* **2016**, *68*, 157–166. [CrossRef] [PubMed]
8. Romero, A.A.; Ramos, I.; Castellano, E.; Martinez, V.; Martinez-Larranaga, M.; Anadon, M.R.; Martinez, M.A. Mycotoxins modify the barrier function of Caco-2 cells through differential gene expression of specific claudin isoforms: Protective effect of illite mineral clay. *Toxicology* **2016**, *353*, 21–33. [CrossRef] [PubMed]
9. Yu, M.L.; Chen, Z.; Peng, A.K.; Nussler, Q.; Wu, L.; Liu, W.Y. Mechanism of deoxynivalenol effects on the reproductive system and fetus malformation: Current status and future challenges. *Toxicol. In Vitro* **2017**, *41*, 150–158. [CrossRef] [PubMed]
10. Pierron, A.; Alassane-Kpembi, I.; Oswald, I.P. Impact of two mycotoxins deoxynivalenol and fumonisin on pig intestinal health. *Porc. Health Manag.* **2016**, *2*, 2–8. [CrossRef] [PubMed]
11. Du, K.; Wang, C.; Liu, P.; Li, Y.; Ma, X. Effects of Dietary Mycotoxins on Gut Microbiome. *Protein Pept. Lett.* **2017**, *24*, 397–405. [CrossRef] [PubMed]
12. Burel, C.; Tanguy, M.; Guerre, P.; Boilletot, E.; Cariolet, R.; Queguiner, M.; Postollec, G.; Pinton, P.; Salvat, G.; Oswald, I.P.; et al. Effect of low dose of fumonisins on pig health: Immune status, intestinal microbiota and sensitivity to *Salmonella*. *Toxins* **2013**, *5*, 841–864. [CrossRef] [PubMed]
13. Wache, Y.J.; Valat, C.; Postollec, G.; Bougeard, S.; Burel, C.; Oswald, I.P.; Fravalo, P. Impact of deoxynivalenol on the intestinal microflora of pigs. *Int. J. Mol. Sci.* **2009**, *10*, 1–17. [CrossRef] [PubMed]
14. Hathout, A.S.; Aly, S.E. Biological detoxification of mycotoxins: A review. *Ann. Microbiol.* **2014**, *64*, 905–919. [CrossRef]
15. Repečkienė, J.L.; Levinskaitė, A.; Paškevičius, V.R. Toxin-producing fungi on feed grains and application of yeasts for their detoxification. *Pol. J. Vet. Sci.* **2013**, *16*, 391–393. [CrossRef]
16. Oliveira, P.B.; Brosnan, F.; Jacob, A.; Furey, A.; Coffey, E.; Zannini, E.; Arendt, K. *Lactic acid bacteria* bioprotection applied to the malting process. Part II: Substrate impact and mycotoxin reduction. *Food Control* **2015**, *51*, 444–452. [CrossRef]
17. Chang, C.; Zhou, S.N.; Wang, X.D.; Wu, J.E. Protective Effect of Saccharomyces boulardii on Deoxynivalenol-Induced Injury of Porcine Macrophage via Attenuating p38 MAPK Signal Pathway. *Appl. Biochem. Biotechnol.* **2017**, *182*, 411–427. [CrossRef] [PubMed]
18. Segata, N.; Waldron, L.; Gevers, D.; Miropolsky, L.; Garrett, W.S.; Huttenhower, C. Metagenomic biomarker discovery and explanation. *Genome Biol.* **2011**, *12*, 2–18. [CrossRef] [PubMed]
19. Dänicke, S.; Valenta, H.; Döll, S. On the toxicokinetics and the metabolism of deoxynivalenol (DON) in the pig. *Arch. Anim. Nutr.* **2004**, *58*, 169–180. [CrossRef] [PubMed]
20. Thanner, S.; Czeglédi, L.; Schwartz-Zimmermann, H.E.; Berthiller, A.F.; Gutzwiller, A. Urinary deoxynivalenol (DON) and zearalenone (ZEA) as biomarkers of DON and ZEA exposure of pigs. *Mycotoxin Res.* **2016**, *32*, 69–75. [CrossRef] [PubMed]
21. Li, W.; Wang, W.; Huang, R.; Cui, Z.; He, L.; Yin, J.; Duan, L.; Li, T.; Wang, J.Q. Deoxynivalenol residues in edible tissue of infested pig. *J. Food Agric. Environ.* **2013**, *11*, 1129–1133.

22. Danicke, S.; Brezina, U. Kinetics and metabolism of the *Fusarium* toxin deoxynivalenol in farm animals: Consequences for diagnosis of exposure and intoxication and carry over. *Food Chem. Toxicol.* **2013**, *60*, 58–75. [CrossRef] [PubMed]

23. Warth, B.S.; Fruhmann, M.; Mikula, P.; Berthiller, H.; Schuhmacher, F.; Hametner, R.; Abia, C.; Adam, W.A.; Frohlich, G.; Krska, J.R. Development and validation of a rapid multi-biomarker liquid chromatography/tandem mass spectrometry method to assess human exposure to mycotoxins. *Rapid Commun. Mass Spectrom.* **2012**, *26*, 1533–1540. [CrossRef] [PubMed]

24. Maresca, M. From the gut to the brain: Journey and pathophysiological effects of the food-associated trichothecene mycotoxin deoxynivalenol (Review). *Toxins* **2013**, *23*, 784–820. [CrossRef] [PubMed]

25. Diesing, A.K.N.; Panther, C.; Walk, P.; Post, N.; Kluess, A.; Kreutzmann, J.; Danicke, P.; Rothkotter, S.H.; Kahlert, J.S. Mycotoxin deoxynivalenol (DON) mediates biphasic cellular response in intestinal porcine epithelial cell lines IPEC-1 and IPEC-J2. *Toxicol. Lett.* **2011**, *200*, 8–18. [CrossRef] [PubMed]

26. Alassane-Kpembi, I.P.; Oswald, I.P. Toxicological interactions between the mycotoxins deoxynivalenol, nivalenol and their acetylated derivatives in intestinal epithelial cells. *Arch. Toxicol.* **2015**, *89*, 1337–1346. [CrossRef] [PubMed]

27. Akbari, P.B.; Gremmels, S.; Koelink, H.; Verheijden, J.; Garssen, K.A.; Fink-Gremmels, J. Deoxynivalenol: A trigger for intestinal integrity breakdown. *FASEB J.* **2014**, *28*, 2414–2429. [CrossRef] [PubMed]

28. Broekaert, N.D.; Demeyere, M.; Berthiller, K.; Michlmayr, F.; Varga, H.; Adam, E.; Meyer, G.; Croubels, E.S. Comparative in vitro cytotoxicity of modified deoxynivalenol on porcine intestinal epithelial cells. *Food Chem. Toxicol.* **2016**, *95*, 103–109. [CrossRef] [PubMed]

29. Barnett, A.M.; Roy, N.C.; McNabb, W.C.; Cookson, A.L. The interactions between endogenous bacteria, dietary components and the mucus layer of the large bowel. *Food Funct.* **2012**, *3*, 690–699. [CrossRef] [PubMed]

30. Osselaere, A.M.; Devreese, J.; Goossens, V.; Vandenbroucke, S.; De Baere, P.; Croubels, S. Toxicokinetic study and absolute oral bioavailability of deoxynivalenol, T-2 toxin and zearalenone in broiler chickens. *Food Chem. Toxicol.* **2013**, *51*, 350–355. [CrossRef] [PubMed]

31. Frey, J.C.; Pell, A.N.; Berthiaume, R.; Lapierre, H.S.; Lee, J.K.; Ha, J.E.; Angert, E.R. Comparative studies of microbial populations in the rumen, duodenum, ileum and faeces of lactating dairy cows. *J. Appl. Microbiol.* **2010**, *108*, 1982–1993. [CrossRef] [PubMed]

32. Rotter, B.A.; Prelusky, D.B.; Pestks, J.J. Toxicology of deoxynivalenol (vomitoxin). *J. Toxicol. Environ. Health* **1996**, *48*, 1–34. [CrossRef] [PubMed]

33. Eriksen, G.S.; Pettersson, H.; Johnsen, K.; Lindberg, J.E. Transformation of trichothecenes in ileal digesta and faeces from pigs. *Arch. Anim. Nutr.* **2002**, *56*, 263–274. [CrossRef]

34. Prelusky, D.B.; Veira, D.M.; Trenholm, H.L. Plasma pharmacokinetics of the mycotoxin deoxynivalenol following oral and intravenous administration to sheep. *J. Environ. Sci. Health B* **1985**, *20*, 603–624. [CrossRef] [PubMed]

35. Lessard, M.C.; Savard, K.; Deschene, K.; Lauzon, V.A.; Pinilla, C.A.; Gagnon, J.; Lapointe, F.; Chorfi, Y. Impact of deoxynivalenol (DON) contaminated feed on intestinal integrity and immune response in swine. *Food Chem. Toxicol.* **2015**, *80*, 7–16. [CrossRef] [PubMed]

36. Papadimitriou, K.; Zoumpopoulou, G.; Folign, B.; Alexandraki, V.; Kazou, M.; Pot, B.; Tsakalidou, E. Discovering probiotic microorganisms: In vitro, in vivo, genetic and omics approaches. *Front. Microbiol.* **2015**, *6*, 58. [CrossRef] [PubMed]

37. Jia, J.; Frantz, N.; Khoo, C.; Gibson, G.R.; Rastall, R.A.; McCartney, A.L. Investigation of the faecal microbiota associated with canine chronic diarrhoea. *FEMS Microbiol. Ecol.* **2010**, *71*, 304–312. [CrossRef] [PubMed]

38. Arqués, J.L.; Rodríguez, E.; Langa, S.; Landete, J.M.; Medina, M. Antimicrobial activity of *lactic acid bacteria* in dairy products and gut: Effect on pathogens. *Biomed. Res. Int.* **2015**, *22*, 584183. [CrossRef] [PubMed]

39. Goyal, N.; Rishi, P.; Shukla, G. *Lactobacillus rhamnosus* GG antagonizes Giardia intestinalis induced oxidative stress and intestinal disaccharidases: An experimental study. *World J. Microbiol. Biotechnol.* **2013**, *29*, 1049–1057. [CrossRef] [PubMed]

40. Zhu, Y.; Wang, C.; Li, F. Impact of dietary fiber/starch ratio in shaping caecal microbiota in rabbits. *Can. J. Microbiol.* **2015**, *61*, 771–784. [CrossRef] [PubMed]

41. Michelland, R.J.S.; Combes, V.; Monteils, L.; Cauquil, T.; Fortun-Lamothe, L. Rapid adaptation of the bacterial community in the growing rabbit caecum after a change in dietary fibre supply. *Animal* **2011**, *5*, 1761–1768. [CrossRef] [PubMed]

42. Wang, C.; Zhu, Y.L.; Huang, L.; Li, F.C. The Effect of *Lactobacillus* isolates on growth performance, immune response, intestinal bacterial community composition of growing Rex Rabbits. *J. Anim. Physiol. Anim. Nutr.* **2017**, *101*, e1–e13. [CrossRef] [PubMed]

43. Jia, H.R.; Geng, L.L.; Li, Y.H.; Wang, Q.; Diao, Q.Y.; Zhou, T.; Dai, P.L. The effects of Bt Cry1Ie toxin on bacterial diversity in the midgut of *Apis mellifera ligustica* (Hymenoptera: Apidae). *Sci. Rep.* **2016**, *6*, 24664. [CrossRef] [PubMed]

44. McGuire, K.L.; Payne, S.G.; Palmer, M.I.; Gillikin, C.M.; Keefe, D.S.; Kim, J.S.; Gedallovich, M.J.; Discenza, R.; Rangamannar, J.A.; Koshner, A.L.; et al. Digging the New York City Skyline: Soil fungal communities in green roofs and city parks. *PLoS ONE* **2013**, *8*, e58020. [CrossRef] [PubMed]

45. Caporaso, J.G.; Lauber, C.L.; Walters, W.A.; Berg-Lyons, D.; Lozupone, C.A.; Turnbaugh, P.J.; Fierer, N.; Knight, R. Global patterns of 16S rRNA diversity at a depth of millions of sequences per sample. *Proc. Natl. Acad. Sci. USA* **2011**, *108*, 4516–4522. [CrossRef] [PubMed]

46. Edgar, R.C. UPARSE: Highly accurate OTU sequences from microbial amplicon reads. *Nat. Methods* **2013**, *10*, 996–999. [CrossRef] [PubMed]

47. Edgar, R.C. MUSCLE: multiple sequence alignment with high accuracy and high throughput. *Nucleic Acids Res.* **2004**, *32*, 1792–1797. [CrossRef] [PubMed]

48. Caporaso, J.G.; Kuczynski, J.; Stombaugh, J.; Bittinger, K.; Bushman, F.D. QIIME allows analysis of high-throughput community sequencing data. *Nat. Methods* **2010**, *7*, 335–336. [CrossRef] [PubMed]

49. Winkler, J.; Kersten, S.; Valenta, H.; Hüther, L.; Engelhardt, U.; Dänicke, S. Simultaneous determination of zearalenone, deoxynivalenol and their metabolites in bovine urine as biomarkers of exposure. *World Mycotoxin J.* **2014**, *8*, 63–74. [CrossRef]

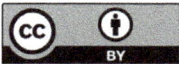

Article

Intestinal Microbiota Ecological Response to Oral Administrations of Hydrogen-Rich Water and Lactulose in Female Piglets Fed a *Fusarium* Toxin-Contaminated Diet

Weijiang Zheng [1], Xu Ji [1], Qing Zhang [1] and Wen Yao [1,2,*]

[1] Laboratory of Gastrointestinal Microbiology, Jiangsu Key Laboratory of Gastrointestinal Nutrition and Animal Health, College of Animal Science and Technology, Nanjing Agricultural University, Nanjing 210095, China; zhengweijiang@njau.edu.cn (W.Z.); jixuchance@gmail.com (X.J.); zhangqingzee@163.com (Q.Z.)
[2] Key Lab of Animal Physiology and Biochemistry, Ministry of Agriculture, Nanjing 210095, China
* Correspondence: yaowen67jp@njau.edu.cn; Tel.: +86-25-84399830

Received: 27 May 2018; Accepted: 13 June 2018; Published: 16 June 2018

Abstract: The objective of the current experiment was to explore the intestinal microbiota ecological response to oral administrations of hydrogen-rich water (HRW) and lactulose (LAC) in female piglets fed a *Fusarium* mycotoxin-contaminated diet. A total of 24 individually-housed female piglets (Landrace × large × white; initial average body weight, 7.25 ± 1.02 kg) were randomly assigned to receive four treatments (six pigs/treatment): uncontaminated basal diet (negative control, NC), mycotoxin-contaminated diet (MC), MC diet + HRW (MC + HRW), and MC diet + LAC (MC + LAC) for 25 days. Hydrogen levels in the mucosa of different intestine segments were measured at the end of the experiment. Fecal scoring and diarrhea rate were recorded every day during the whole period of the experiment. Short-chain fatty acids (SCFAs) profiles in the digesta of the foregut and hindgut samples were assayed. The populations of selected bacteria and denaturing gradient gel electrophoresis (DGGE) profiles of total bacteria and methanogenic *Archaea* were also evaluated. Results showed that *Fusarium* mycotoxins not only reduced the hydrogen levels in the caecum but also shifted the SCFAs production, and populations and communities of microbiota. HRW treatment increased the hydrogen levels of the stomach and duodenum. HRW and LAC groups also had higher colon and caecum hydrogen levels than the MC group. Both HRW and LAC protected against the mycotoxin-contaminated diet-induced higher diarrhea rate and lower SCFA production in the digesta of the colon and caecum. In addition, the DGGE profile results indicated that HRW and LAC might shift the pathways of hydrogen-utilization bacteria, and change the diversity of intestine microbiota. Moreover, HRW and LAC administrations reversed the mycotoxin-contaminated diet-induced changing of the populations of *Escherichia coli* (*E. coli*) and *Bifidobacterium* in ileum digesta and hydrogen-utilizing bacteria in colon digesta.

Keywords: intestinal microbiota; hydrogen-rich water; lactulose; *Fusarium* mycotoxins; piglets

Key contribution: Our results showed that both hydrogen-rich water and lactulose administrations protected against the imbalance of intestinal microbiota, reduction of SCFAs production and higher diarrhea rate induced by a *Fusarium* mycotoxin diet, partly through affecting the communities/populations of microbiota and the evaluation of hydrogen gas.

1. Introduction

Fusarium mycotoxins are secondary metabolites of fungi, produced by several kinds of *Fusarium* species that occur naturally worldwide in cereal grains and animal feed [1]. Among the *Fusarium*

mycotoxins, deoxynivalenol (DON) and zearalenone (ZEN) are of special importance as they are formed under predisposing environmental conditions in the field prior to harvest and cannot be completely avoided by strategies [2]. Consumption of *Fusarium* mycotoxins is widely considered as a serious health hazard issue for both animals and human beings, due to their potent toxicity on the gastrointestinal (GI) tract, with symptoms including nausea, vomiting, diarrhea, and oxidative damage [3]. The GI tract is the place where mycotoxin absorption and metabolism occur. Therefore, interactions between the mycotoxins and intestinal microbiota play a major role in the toxicology of mycotoxins [4]. It has been shown that intestinal bacteria are able to bind, transform, degrade, and transfer mycotoxins *in vivo* and *in vitro* [5]. Increasingly attention has been paid on how mycotoxin exposure impacts the intestinal microbiota. Previous studies have shown that the profiles and biodiversity of intestinal microbiota were rapidly and clearly modified in pig exposure to a mycotoxin-contaminated diet [6,7]. Considering the functional effects of microbiota, many methods have been attempted to balance gut microbiota to normalize microbiota in intestinal tracts and keep the host healthy. For example, supplementation of nutritional elements, probiotics, and prebiotics or symbiotic, etc.

Hydrogen gas is one of the metabolites of bacterial fermentation in the gut, which has been proven to act as a novel antioxidant [8]. It has been demonstrated that H_2 could penetrate cytoplasmic membranes, targets intracellular organelles, and selectively neutralizes cytotoxic reactive oxygen species (ROS) [9]. As a result, hydrogen gas has been applied in many disease models, such as dextran sodium sulfate (DSS)-induced colon inflammatory [10] and intestinal ischemia-reperfusion injuries [11]. A recent report described that 70% of GI microbial species that encoded genetic capacity to metabolize H_2 [12], indicating that H_2 levels might affect the gut microbial activity, population, or community. Interestingly, one recent study reported that molecular hydrogen-dissolved alkaline electrolyzed water (AEW) had a strong antimicrobial effect and significantly reduced populations of pathogenic bacteria, such as *Escherichia coli* O157 and *Salmonella* [13]. Xiao et al. also reported that HRW oral gavage resulted in retention of the total abdominal irradiation (TAI)-shifted intestinal bacterial composition in mice [14]. As we know, H_2 is produced continuously under a normal physiological condition in mammalian animals, primarily during the fermentation of non-digestible carbohydrates by bacteria in the large intestine. Therefore, administration of hydrogen-producing prebiotics might also be a viable method to provide functional H_2 to animals and humans. Lactulose is a synthetic non-absorbable disaccharide consisting of fructose and galactose [15]. It has been reported that microbial fermentation of lactulose in the hindgut could induce dramatic amounts of endogenous H_2, providing beneficial effects on liver regeneration [16] and cerebral ischemia-reperfusion injury [17] in rats. In addition, lactulose administration could also lead to the production of short-chain fatty acids (SCFAs) and methane, increasing the diversity and creating a distinct microbiota community in piglets [18,19].

Although HRW and LAC have shown the modifications of microbiota, the effects of HRW or LAC on mycotoxin-induced microbiota imbalance in piglets have not ever been studied. Here, the rationale underlying this study is that HRW or LAC might maintain the intestinal microbiota communities and bacteria populations, thus affecting SCFAs production and eventually improving the health status of female weaning piglets. Therefore, the impacts of HRW and LAC on fecal scoring, diarrhea rate, SCFAs production, intestinal microbiota communities, and populations in piglets fed a *Fusarium* mycotoxin-contaminated diet were explored in this study.

2. Results

2.1. Hydrogen Levels in Intestinal Segments

At the end of the experiment, that is, day 25 of the experiment, hydrogen concentrations in the mucosa of stomach, duodenum, jejunum, ileum, colon, and caecum are presented in Figure 1. Results showed that stomach and duodenum in the MC + HRW group had the highest hydrogen levels among the four groups ($p < 0.05$), while no difference was found among the other three groups ($p > 0.05$). No difference was found in the jejunum and ileum hydrogen concentrations among the four groups ($p > 0.05$). *Fusarium* mycotoxin-contaminated diet was found to reduce the hydrogen levels in the caecum ($p < 0.05$), but have no impact on the hydrogen levels in the colon ($p > 0.05$). Interestingly, both LAC and HRW treatments significantly increased the hydrogen levels either in the colon or caecum when they compared with the MC group ($p < 0.05$). Furthermore, the MC + LAC group had higher hydrogen levels than the MC + HRW group in the colon and caecum samples ($p < 0.05$).

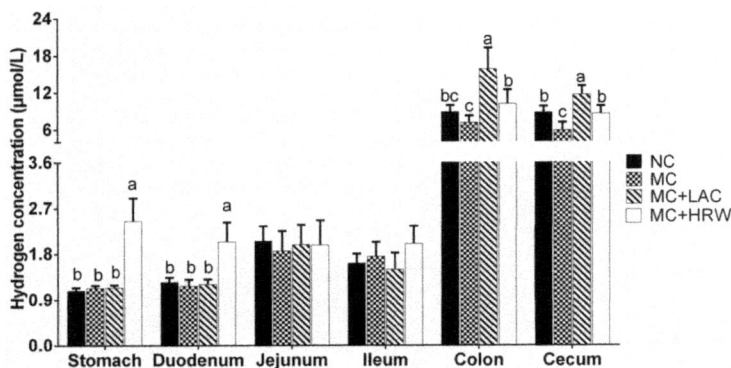

Figure 1. Effects of hydrogen-rich water and lactulose on hydrogen concentrations in different intestinal segments of female piglets fed a *Fusarium* mycotoxin-contaminated diet. Each column represents the mean hydrogen levels with five independent replications, mean ± SD. Letters a–c above the bars indicate statistical significance ($p < 0.05$) among the four treatments. NC (negative control), basal diet; MC, *Fusarium* mycotoxin-contaminated diet; MC + LAC, MC diet + lactulose treatment; and MC + HRW, MC diet + hydrogen-rich water treatment.

2.2. Fecal Scoring and Diarrhea Rate

The effects of HRW and LAC on fecal scoring and diarrhea rate in piglets fed a *Fusarium* mycotoxin-contaminated diet are shown in Table 1. From days 0 to 7 and days 7 to 14, the *Fusarium* mycotoxin diet was found to significantly increase the fecal score ($p < 0.05$), while HRW and LAC treatments lowered the fecal score from days 0 to 7 and days 7 to 14, respectively ($p < 0.05$). From days 14 to 21, days 21 to 25, and days 0 to 25, no significant difference was found on fecal scoring among the four groups ($p > 0.05$). No difference was found on the diarrhea rate from different time periods except from days 0 to 7 ($p > 0.05$). Compared with the NC group, the diarrhea rate was significantly increased in both MC and MC + LAC from days 0 to 7 ($p < 0.05$), while HRW treatment decreased the diarrhea rate compared with the MC group ($p < 0.05$). Additionally, there was no difference between the MC and MC + LAC groups ($p > 0.05$).

Table 1. Effects of hydrogen-rich water and lactulose on fecal scoring and diarrhea rate of female piglets fed a *Fusarium* mycotoxin-contaminated diet [1,2].

Item	NC	MC	MC + LAC	MC + HRW	SEM	*p*-Value
			Fecal score			
Days 0–7	2.64 [c]	3.60 [a]	3.17 [b]	2.64 [c]	0.10	<0.001
Days 7–14	2.84 [b]	3.74 [a]	3.12 [b]	3.02 [b]	0.12	0.037
Days 14–21	2.78	3.00	2.82	2.95	0.11	0.909
Days 21–25	2.79	2.53	2.82	3.00	0.15	0.758
Days 0–25	2.76	3.30	3.02	2.91	0.09	0.163

Table 1. *Cont.*

Item	NC	MC	MC + LAC	MC + HRW	SEM	*p*-Value
			Diarrhea rate %			
Days 0–7	5.00 [b]	30.00 [a]	25.00 [a]	5.00 [b]	3.64	0.008
Days 7–14	5.00	30.00	22.50	15.00	5.00	0.353
Days 14–21	7.50	17.50	15.00	12.50	5.09	0.927
Days 21–25	12.00	0.00	12.00	16.00	5.53	0.788
Days 0–25	6.92	22.31	20.00	12.31	3.65	0.449

[a,b,c] Values with different letters within the same row are different ($p < 0.05$).[1] NC (negative control), basal diet; MC, *Fusarium* mycotoxin-contaminated diet; MC + LAC, MC diet + lactulose treatment; and MC + HRW, MC diet + hydrogen-rich water treatment. [2] $n = 5$.

2.3. Short-Chain Fatty Acids (SCFAs) Levels in the Digesta of Jejumun, Ileum, Colon, and Caecum

There was no difference ($p > 0.05$) in the pH value of different intestine segments among the four groups (Table S1). The concentrations of SCFAs levels in different intestinal segments among the treatments are shown in Table 2. In the jejunum and ileum, the levels of acetate, propionate, butyrate, and total SCFAs were found to be no different among the four groups ($p > 0.05$). In the colon, the acetate levels were not influenced by treatments ($p > 0.05$), but the propionate, butyrate, valeric acid, and total SCFAs concentrations in the MC group were lower than the NC group ($p < 0.05$). Compared with the MC group, HRW treatment had higher levels of butyrate ($p < 0.05$) and no effects on colon propionate, valeric acid, and total SCFAs status ($p > 0.05$). However, LAC administration significantly increased the levels of propionate, butyrate, valeric acid, and total SCFAs ($p < 0.05$) when they compared with the MC group. In the caecum, the *Fusarium* mycotoxin-contaminated diet significantly reduced the concentrations of acetate, propionate, butyrate, valeric acid, and total SCFAs ($p < 0.05$). Compared with the MC group, the LAC group had higher concentrations of acetate, propionate, butyrate, and total SCFAs ($p < 0.05$), and the HRW group had higher levels of acetate, butyrate, and total SCFAs ($p < 0.05$).

Table 2. Effects of hydrogen-rich water and lactulose on short-chain fatty acids (SCFAs) profiles in the jejunum, ileum, colon, and caecum digesta of female piglets fed a *Fusarium* mycotoxin-contaminated diet [1,2].

Item	NC	MC	MC + LAC	MC + HRW	SEM	*p*-Value
			Jejunum (µmol/g wt digesta)			
Acetate	4.30	3.80	4.48	4.14	0.27	0.819
Propionate	2.08	1.58	1.83	1.99	0.12	0.486
Butyrate	0.94	0.72	0.84	1.00	0.06	0.425
Total SCFAs	7.45	6.10	7.15	7.13	0.43	0.737
			Ileum (µmol/g wt digesta)			
Acetate	10.50	10.64	10.58	10.29	0.41	0.993
Propionate	5.09	5.56	5.65	5.16	0.27	0.660
Butyrate	0.49	0.50	0.52	0.54	0.03	0.932
Total SCFAs	16.08	16.69	16.75	15.99	0.66	0.971
			Colon (µmol/g wt digesta)			
Acetate	44.28	39.83	49.94	43.78	1.48	0.102
Propionate	19.13 [a]	11.19 [b]	20.13 [a]	14.62 [ab]	1.17	0.010
Butyrate	8.25 [a]	4.00 [b]	7.55 [a]	7.35 [a]	0.53	0.008
Valeric acid	4.40 [a]	1.00 [c]	2.55 [b]	0.91 [c]	0.40	<0.001
Total SCFAs	76.06 [a]	56.02 [b]	80.18 [a]	66.66 [ab]	2.99	0.008

Toxins 2018, 10, 246

Table 2. *Cont.*

Item	NC	MC	MC + LAC	MC + HRW	SEM	*p*-Value
	Caecum (μmol/g wt digesta)					
Acetate	57.29 [a]	51.47 [b]	60.45 [a]	60.91 [a]	1.14	0.003
Propionate	26.20 [a]	19.12 [b]	25.97 [a]	22.50 [ab]	0.99	0.020
Butyrate	12.43 [a]	6.02 [c]	9.89 [b]	10.04 [b]	0.59	<0.001
Valeric acid	9.84 [a]	2.49 [b]	2.22 [b]	3.01 [b]	0.77	<0.001
Total SCFAs	105.76 [a]	79.10 [c]	98.53 [ab]	96.46 [b]	2.60	<0.001

[a,b,c] Values with different letters within the same row are different (*p* < 0.05). [1] NC (negative control), basal diet; MC, *Fusarium* mycotoxin-contaminated diet; MC + LAC, MC diet + lactulose treatment; and MC + HRW, MC diet + hydrogen-rich water treatment. [2] *n* = 5.

2.4. Microbiota Communities of Total Bacteria and Methanogenic Archaea in the Digesta of Intestinal Segments

Representative DGGE analysis of total bacteria in foregut (jejunum and ileum) and hindgut (colon and caecum) are shown in Figure 2A,C and Figure 3A,C, respectively. DGGE profiles of PCR products in the V6–V8 regions of the 16S rRNA gene from the four groups revealed some difference among different treatments at the foregut and hindgut. It is shown that jejunum (Figure 2A), ileum (Figure 2C), and colon (Figure 3A) amplicons migrating to the top of the gel were predominant in the samples of all groups, and caecum amplicons (Figure 3C) migrating to the middle of the gel were predominant in the samples of all treatment.

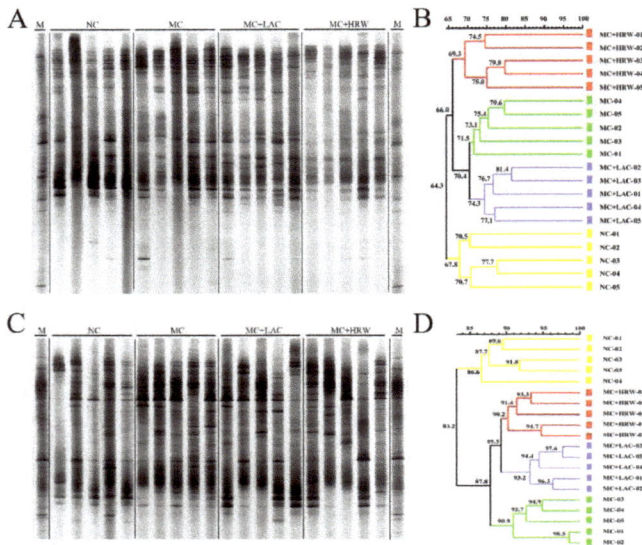

Figure 2. Effects of hydrogen-rich water and lactulose on jejunum and ileum digesta PCR-DGGE profiles of V6–V8 amplicons and similarities index of female piglets fed a *Fusarium* mycotoxin-contaminated diet. (**A**) DGGE profile of bacteria community in the jejunum digesta of four groups; (**B**) Similarity index of bacteria DGGE profile obtained from jejunum digesta of four groups; (**C**) DGGE profile of bacteria community in the ileum digesta of four groups; (**D**) Similarity index of bacteria DGGE profile obtained from ileum digesta of four groups. NC (negative control), basal diet; MC, *Fusarium* mycotoxin-contaminated diet; MC + LAC, MC diet + lactulose treatment; and MC + HRW, MC diet + hydrogen-rich water treatment.

226

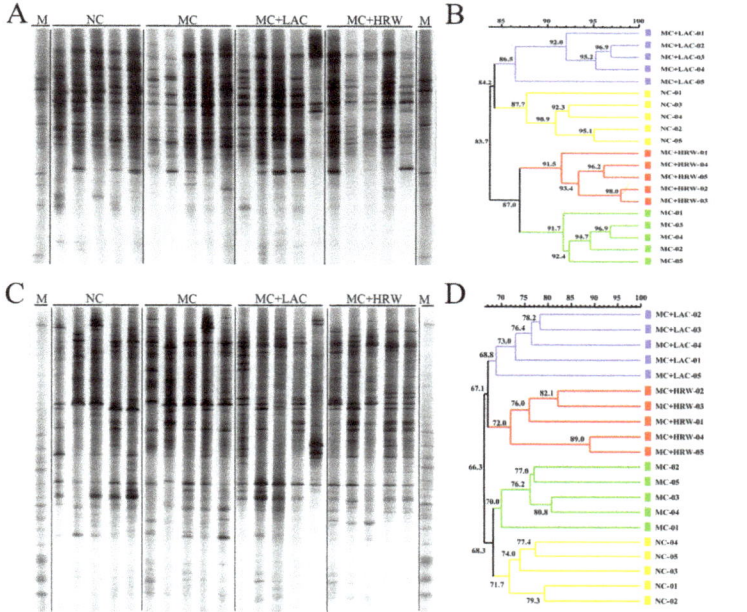

Figure 3. Effects of hydrogen-rich water and lactulose on colon and caecum digesta PCR-DGGE profiles of V6–V8 amplicons and similarities index of female piglets fed a *Fusarium* mycotoxin-contaminated diet. (**A**) DGGE profile of bacteria community in the colon digesta of four groups; (**B**) Similarity index of bacteria DGGE profile obtained from colon digesta of four groups; (**C**) DGGE profile of bacteria community in the caecum digesta of four groups; (**D**) Similarity index of bacteria DGGE profile obtained from caecum digesta of four groups. NC (negative control), basal diet; MC, *Fusarium* mycotoxins-contaminations diet; MC + LAC, MC diet + lactulose treatment; and MC + HRW, MC diet + hydrogen-rich water treatment.

Cluster analysis revealed that the overall similarity of total bacteria DGGE patterns in the jejunum, ileum, colon, and caecum were 64.3%, 83.2%, 83.7%, and 66.3%, respectively (Figure 2B,D, Figure 3B,D, respectively). In the jejunum and ileum, the NC group samples formed in one cluster with a similarity of 67.8% and 86.6%, while MC, MC + LAC, and MC + HRW groups were in another cluster with a similarity of 66.0% and 87.8%, respectively. In the colon, NC and MC + HRW groups formed in one cluster with 84.2% similarity, and MC formed another cluster with the MC + LAC group. However, the cluster pattern in the caecum was quite different, in which NC and MC groups were found in one coherent cluster with 68.3% similarity, and MC + LAC with MC + HRW groups formed another cluster with 67.1% similarity.

For the methanogenic *Archaea* compositions, the ileum (Figure 4A), colon (Figure 4C), and caecum (Figure 4E) amplicons migrating to the top of gels were predominant in the samples of all groups. DGGE cluster analysis showed that the overall similarity in the ileum, colon, and caecum were 39.7%, 83.7%, and 43.0%, respectively. In the ileum (Figure 4B), the NC group formed one cluster with a similarity of 44.1%, while MC, MC + LAC, and MC + HRW groups formed another cluster with a similarity of 43.6%. In the colon (Figure 4D), the methanogenic *Archaea* pattern is different than the ileum, in which NC and MC + LAC treatments formed one cluster with 84.2% similarity, while MC and MC + HRW groups formed another cluster with 87.2% similarity. In the caecum (Figure 4F), the NC group formed one cluster with 58.3% similarity. Except for one sample from the MC + LAC group, the MC, MC + HRW, and MC + LAC groups formed another cluster with 55.1% similarity.

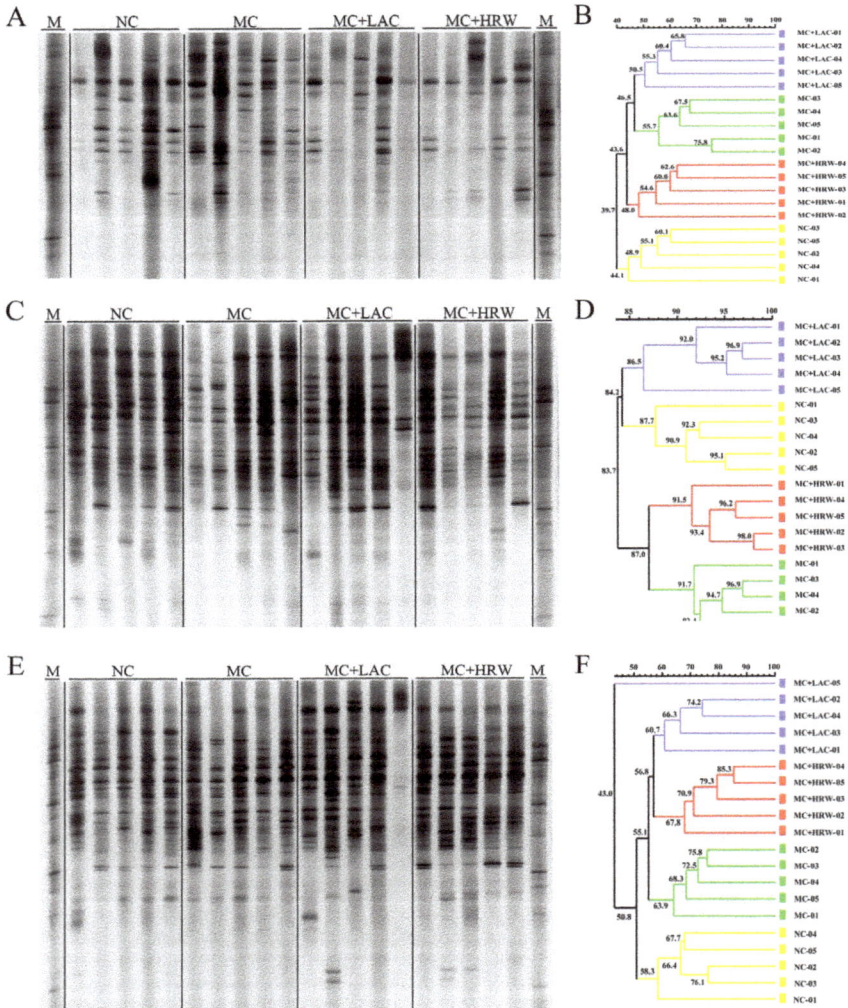

Figure 4. Effects of hydrogen-rich water and lactulose on the ileum, colon and caecum digesta PCR-DGGE profiles of methanogenic *Archaea* and the similarities index of female piglets fed a *Fusarium* mycotoxin-contaminated diet. (**A**) DGGE profile of methanogenic *Archaea* community in the ileum digesta of four groups; (**B**) Similarity index of methanogenic *Archaea* DGGE profile obtained from ileum digesta of four groups; (**C**) DGGE profile of methanogenic *Archaea* community in the colon digesta of four groups; (**D**) Similarity index of methanogenic *Archaea* DGGE profile obtained from colon digesta of four groups; (**E**) DGGE profile of methanogenic *Archaea* community in the caecum digesta of four groups; (**F**) Similarity index of methanogenic *Archaea* DGGE profile obtained from caecum digesta of four groups. NC (negative control), basal diet; MC, *Fusarium* mycotoxins-contaminations diet; MC + LAC, MC diet + lactulose treatment; and MC + HRW, MC diet + hydrogen-rich water treatment.

The band number and Shannon diversity index of total bacteria and methanogenic *Archaea* were also analyzed and are shown in Table 3. For total bacteria, the band numbers and Shannon diversity in the jejunum were not affected by treatments ($p > 0.05$). In the ileum, *Fusarium* mycotoxins did not affect the band numbers ($p > 0.05$), but MC + LAC group had more band numbers than the MC group ($p < 0.05$). The Shannon diversity was found to be significantly increased by *Fusarium* mycotoxin treatment, while neither LAC nor HRW influenced the Shannon diversity ($p > 0.05$). In the colon, Shannon diversity found no differences among the treatments ($p > 0.05$). MC and MC + LAC groups were found to have higher band numbers than the NC and MC + HRW groups ($p < 0.05$), and no difference was found neither between the MC and MC + LAC groups nor between the NC and MC + HRW groups ($p > 0.05$). In the caecum, Shannon diversity did not find any differences among the four groups. Band numbers in the MC, MC + LAC, and MC + HRW groups were significantly higher than the NC group ($p > 0.05$), while no difference was found among the MC, MC + LAC, and MC + HRW groups ($p < 0.05$).

Table 3. Effects of hydrogen-rich water and lactulose on the number of DGGE bands and Shannon diversity of the jejunum, ileum, colon, and caecum digesta of female piglets fed a *Fusarium* mycotoxin-contaminated diet [1,2].

Target Group	DNA Sample	Item	NC	MC	MC + LAC	MC + HRW	SEM	*p*-Value
Total bacteria	Jejunum	Band number	59.20	60.60	64.60	59.60	1.34	0.498
		Shannon diversity	3.40	3.64	3.68	3.60	0.05	0.278
	Ileum	Band number	34.40 [c]	37.70 [bc]	44.40 [a]	38.40 [b]	1.00	<0.001
		Shannon diversity	3.00 [b]	3.27 [a]	3.49 [a]	3.34 [a]	0.06	0.006
	Colon	Band number	40.00 [b]	50.40 [a]	52.00 [a]	40.00 [b]	1.60	0.001
		Shannon diversity	3.14	3.15	3.14	3.19	0.04	0.948
	Caecum	Band number	61.60 [b]	72.60 [a]	72.80 [a]	71.60 [a]	4.23	0.036
		Shannon diversity	3.55	3.76	3.75	3.81	0.04	0.070
Methanogens	Ileum	Band number	15.20 [b]	26.80 [a]	17.20 [b]	18.40 [b]	1.14	<0.001
		Shannon diversity	2.27 [b]	2.91 [a]	2.27 [b]	2.28 [b]	0.09	0.015
	Colon	Band number	29.80 [bc]	36.20 [a]	32.20 [b]	27.40 [c]	0.89	<0.001
		Shannon diversity	2.99	3.23	2.87	2.89	0.07	0.208
	Caecum	Band number	31.40 [b]	41.00 [a]	32.80 [b]	34.60 [b]	1.27	0.023
		Shannon diversity	3.06	3.34	2.92	3.22	0.08	0.234

[a,b,c] Values with different letters within the same row are different ($p < 0.05$). [1] NC (negative control), basal diet; MC, *Fusarium* mycotoxin-contaminated diet; MC + LAC, MC diet + lactulose treatment; and MC + HRW, MC diet + hydrogen-rich water treatment. [2] $n = 5$.

For methanogenic *Archaea*, the band number from the ileum, colon, and caecum digesta in the MC group were significantly higher than the NC group ($p < 0.05$), and both LAC and HRW were found to reduce those band number compared with MC group ($p < 0.05$). The Shannon diversity of ileum digesta in the MC group was significantly higher than the NC group ($p < 0.05$), and MC + LAC and MC + HRW were found to have lower Shannon diversity than the MC group ($p < 0.05$). The Shannon diversity of colon and caecum digesta showed no significant differences among the four groups ($p > 0.05$).

2.5. Populations of Selected Bacteria in the Digesta of Different Intestinal Segments

Table 4 shows the populations of selected microbiota in the digesta of the jejunum, ileum, colon, and caecum in piglets fed a *Fusarium* mycotoxin-contaminated diet. In the jejunum and caecum, no difference was found on the abundance of selected bacteria among the four treatments ($p > 0.05$). In the ileum, the populations of total bacteria, *Lactobacillus*, and *Enterococcus* were not impacted by treatments, but the abundance of *E. coli* in the MC group was higher than NC, MC + LAC, and MC + HRW groups ($p < 0.05$). The MC group also had a lower ($p < 0.05$) *Bifidobacterium* abundance than the NC, MC + LAC, and MC + HRW groups, while no difference was found among the latter three groups ($p > 0.05$). In the colon, the populations of total bacteria and acetogenic bacteria showed no significant difference among the four groups ($p > 0.05$). However, the abundance of methanogenic *Archaea* and sulfate-reducing bacteria (SRB) was lower in the MC group than the NC group ($p < 0.05$). In addition, MC + HRW and MC + LAC groups were found to have higher populations of these two selected species than the MC group ($p < 0.05$).

Table 4. Effects of hydrogen-rich water and lactulose on the populations (log copies number/g) of selected bacteria in the digesta of the jejunum, ileum, colon and caecum of female piglets fed a *Fusarium* mycotoxin-contaminated diet [1,2].

Sample	Item	NC	MC	MC + LAC	MC + HRW	SEM	p-Value
Jejunum	All bacteria	8.75	8.66	8.67	8.20	0.13	0.486
	Lactobacillus	7.96	7.43	7.25	7.28	0.19	0.552
	Bifidobacterium	4.90	4.76	5.26	5.14	0.08	0.124
	Escherichia coli	4.87	5.78	5.53	5.31	0.14	0.127
	Enterococcus	3.30	3.45	3.21	3.06	0.11	0.685
Ileum	All bacteria	9.04	9.64	9.43	9.53	0.14	0.221
	Lactobacillus	8.85	8.60	8.75	8.86	0.25	0.906
	Bifidobacterium	5.07 [a]	4.23 [b]	5.26 [a]	5.13 [a]	0.13	0.009
	Escherichia coli	5.67 [b]	7.25 [a]	6.14 [b]	6.21 [b]	0.16	0.005
	Enterococcus	3.08	3.66	3.39	3.32	0.58	0.488
Colon	All bacteria	11.04	11.09	11.17	10.93	0.07	0.704
	Methanogens	4.49 [a]	3.47 [c]	5.52 [a]	4.58 [b]	0.20	0.001
	SRB [3]	4.54 [a]	3.27 [b]	4.68 [a]	4.12 [a]	0.18	0.011
	Acetogenic bacteria	6.87	6.85	7.17	6.54	0.11	0.297
Caecum	All bacteria	11.57	11.34	11.69	11.60	0.05	0.119
	Methanogens	5.14	5.55	5.44	5.36	0.28	0.969
	SRB [3]	2.89	3.39	3.02	2.88	0.12	0.470
	Acetogenic bacteria	6.21	6.31	6.32	6.19	0.16	0.992

[a,b,c] Values with different letters within the same row are different ($p < 0.05$). [1] NC (negative control), basal diet; MC, *Fusarium* mycotoxin-contaminated diet; MC + LAC, MC diet + lactulose treatment; and MC + HRW, MC diet + hydrogen-rich water treatment. [2] $n = 5$. [3] SRB = Sulfate-reducing bacteria.

3. Discussion

The gut microbiota ecological system represents an abundant community of organisms, including bacteria, archaea, fungi, and viruses, that colonized within the GI tract [20]. The complex and large diverse communities of the microbiota play important roles in nutrition decomposition and transformation, immunity intrusion, and gut villous structure development through a symbiotic relationship with the host [20]. Diet is a major factor that influences the makeup and activity of colonized microbes in the intestinal gut, and we had hypothesized that *Fusarium* mycotoxins could induce compositions and/or metabolites changes in the gut microbiota, and eventually affect the health of female piglets. In addition, oral HRW or lactulose administrations may partly spare the harmful activity of *Fusarium* mycotoxins on the intestinal microbiota ecosystem of female weaning piglets. These results partly support our hypothesis.

3.1. Hydrogen Levels in Intestinal Segments

One major function of microbiota in the gut lumen is the fermentation of indigestible polysaccharides, dietary fiber, and resistant starch, which generates large quantities of H_2 [21]. In this study, our data showed that administration of HRW increased concentrations of H_2 in the stomach, duodenum, colon, and caecum. However, lactulose treatment was found to have no impact on the H_2 levels in the foregut, but significantly increased the concentrations of H_2 in the hindgut (colon and caecum). The communities, species, and population of microbiota in the hindgut were more complex than the foregut and might contribute to this difference [22]. In fact, these observed H_2 concentrations in the intestine were similar to those in a study reported by Liu et al. [23], who recently developed a conventional gas chromatography method to measure the hydrogen levels in the tissue following administration of HRW, hydrogen-rich saline and inhalation of hydrogen gas at different time points. Their data indicated that after 30 min of administration, hydrogen gas could also be detected at around 10–20 ppb/g intestine tissue. Moreover, oral administration of HRW had the highest C_{max} compared with other methods [23]. Watanabe et al. found that inhalation of hydrogen gas resulted in slower elevation than that achieved with intraperitoneal administration [24], indicating that different administration ways of providing hydrogen may result in different hydrogen distributions in blood and tissues. On the other hand, previous studies also indicated that oral administration of hydrogen-rich water/saline had very short lasting time [25]. Thus, the protective effects of HRW in this study may not yet be fully exerted. Therefore, the search for an ideal hydrogen-producing prebiotic may be an interesting method to solve this concern.

Lactulose is a semisynthetic disaccharide and cannot be metabolized nor absorbed in the intestine [15]. Like other polysaccharides, lactulose is fermented in the gastrointestinal gut by bacteria, producing SCFAs. Hydrogen gas is one of its metabolites, which may act as an effective ideal agent [26]. A higher breath H_2 can be detected after oral administration of lactulose [17]. After lactulose administration, the exhaled breath H_2 concentration was found to be increased after 15 min and reaching a peak at 45 min in mice; meanwhile, lactulose with antibiotic treatment did not find an improvement of breath hydrogen levels [27]. On one hand, a proportion of hydrogen gas may pass through the gut mucosa wall into the blood and be transported to other organs. On the other hand, hydrogen also can be metabolized by intestinal microbiota. Yu et al. also demonstrated that lactulose significantly increased the accumulated hydrogen levels, and antibiotic administration induced a smaller amount of H_2 in rats [16]. These results indicate that bacterial fermentation may play a curial role in the beneficial effects of lactulose in animals. Considering the features of LAC, it is broadly in line with our expectations that lactulose administration had a continual improvement in the hydrogen concentrations in the mucosa of the hindgut (colon and caecum). Although higher hydrogen levels were both observed in HRW (stomach and duodenum) and LAC (colon and caecum) treatments compared with MC group, it is not representative of all H_2 production of HRW or LAC. Thus, more research needs to be carried out to demonstrate the dynamic changes of hydrogen gas in the intestine after receiving hydrogen-rich water or lactulose in piglets.

3.2. Fecal Scoring and Diarrhea Rate

Disruptions of the microbiota ecological system under abnormal conditions is recognized as a major risk factor for various diseases, such as diarrhea and inflammatory bowel disease. In the swine industry, weaning piglets face enormous stress, leading to perturbations in gut microbiota, and host physiological and mucosal immune function, such as microbiological, environmental, and dietary factors. The transition from liquid to solid feeding is expected to result in decreased feed intake and daily weight gain, and increased diarrhea incidence [28]. Corn and soybean meal represent over 50% of the total dietary ingredients, which are often contaminated with mycotoxins [29]. Thus, post-weaning piglets are always associated with diarrhea or loose feces [30]. Consumption of DON- and ZEN-contaminated feeds will induce intoxication symptoms, including vomiting, abdominal distress, malaise, diarrhea emesis, and even shock or death [3]. In the present study, lower feed intake and weight gain [31], fever, and severe diarrhea were observed in piglets fed a *Fusarium* mycotoxin-contaminated diet. A lower fecal score has been considered a good indicator of gut health [32]. Feces scoring was decreased in piglets fed a *Fusarium* mycotoxin-contaminated diet in the critical period of days 0 to 7 and days 7 to 14 after weaning. In addition, the MC group had higher diarrhea rates than the NC group in the first week. These results are consistent with previous studies in which DON has the capacity to increase intestinal permeability, and cause microbiota dysfunctions which promote intestinal disorders [3,33]. It is also reported that DON ingestion was associated with the reduction of mRNA expression of Na^+-dependent glucose transport sodium-dependent glucose cotransporter 1 (SGLT1) [34]. Since SGLT1 is responsible for water reabsorption, inhibition of SGLT1 could also cause diarrhea, which might be the underlying cause of diarrhea in animals exposed to mycotoxins [34].

A number of studies have demonstrated that prebiotics may selectively increase the population and/or activity of beneficial bacteria [35], decreasing the incidence of diarrhea. Lactulose is always used in the treatment of constipation and hepatic encephalopathy in humans [15]. However, at low doses, lactulose acts as a prebiotic that improves growth performance and intestinal morphology in pigs [36]. A previously study on piglets showed that 1% lactulose supplementation had higher growth performance [37]. Additionally, our previous study also suggested that lactulose could improve anti-oxidant capacity of piglets fed a mycotoxin-contaminated diet [31]. Although no studies explored the effects of HRW on diarrhea, a protective effect of HRW was found on DSS-induced inflammatory bowel disease (IBD) in rats, and intestinal villi damage in mice [10]. The exact mechanisms underlying the protective effects of HRW and LAC on diarrhea is still unclear, but might be attributed to the ability of both HRW and lactulose could remedy mycotoxin-induced intestine damage through the anti-oxidant and anti-inflammatory properties. Therefore, it is not surprising that piglets orally administered HRW or lactulose had a lower fecal score and incidence of diarrhea than the MC group.

3.3. SCFAs Levels in the Digesta of Jejumun, Ileum, Colon, and Caecum

Shifting of the microbiota composition and quality of intestinal microbiota, followed by the alternation in SCFAs levels and other metabolites, may have a role in ensuring animal health and disease [38]. Here, we found a significant inhibitory effect of *Fusarium* mycotoxins on the production of SCFAs in the colon and caecum, which have not been previously reported. Ingestion of DON contaminated diet was found to significantly reduce feed intake and increase diarrhea [3], which would increase the water levels and reduce the dry matter content in the digesta. In fact, compared with the NC group, a lower caecum relative weight was observed in the MC group (Figure S1). Therefore, it is conceivable that *Fusarium* mycotoxins (DON and ZEN) may have modified the microbiota fermentation in the hindgut due to changes in the colon and caecum nutrient flow and water content. In addition, the hydrogen levels in the hindgut were also reduced by *Fusarium* mycotoxin treatment, which may support the changes of SCFAs production.

As a prebiotic, lactulose is not broken down by mammalian intestine enzymes, but can be metabolized by gut microbiota to SCFAs. A previous study in pigs revealed that the inclusion of lactulose in the diet increased the SCFAs concentration in the large intestine [39]. Increased SCFAs concentrations were also observed in broiler chickens provided with lactulose supplementation [40]. However, Martin-Pelaez et al. found that 1% dietary lactulose supplementation did not affect caecum butyric acid concentration in piglets that were orally challenged with *Salmonella* [41]. Recently, it has been shown that the dietary inclusion of 1% lactulose did not change the branched-chain fatty acids (BCFA) levels in piglets [37]. Our data suggests that lactulose modified the hindgut microbiota fermentation, resulting in higher SCFAs production. So far, the relationship of hydrogen-rich water on short-chain fatty acid production in vivo and in vitro are unknown. Further studies are warranted to explore the effects of HRW and lactulose on bacteria fermentation in piglets.

3.4. Microbiota Communities and Populations

It is well known that the dynamic complex intestinal microbial ecosystem plays key roles in maintaining host nutritional, physiological, and immunological functions [38]. Thus, impairment of microbiota balance could have many adverse effects on the health of the host. Mycotoxins not only undergo microbial metabolism in the gastrointestinal tract, but may also affect the communities due to some toxins exhibiting antimicrobial properties [34,42]. *In vitro* studies showed that DON did not influence the growth of *Staphylococcus aureus*, *E. coli*, and *Yersinia enterocolitica* [43]. It has been reported that consumption of feed contaminated with a moderate level of DON had a slight effect on cultivable bacteria in pig intestines, and the composition of intestinal microbiota was also observed in DON-exposed animals [44]. Feeding pigs with T-2 toxin led to a substantial increase of aerobic bacterial counts in the intestine [45]. Similarly, chronic exposure of pigs to low doses of DON caused an increase in the number of intestinal aerobic bacteria and modified the dynamics of intestinal bacteria communities [6]. Piotrowska et al. also reported the effect of exposure of pigs to the *Fusarium* mycotoxins ZEN and DON, administered together and separately, on the colon microbiota [7]. After 42 days of experiment, their data found that ZEN alone, and together with DON, had an adverse effect on mesophilic aerobic bacteria. The concentration of *C. perfringens*, *E. coli*, and other bacteria in the family *Enterobacteriaceae* was significantly reduced by ZEN alone, and together with DON. The functional biodiversity of microorganisms was also affected by mycotoxins, which Shannon's diversity index was higher [7]. In our study, cluster results of DGGE profiles obtained from the jejunum, ileum, colon, and caecum showed that the mycotoxin-contaminated diet drastically affected the communities, diversity, and population of gastrointestinal microbiota (especially in the ileum and colon). Moreover, our data also indicated that hydrogen-utilizing bacteria (methanogenic *Archaea* and SRB) were also involved in the mycotoxincosis-induced intestinal microbiota dysbiosis.

Previous *in vivo* studies demonstrated positive protective effects of lactulose on colon fermentation [46]. Lactulose was reported to increase the number of *Bifidobacteria* and *Lactobacilli* while reducing the numbers of *Clostridium* spp., *Salmonella* spp., or *E. coli* in the pig gastrointestinal tract [36]. Guerra-Ordaz et al. demonstrated that lactulose significantly improved the performance and colonic microbial activity of weaning piglets [37]. In a previous study, lactulose was included in the diet at 1%, 0.2%, 0.4%, 0.6%, or 0.8% at the expense of corn and/or soybean meal. A significant quadratic response in the *Lactobacillus* count was observed at 42 days on increasing the level of lactulose [40]. However, the effects of HRW on intestinal microbiota in piglets are quite limited. In a mouse study, 16S rRNA gene sequencing analysis was introduced to explore the effects of AEW on the microbial composition of C57BL/6N mice. After four weeks of treatment, the relative abundance of 20 taxa differed significantly in AEW-administered mice [47]. Xiao et al. also reported that hydrogen-water oral gavage resulted in retention of TAI–shifted intestinal bacterial composition in mice by high-throughput sequencing [14], which is consistent with our results. In the present, our data showed that both lactulose supplemental could influence the communities and diversity of bacteria and methanogenic *Archaea* in different segments of piglets fed a mycotoxin-contaminated diet. In addition, the shifts of the abundance of *Bifidobacterium* and *E. coli* in the ileum digesta, and hydrogen-utilizing bacteria in the colon were also attenuated by both HRW and LAC treatments.

4. Conclusions

In this study, we found that *Fusarium* mycotoxin significantly affected the metabolism, activities, and communities of gut microbiota, and eventually caused a higher diarrhea rate in female piglets. Most importantly, both hydrogen-rich water and lactulose have shown protective effects on the imbalance of intestinal microbiota, reducing the SCFAs production and the higher diarrhea rate induced by *Fusarium* mycotoxin-contaminated diet, partly through affecting the communities/populations of microbiota and the evaluation of hydrogen gas. These results partly support our original hypothesis.

5. Materials and Methods

5.1. Preparation of Fusarium Mycotoxin-Contaminated Maize

The *Fusarium graminearum* strain 2021 was cultured and conidia were prepared as previously described [48]. Commercial maize was soaked in tap water for 72 h, and autoclaved at 121 °C for 30 min. Then, the maize was incubated in plastic storage boxes with 1×10^6 conidia/kg for 30 days (15–25 °C and 50–85% humidity). The cool autoclaved maize without conidia was used as the control maize. Finally, uncontaminated and *Fusarium graminearum*-contaminated maize were dried in an oven at 70 for 24 h, respectively.

5.2. Experimental Diets and Mycotoxins Analyusis

Fusarium mycotoxin-contaminated maize and uncontaminated control maize were used at 44.5% at the expense of normal maize for the manufacturing of two experimental diets, respectively. The experimental diets (negative control (NC) and mycotoxin-contaminated diet (MC), respectively) were formulated according to the recommendation of the nutrient requirement of swine by the National

Research Council [49] and based on a previous study [50] with minor modifications to the vitamin and mineral premix.

No antibiotic, hormone, and preservatives were added to the diets. Table S2 shows the ingredients of the two experimental diets used in this study. The analysis of *Fusarium* mycotoxin levels in the two experimental diets were described in our previous study [31]. The NC diet contained 221.10 µg/kg DON, 12.12 µg/kg 3-acetyl DON, 32.95 µg/kg 15-acetyl DON, and 266.26 µg/kg total DON. The MC diet contained 825.46 µg/kg DON, 212.79 µg/kg 3-acetyl DON, 59.45 µg/kg 15-acetyl DON, 1097.99 µg/kg total DON, and 501.56 µg/kg ZEN, which were each significantly higher ($p < 0.05$) than in the NC diet. In the current study, the levels of DON in the contaminated diet were expected in natural conditions, which is similar with a previous Chinese report showing the mean DON levels were 753.1–1194.0 µg/kg and the maximum levels reached to 4279.3 µg/kg in complete pig feed between 2016 and 2017 [51].

5.3. Animals

In the swine industry, weaning piglets face enormous stress, which leads to perturbations in gut microbiota, host physiological, and mucosal immune function, such as microbiological, environmental, and dietary factors [28]. In addition, corn and soybean meal represent over 50% of the total dietary ingredients, which is often contaminated with mycotoxins [29], which will aggravate the post-weaning stress and induce higher economic losses. Therefore, piglets are a good model to explore the effects of *Fusarium* mycotoxins on microbiota. Furthermore, finding a way to minimize the side effects of mycotoxins on piglets should be valuable for swine production.

Therefore, a total of 24 clinically-healthy female weaning piglets (Landrace × large × white; initial average body weight, 7.25 ± 1.02 kg) from six litters (four pigs/little) were individually housed in pens (1.2 by 2.0 m) with one feeder and one nipple drinker. The piglets had ab libitum access to feed and water. This protocol was approved by the Committee of Animal Research Institute (Certification No. SYXK(Su)2011-0036, 11 August 2015), Nanjing Agricultural University, China.

5.4. Experimental Design and Sampling

After a six day adaption period, the animals were randomly assigned to four treatment groups (NC, MC, MC + HRW and MC + LAC, respectively), with six piglets in each group. The piglets were fed their corresponding experimental diets for 25 days. The piglets in the NC group were fed an uncontaminated control diet, while piglets in the MC, MC + HRW, and MC + LAC groups were fed *Fusarium* mycotoxin-contaminated diets.

Piglets in each group received oral administration with their corresponding treatment twice a day (1000 and 1400 h) through a 6 × 200 mm nasogastric tube (Jiangsu Huatai Medical Devices Company, Yangzhou, China). The hydrogen-free water was orally administered at 10 mL/kg body weight (BW) to piglets in both NC and MC groups. While piglets in the MC + HRW group received 10 mL/kg BW HRW (Beijing Hydrovita Biotechnology Company, Beijing, China). The HRW was produced by dissolving high-pressure hydrogen gas into pure water, and kept in 300 mL aluminum pouches at room temperature. At least 0.6 mM levels of hydrogen were detected in the HRW, and they were administered to piglets within 15 min after opening. Lactulose (4-*O*-β-D-galactosyl-D-fructose; formula, $C_{12}H_{22}O_{11}$; CAS number, 4618-18-2) was used in this study. A dose of 500 mg/kg BW of LAC oral solution (Abbott Healthcare Products, Weesp, The Netherlands) was dissolved in 10 mL/kg BW of hydrogen-free water, and administrated to piglets in the MC + LAC group.

The amounts of LAC and HRW were dependent on the body weight and updated weekly. One piglet was removed from the MC, MC + LAC, and MC + HRW groups fed with a *Fusarium* mycotoxin diet due to poor health condition. Therefore, five independent replicates from each group were used in this study. On day 25, 30 min after administration of different treatments, piglets were euthanized by an intramuscular injection of sodium pentobarbital (40 mg/kg BW). The whole cecum and colon were obtained and weighted. Digesta samples from jejunum, ileum, colon, and caecum were collected and stored at −70 °C for further analysis.

5.5. Feces Scoring

Piglets were closely observed daily for clinical signs of diarrhea and a scoring system was applied to indicate the presence and severity of diarrhea as previously described [52]. Feces scoring began on day 0 on the experimental diets and continued until day 25. Scores were given daily watch and the average fecal score value per piglets was given. The following feces scoring system was used: 1 = hard feces, 2 = slightly soft feces, 3 = soft, partially formed feces, 4 = loose, semiliquid feces, and 5 = watery, mucous-like feces.

5.6. Hydrogen Gas Measurement in Different Intestine Segments

Hydrogen levels in the mucosa samples from different intestine segments were analyzed using a hydrogen sensor (Unisense, Aarhus, Denmark) as previously described [53]. Briefly, piglets were euthanized with sodium pentobarbital and placed in supine position. Incisions were made in the segments of stomach, duodenum, jejunum, ileum, colon and cecum. The digesta were removed and hydrogen microelectrode (diameter, 50 µm) was penetrated into the mucosa at a depth of 200 µm.

5.7. SCFA Detection in the Digesta of Different Intestine Segments

The digesta samples (0.3 g) was weighed and mixed with 0.9 mL of meta-phosphoric acid (25%, *w/v*) and crotonic acid (75 mM) solution. The mixture was vortexed and centrifuged at $12,000\times g$ for 10 min at 4 °C, and the supernatant was stored at −20 °C until assay. After thawing, the supernatant was centrifuged at $12,000\times g$ for 5 min, and the supernatant was used for SCFA detection. The supernatant was detected by using a capillary column gas chromatograph (GC-14A with an FID detector; Shimadzu, Japan; capillary column: 30 m × 0.32 mm × 0.25 µm film thickness) with a H_2 flame ionization detector and split injection as previously described [54]. The column, injector, and detector temperature were 140 °C, 180 °C, and 180 °C, respectively.

5.8. DNA Isolation, PCR Amplification, and DGGE Analysis

Total DNA of the jejunum, ileum, colon, and caecum digesta samples were extracted by a QIAamp® DNA Stool Mini Kit (Qiagen, Germany) according to the manufacturer's instructions. PCR products of the total bacteria and methanogenic *Archaea* for denaturing gradient gel electrophoresis (DGGE) analysis were amplified with specific primers (Table S3) and separated in denaturing gradient polyacrylamide gels as previously described [55].

5.9. Real-Time PCR Assays for Quantification of the Selected Bacteria

The abundance of total bacteria, *Lactobacillus*, *Bifidobacterium*, *Escherichia coli*, *Enterococcus*, methanogenic *Archaea*, sulfate-reducing bacteria, and acetogenic bacteria were quantified by real-time PCR using specific primers (Table S3). Standard curves of each bacterial group were generated using triplicate ten-fold dilutions of known copy numbers of a target gene cloned into a plasmid vector. Real-time PCR was carried out on SetpOnePlusTM Real-Time PCR System (Life Technologies, Carlsbad, CA, USA) by using SYBR Premix Ex Taq (Takara, Dalian, China).

5.10. Statistical Analyses

Data from DGGE gels were calculated as previously described [55]. All statistical analyses were performed by one-way ANOVA with SPSS statistical software (version 18.0 for Windows, SPSS Inc., Chicago, IL, USA, 2009). The differences among treatments were considered significant at $p < 0.05$. Differences among treatments were determined using the Tukey-Kramer test.

Supplementary Materials: The following are available online at http://www.mdpi.com/2072-6651/10/6/246/s1, Table S1: Effects of hydrogen-rich water and lactulose on pH values in different intestine segments in piglets fed *Fusarium* mycotoxins contaminated diets, Table S2: Ingredient composition and nutrient contents of control and experimental diets, Table S3: Primers sequences used in this study, Figure S1: Effects of lactulose and hydrogen water on the relative colon and caecum weights of piglets fed *Fusarium* mycotoxins contaminated diet.

Author Contributions: W.Z. and W.Y. have contributed to the conception and the design of the study; X.J., and Q.Z., carried out the experiments; X.J. and Q.Z. analyzed the data; W.Z., and W.Y. contributed the reagents/materials/analysis tools; W.Z. drafted the manuscript; W.Z. and W.Y. revised the article. All authors read and approved final manuscript.

Funding: This work was funded by the National Nature Science Foundation of China (31501986), the Fundamental Research Funds for Central Universities (KJQN201611) and Jiangsu Modern Agricultural (Pig) Industrial Technology System (SXGC(2017)286).

Acknowledgments: The authors would like to thank Dr. Ming-Guo Zhou and Dr. Ya-bing Duan for providing the *Fusarium graminearum* strain 2021 and preparing the conidia. We thank Dr. Jin Cui for her kindly aid with hydrogen measurements in the samples from the piglets. We also would like thank Dr. Tao Shao and Dr. Xianjun Yan for their kindly aid with SCFAs detection.

Conflicts of Interest: The authors declare no conflict of interest.

References

1. Cortinovis, C.; Pizzo, F.; Spicer, L.J.; Caloni, F. Fusarium mycotoxins: Effects on reproductive function in domestic animals—A review. *Theriogenology* **2013**, *80*, 557–564. [CrossRef] [PubMed]

2. Doll, S.; Danicke, S. The fusarium toxins deoxynivalenol (don) and zearalenone (zon) in animal feeding. *Prev. Vet. Med.* **2011**, *102*, 132–145. [CrossRef] [PubMed]

3. Antonissen, G.; Martel, A.; Pasmans, F.; Ducatelle, R.; Verbrugghe, E.; Vandenbroucke, V.; Li, S.; Haesebrouck, F.; Van Immerseel, F.; Croubels, S. The impact of fusarium mycotoxins on human and animal host susceptibility to infectious diseases. *Toxins* **2014**, *6*, 430–452. [CrossRef] [PubMed]

4. Kollarczik, B.; Gareis, M.; Hanelt, M. In vitro transformation of the fusarium mycotoxins deoxynivalenol and zearalenone by the normal gut microflora of pigs. *Nat. Toxins* **1994**, *2*, 105–110. [CrossRef] [PubMed]

5. Karlovsky, P. Biological detoxification of the mycotoxin deoxynivalenol and its use in genetically engineered crops and feed additives. *Appl. Microbiol. Biotechnol.* **2011**, *91*, 491–504. [CrossRef] [PubMed]

6. Wache, Y.J.; Valat, C.; Postollec, G.; Bougeard, S.; Burel, C.; Oswald, I.P.; Fravalo, P. Impact of deoxynivalenol on the intestinal microflora of pigs. *Int. J. Mol. Sci.* **2009**, *10*, 1–17. [CrossRef] [PubMed]

7. Piotrowska, M.; Slizewska, K.; Nowak, A.; Zielonka, L.; Zakowska, Z.; Gajecka, M.; Gajecki, M. The effect of experimental fusarium mycotoxicosis on microbiota diversity in porcine ascending colon contents. *Toxins* **2014**, *6*, 2064–2081. [CrossRef] [PubMed]

8. Ge, L.; Yang, M.; Yang, N.N.; Yin, X.X.; Song, W.G. Molecular hydrogen: A preventive and therapeutic medical gas for various diseases. *Oncotarget* **2017**, *8*, 102653–102673. [CrossRef] [PubMed]

9. Ohsawa, I.; Ishikawa, M.; Takahashi, K.; Watanabe, M.; Nishimaki, K.; Yamagata, K.; Katsura, K.; Katayama, Y.; Asoh, S.; Ohta, S. Hydrogen acts as a therapeutic antioxidant by selectively reducing cytotoxic oxygen radicals. *Nat. Med.* **2007**, *13*, 688–694. [CrossRef] [PubMed]

10. Kajiya, M.; Silva, M.J.B.; Sato, K.; Ouhara, K.; Kawai, T. Hydrogen mediates suppression of colon inflammation induced by dextran sodium sulfate. *BBRC* **2009**, *386*, 11–15. [CrossRef] [PubMed]

11. Zheng, X.; Mao, Y.; Cai, J.; Li, Y.; Liu, W.; Sun, P.; Zhang, J.H.; Sun, X.; Yuan, H. Hydrogen-rich saline protects against intestinal ischemia/reperfusion injury in rats. *Free Radic. Res.* **2009**, *43*, 478–484. [CrossRef] [PubMed]

12. Wolf, P.G.; Biswas, A.; Morales, S.E.; Greening, C.; Gaskins, H.R. H2 metabolism is widespread and diverse among human colonic microbes. *Gut Microbes* **2016**, *7*, 235–245. [CrossRef] [PubMed]

13. Shimamura, Y.; Shinke, M.; Hiraishi, M.; Tsuchiya, Y.; Masuda, S. The application of alkaline and acidic electrolyzed water in the sterilization of chicken breasts and beef liver. *Food Sci. Nutr.* **2016**, *4*, 431–440. [CrossRef] [PubMed]

14. Xiao, H.W.; Li, Y.; Luo, D.; Dong, J.L.; Zhou, L.X.; Zhao, S.Y.; Zheng, Q.S.; Wang, H.C.; Cui, M.; Fan, S.J. Hydrogen-water ameliorates radiation-induced gastrointestinal toxicity via myd88's effects on the gut microbiota. *Exp. Mol. Med.* **2018**, *50*, e433. [CrossRef] [PubMed]

15. Panesar, P.S.; Kumari, S. Lactulose: Production, purification and potential applications. *Biotechnol. Adv.* **2011**, *29*, 940–948. [CrossRef] [PubMed]

16. Yu, J.; Zhang, W.; Zhang, R.; Ruan, X.; Ren, P.; Lu, B. Lactulose accelerates liver regeneration in rats by inducing hydrogen. *J. Surg. Res.* **2015**, *195*, 128–135. [CrossRef] [PubMed]
17. Zhai, X.; Chen, X.; Shi, J.; Shi, D.; Ye, Z.; Liu, W.; Li, M.; Wang, Q.; Kang, Z.; Bi, H.; et al. Lactulose ameliorates cerebral ischemia-reperfusion injury in rats by inducing hydrogen by activating nrf2 expression. *Free Radic. Biol. Med.* **2013**, *65*, 731–741. [CrossRef] [PubMed]
18. Chae, J.P.; Pajarillo, E.A.B.; Park, C.-S.; Kang, D.-K. Lactulose increases bacterial diversity and modulates the swine faecal microbiome as revealed by 454-pyrosequencing. *Anim. Feed Sci. Technol.* **2015**, *209*, 157–166. [CrossRef]
19. Zheng, W.; Hou, Y.; Su, Y.; Yao, W. Lactulose promotes equol production and changes the microbial community during in vitro fermentation of daidzein by fecal inocula of sows. *Anaerobe* **2014**, *25*, 47–52. [CrossRef] [PubMed]
20. Sommer, F.; Backhed, F. The gut microbiota—Masters of host development and physiology. *Nat. Rev. Microbiol.* **2013**, *11*, 227–238. [CrossRef] [PubMed]
21. Slavin, J. Fiber and prebiotics: Mechanisms and health benefits. *Nutrients* **2013**, *5*, 1417–1435. [CrossRef] [PubMed]
22. Zhao, W.J.; Wang, Y.P.; Liu, S.Y.; Huang, J.J.; Zhai, Z.X.; He, C.; Ding, J.M.; Wang, J.; Wang, H.J.; Fan, W.B.; et al. The dynamic distribution of porcine microbiota across different ages and gastrointestinal tract segments. *PLoS ONE* **2015**, *10*. [CrossRef] [PubMed]
23. Liu, C.; Kurokawa, R.; Fujino, M.; Hirano, S.; Sato, B.; Li, X.K. Estimation of the hydrogen concentration in rat tissue using an airtight tube following the administration of hydrogen via various routes. *Sci. Rep.* **2014**, *4*. [CrossRef]
24. Watanabe, M.; Kamimura, N.; Iuchi, K.; Nishimaki, K.; Yokota, T.; Ogawa, R.; Ohta, S. Protective effect of hydrogen gas inhalation on muscular damage using a mouse hindlimb ischemia-reperfusion injury model. *Plast. Reconstr. Surg.* **2017**, *140*, 1195–1206. [CrossRef]
25. Hong, Y.; Chen, S.; Zhang, J. Hydrogen as a selective antioxidant: A review of clinical and experimental studies. *J. Int. Med. Res.* **2010**, *38*, 1893–1903. [CrossRef] [PubMed]
26. Chen, X.; Zuo, Q.; Hai, Y.; Sun, X.J. Lactulose: An indirect antioxidant ameliorating inflammatory bowel disease by increasing hydrogen production. *Med. Hypotheses* **2011**, *76*, 325–327. [CrossRef] [PubMed]
27. Chen, X.; Zhai, X.; Shi, J.; Liu, W.W.; Tao, H.; Sun, X.; Kang, Z. Lactulose mediates suppression of dextran sodium sulfate-induced colon inflammation by increasing hydrogen production. *Dig. Dis. Sci.* **2013**, *58*, 1560–1568. [CrossRef] [PubMed]
28. Campbell, J.M.; Crenshaw, J.D.; Polo, J. The biological stress of early weaned piglets. *J. Anim. Sci. Biotechnol.* **2013**, *4*. [CrossRef] [PubMed]
29. Daga, A.; Horn, M.B.; Kottwitz, L.B.M.; de Farina, L.O. Bromatological and mycotoxin analysis on soybean meal before and after the industrial process of micronization. *Cienc. Rural* **2015**, *45*, 1336–1341. [CrossRef]
30. Heo, J.M.; Opapeju, F.O.; Pluske, J.R.; Kim, J.C.; Hampson, D.J.; Nyachoti, C.M. Gastrointestinal health and function in weaned pigs: A review of feeding strategies to control post-weaning diarrhoea without using in-feed antimicrobial compounds. *J. Anim. Physiol. Anim. Nutr.* **2013**, *97*, 207–237. [CrossRef] [PubMed]
31. Zheng, W.; Ji, X.; Zhang, Q.; Du, W.; Wei, Q.; Yao, W. Hydrogen-rich water and lactulose protect against growth suppression and oxidative stress in female piglets fed fusarium toxins contaminated diets. *Toxins* **2018**, *10*, 228. [CrossRef] [PubMed]
32. Gahan, D.A.; Lynch, M.B.; Callan, J.J.; O'Sullivan, J.T.; O'Doherty, J.V. Performance of weanling piglets offered low-, medium- or high-lactose diets supplemented with a seaweed extract from laminaria spp. *Animal* **2009**, *3*, 24–31. [CrossRef] [PubMed]
33. Maresca, M. From the gut to the brain: Journey and pathophysiological effects of the food-associated trichothecene mycotoxin deoxynivalenol. *Toxins* **2013**, *5*, 784–820. [CrossRef] [PubMed]
34. Grenier, B.; Applegate, T.J. Modulation of intestinal functions following mycotoxin ingestion: Meta-analysis of published experiments in animals. *Toxins* **2013**, *5*, 396–430. [CrossRef] [PubMed]
35. Roberfroid, M.; Gibson, G.R.; Hoyles, L.; McCartney, A.L.; Rastall, R.; Rowland, I.; Wolvers, D.; Watzl, B.; Szajewska, H.; Stahl, B.; et al. Prebiotic effects: Metabolic and health benefits. *Br. J. Nutr.* **2010**, *104* (Suppl. 2), S1–S63. [CrossRef] [PubMed]
36. Krueger, M.; Schroedl, W.; Isik, W.; Lange, W.; Hagemann, L. Effects of lactulose on the intestinal microflora of periparturient sows and their piglets. *Eur. J. Nutr.* **2002**, *41* (Suppl. 1), I26–I31. [CrossRef] [PubMed]

37. Guerra-Ordaz, A.A.; Molist, F.; Hermes, R.G.; de Segura, A.G.; La Ragione, R.M.; Woodward, M.J.; Tchorzewska, M.A.; Collins, J.W.; Pérez, J.F.; Martín-Orúe, S.M. Effect of inclusion of lactulose and lactobacillus plantarum on the intestinal environment and performance of piglets at weaning. *Anim. Feed Sci. Technol.* **2013**, *185*, 160–168. [CrossRef]
38. Richards, J.D.; Gong, J.; de Lange, C.F.M. The gastrointestinal microbiota and its role in monogastric nutrition and health with an emphasis on pigs: Current understanding, possible modulations, and new technologies for ecological studies. *Can. J. Anim. Sci.* **2005**, *85*, 421–435. [CrossRef]
39. Kamphues, J.; Tabeling, R.; Stuke, O.; Bollmann, S.; Amtsberg, G. Investigations on potential dietetic effects of lactulose in pigs. *Livest. Sci.* **2007**, *109*, 93–95. [CrossRef]
40. Calik, A.; Ergun, A. Effect of lactulose supplementation on growth performance, intestinal histomorphology, cecal microbial population, and short-chain fatty acid composition of broiler chickens. *Poult. Sci.* **2015**, *94*, 2173–2182. [CrossRef] [PubMed]
41. Martín-Peláez, S.; Costabile, A.; Hoyles, L.; Rastall, R.A.; Gibson, G.R.; La Ragione, R.M.; Woodward, M.J.; Mateu, E.; Martín-Orúe, S.M. Evaluation of the inclusion of a mixture of organic acids or lactulose into the feed of pigs experimentally challenged with salmonella typhimurium. *Vet. Microbiol.* **2010**, *142*, 337–345. [CrossRef] [PubMed]
42. Danicke, S.; Matthaus, K.; Lebzien, P.; Valenta, H.; Stemme, K.; Ueberschar, K.H.; Razzazi-Fazeli, E.; Bohm, J.; Flachowsky, G. Effects of fusarium toxin-contaminated wheat grain on nutrient turnover, microbial protein synthesis and metabolism of deoxynivalenol and zearalenone in the rumen of dairy cows. *J. Anim. Physiol. Anim. Nutr.* **2005**, *89*, 303–315. [CrossRef] [PubMed]
43. Ali-Vehmas, T.; Rizzo, A.; Westermarck, T.; Atroshi, F. Measurement of antibacterial activities of t-2 toxin, deoxynivalenol, ochratoxin a, aflatoxin b1 and fumonisin b1 using microtitration tray-based turbidimetric techniques. *Zentralbl. Veterinarmed. A* **1998**, *45*, 453–458. [CrossRef] [PubMed]
44. Burel, C.; Tanguy, M.; Guerre, P.; Boilletot, E.; Cariolet, R.; Queguiner, M.; Postollec, G.; Pinton, P.; Salvat, G.; Oswald, I.P.; et al. Effect of low dose of fumonisins on pig health: Immune status, intestinal microbiota and sensitivity to salmonella. *Toxins* **2013**, *5*, 841–864. [CrossRef] [PubMed]
45. Maresca, M.; Fantini, J. Some food-associated mycotoxins as potential risk factors in humans predisposed to chronic intestinal inflammatory diseases. *Toxicon* **2010**, *56*, 282–294. [CrossRef] [PubMed]
46. Guerra-Ordaz, A.A.; Gonzalez-Ortiz, G.; La Ragione, R.M.; Woodward, M.J.; Collins, J.W.; Perez, J.F.; Martin-Orue, S.M. Lactulose and lactobacillus plantarum, a potential complementary synbiotic to control postweaning colibacillosis in piglets. *Appl. Environ. Microbiol.* **2014**, *80*, 4879–4886. [CrossRef] [PubMed]
47. Naito, Y.; Higashimura, Y.; Baba, Y.; Inoue, R.; Takagi, T.; Uchiyama, K.; Mizushima, K.; Hirai, Y.; Ushiroda, C.; Tanaka, Y. Effects of molecular hydrogen-dissolved alkaline electrolyzed water on intestinal environment in mice. *Med. Gas Res.* **2018**, *8*, 6. [CrossRef] [PubMed]
48. Liu, S.; Duan, Y.; Ge, C.; Chen, C.; Zhou, M. Functional analysis of the beta2-tubulin gene of fusarium graminearum and the beta-tubulin gene of botrytis cinerea by homologous replacement. *Pest Manag. Sci.* **2013**, *69*, 582–588. [CrossRef] [PubMed]
49. National Research Council (U.S.). Committee on Nutrient Requirements of Swine. In *Nutrient Requirements of Swine*, 11th ed.; National Academies Press: Washington, DC, USA, 2012.
50. Xiao, H.; Wu, M.M.; Tan, B.E.; Yin, Y.L.; Li, T.J.; Xiao, D.F.; Li, L. Effects of composite antimicrobial peptides in weanling piglets challenged with deoxynivalenol: I. Growth performance, immune function, and antioxidation capacity. *J. Anim. Sci.* **2013**, *91*, 4772–4780. [CrossRef] [PubMed]
51. Ma, R.; Zhang, L.; Liu, M.; Su, Y.T.; Xie, W.M.; Zhang, N.Y.; Dai, J.F.; Wang, Y.; Rajput, S.A.; Qi, D.S.; et al. Individual and combined occurrence of mycotoxins in feed ingredients and complete feeds in China. *Toxins* **2018**, *10*, 113. [CrossRef] [PubMed]
52. Walsh, A.M.; Sweeney, T.; O'Shea, C.J.; Doyle, D.N.; O'Doherty, J.V. Effect of supplementing different ratios of laminarin and fucoidan in the diet of the weanling piglet on performance, nutrient digestibility, and fecal scoring. *J. Anim. Sci.* **2012**, *90*, 215–217. [CrossRef] [PubMed]
53. Sun, H.; Chen, L.; Zhou, W.; Hu, L.; Li, L.; Tu, Q.; Chang, Y.; Liu, Q.; Sun, X.; Wu, M.; et al. The protective role of hydrogen-rich saline in experimental liver injury in mice. *J. Hepatol.* **2011**, *54*, 471–480. [CrossRef] [PubMed]

54.	Mao, S.Y.; Zhu, W.Y.; Wang, Q.J.; Yao, W. Effect of daidzein on in vitro fermentation by microorganisms from the goat rumen *Anim. Feed Sci. Technol.* **2007**, *136*, 154–163. [CrossRef]

55.	Zheng, W.; Hou, Y.; Yao, W. Lactulose increases equol production and improves liver antioxidant status in barrows treated with daidzein. *PLoS ONE* **2014**, *9*, e93163. [CrossRef] [PubMed]

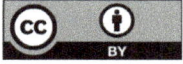

![toxins logo] *toxins*

MDPI

Article

Low Levels of Chito-Oligosaccharides Are Not Effective in Reducing Deoxynivalenol Toxicity in Swine Jejunal Explants

Juliana Gerez [1], Letícia Buck [1], Victor Hugo Marutani [1], Caroline Maria Calliari [2] and Ana Paula Bracarense [1,*]

[1]   Laboratory of Animal Pathology, Universidade Estadual de Londrina, Campus Universitário, Rodovia Celso Garcia Cid, Km 380, Londrina, Paraná 86057-970, Brazil; julianarubira@hotmail.com (J.G.); leleyamasaki26@gmail.com (L.B.); vhbmarutani@gmail.com (V.H.M.)
[2]   Academic Department of Food, Universidade Tecnológica Federal do Paraná, Avenida dos Pioneiros, 3131, Londrina, Paraná 86036-370, Brazil; calliari@utfpr.edu.br
*   Correspondence: ana.bracarense@pq.cnpq.br; Tel.: +55-043-3371-4485

Received: 29 May 2018; Accepted: 26 June 2018; Published: 4 July 2018

Abstract: Deoxynivalenol (DON) is a mycotoxin that affects the intestinal morphology of animals, impairing nutrient intake and growth. On the other hand, dietary supplementation with functional oligosaccharides as chito-oligosaccharides (COS) has shown positive effects on the intestinal health of piglets. Therefore, the objective of the present study was to evaluate the effect of low doses of COS in preventing DON-induced intestinal histological changes, using a swine jejunal explant technique. The intestinal explants were incubated at 37 °C in culture medium for 4 h and exposed to the following treatments: (a) control (only culture medium), (b) DON (10 µM), (c) 25COS (0.025 mg·mL^{-1} of COS); (d) 50COS (0.05 mg·mL^{-1} of COS); (e) 25COS plus DON (25COS + DON); (f) 50COS plus DON (50COS + DON). Explants exposed to COS presented intestinal morphology similar to control samples. DON induced a significant decrease in the histological score as a consequence of moderate to severe histological changes (apical necrosis, villi atrophy, and fusion) and a significant decrease in morphometric parameters (villi height, crypt depth, villi height:crypt depth ratio, and goblet cells density). The intestinal morphology of samples exposed to COS + DON remained similar to DON treatment. In conclusion, low levels of COS did not counteract DON-induced intestinal lesions.

Keywords: functional oligosaccharides; mycotoxins; swine; explant technique; intestinal morphology; goblet cells

Key contribution: Chito-oligosaccharides exposure does not prevent the deleterious effects of DON on piglets' intestinal tissue.

1. Introduction

Deoxynivalenol (DON) is produced mainly by *Fusarium graminearum* and *Fusarium culmorum* in cereals as wheat, barley, and maize [1]. Processing methods may reduce the amount of DON in cereals, however, this mycotoxin is not completely eliminated in grains intended for animal and human consumption [2,3]. In a survey including 15,549 samples of cereals from European and Asian countries, DON was the most prevalent mycotoxin, with concentrations ranging from 0.250 to 50.289 mg·kg^{-1} and a mean level of 0.967 mg·kg^{-1} [4]. This fusariotoxin is known to affect the functional morphology of the intestinal tract in animals, compromising the absorption of nutrients by the intestinal epithelium [5,6]. Consequently, DON can result in significant economic losses in animal production due to the adversely altered animal performance [7,8].

On the other hand, the gut health-promoting effects of chitosan oligosaccharides in swine nutrition have been broadly acknowledged [9]. Chito-oligosaccharides (COS) are obtained by depolymerization of chitin or chitosan by the action of acids, enzymes, or even physical methods [10]. Chitosan is initially extracted from the shells of crustaceans (e.g., shrimp and crabs) or from the cell walls of fungi. However, it has been suggested that COS produced through fermentation of microorganisms such as *Bacillus* spp. [11], using chitosan as a carbon source, can lead to more standardized results since this biotechnological means of obtaining it is independent of climate and environmental changes [12]. Radicals of *N*-acetylglucosamine present in the molecule of chitosan, and in its derivatives are responsible for diverse biological activities [13]. The results of many studies point to antibacterial [14] and anti-inflammatory properties [15] in COS in addition to anti-oxidative, antitumor, and immunostimulatory effects [16]. In pigs, COS modulates the gut microbiota, favoring the growth of beneficial bacteria [17,18]. In addition, diets supplemented with COS result in beneficial effects on small intestinal morphology, barrier function, nutrient digestibility, and zootechnical parameters of weanling pigs [18,19]. Due to these properties, chitosan and COS have been considered as an effective prebiotic and a potential alternative to antibiotics in pig nutrition [17,20–22].

Although COS-treatment has shown beneficial effects in weaners, so far, there have been few reports on the action of oligosaccharide derivatives during intestinal exposure to mycotoxins [23]. Given the need to broaden the knowledge about the possible protective effect of functional oligosaccharides on DON-induced intestinal toxicity in piglets, the objective of the present study was to evaluate the effects of different doses of COS in pig jejunal explants exposed to DON.

2. Results

2.1. Histological Evaluation of the Explants Exposed to COS and DON

The treatments with 25COS and 50COS resulted in no significant change on the histological score (Figure 1a). Explants exposed to COS showed moderate edema of the lamina propria and simple columnar epithelium was preserved (Figure 1c,d). After 4 h of exposure to DON, explants presented a significant decrease of 21.22% in the histological score in relation to control samples ($p = 0.044$) (Figure 1a). Explants submitted to DON showed fusion and atrophy of villi with discontinuous epithelium exhibiting severely flattened enterocytes with necrotic debris (Figure 1e). COS did not affect DON-induced lesions, and a significant reduction in histological scores of 31.25% ($p = 0.013$) and 36.64% ($p = 0.003$) was also observed in the intestinal tissue exposed to 25COS + DON and 50COS + DON when compared with the control, respectively (Figure 1a,f,g).

Villi height was a sensitive parameter of intestinal health; a decrease around 37.29%, 41.45%, and 37.87% in this parameter was observed after exposure to DON ($p = 0.003$), 25COS + DON ($p < 0.0001$), and 50COS + DON ($p < 0.0001$) in relation to control samples, respectively. Mitotic figures were observed in crypt epithelium, and crypt depth was maintained in all experimental groups. In accordance with the above results, the villi height:crypt depth ratio was significantly reduced in DON-treated samples and COS + DON-treated explants in comparison to control explants ($p < 0.05$). The samples exposed to treatments with COS showed no significant changes on morphometrical parameters (Table 1).

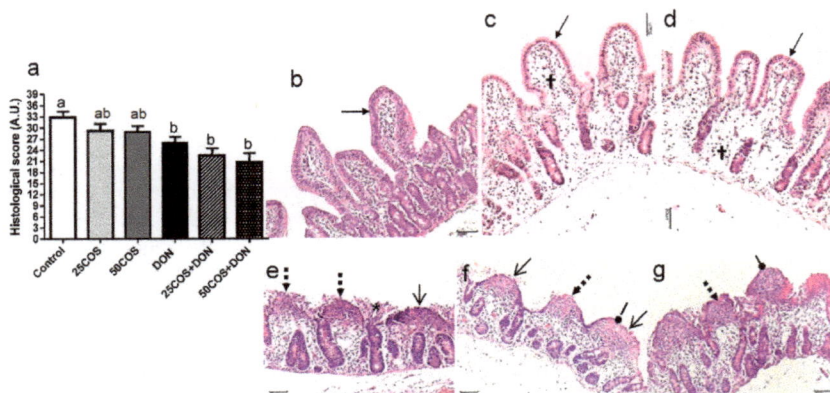

Figure 1. Histological evaluation of the explants exposed to chito-oligosaccharides (COS) and deoxynivalenol (DON). (**a**) Values of histological scores of swine jejunal explants exposed to control treatment (□), 0.025 mg·mL^{-1} of COS (25COS) (▨), 0.05 mg·mL^{-1} of COS (50COS) (■), DON (10 μM) (▮), 25COS plus DON (25COS + DON) (▨), and 50COS plus DON (50COS + DON) (▨). Values are mean ± SEM. Means with unlike letters ($^{a, b}$) differ significantly by Tukey's test ($p \leq 0.05$). Maximum histological score of 39 points in A.U. (arbitrary units); (**b**) Explants exposed to control (n = 30); (**c**) 25COS-exposed explant (n = 30); (**d**) 50COS-exposed explant (n = 30); (**e**) DON-exposed explant (n = 30); (**f**) Explant exposed to treatment 25COS + DON (n = 30); (**g**) Explant exposed to treatment 50COS + DON (n = 30). Histological endpoints with different arrows: simple columnar epithelium (→), moderate edema of the lamina propria (†), multifocal to diffuse fusion and atrophy of villi (→), discontinuous epithelium (••), necrotic debris (*), and severely flattened epithelial cells (→) (Bar = 50 μm; Hematoxylin and eosin staining).

Table 1. Morphometrical evaluation of the swine jejunal explants exposed to COS and DON (mean ± SEM).

Treatments	Villi Height, μm	Crypt Depth, μm	Villi Height:Crypt Depth, μm:μm
Control	139.68 ± 8.48 [a]	129.21 ± 8.53 [a]	1.09 ± 0.07 [a]
25COS	121.74 ± 10.50 [ab]	136.69 ± 16.11 [a]	0.90 ± 0.05 [ab]
50COS	116.56 ± 13.71 [ab]	110.77 ± 3.34 [a]	1.04 ± 0.09 [a]
DON	87.60 ± 4.01 [b]	140.86 ± 18.60 [a]	0.64 ± 0.06 [b]
25COS + DON	81.79 ± 9.99 [b]	131.09 ± 8.18 [a]	0.63 ± 0.09 [b]
50COS + DON	86.78 ± 7.50 [b]	132.34 ± 13.39 [a]	0.65 ± 0.02 [b]

Means (n = 30) within a column followed by the different superscripts ($^{a, b}$) differ significantly by Tukey's test ($p < 0.05$). Explants exposed to Dulbecco's modified Eagle's medium (Control), 0.025 mg·mL^{-1} of COS (25COS), 0.05 mg·mL^{-1} of COS (50COS), DON (10 μM), 25COS plus DON (25COS + DON), or 50COS plus DON (50COS + DON).

2.2. Goblet Cell Density of the Explants Exposed to COS and DON

Goblet cells are present in the intestinal epithelium and are responsible for synthesis and secretion of mucins. Explants exposed to COS presented a number of goblet cells similar to control treatment. The goblet cell density in explants exposed to DON was significantly decreased in the villi region compared to the control samples ($p = 0.003$). The reduction was more pronounced in the samples exposed to 25COS + DON (43.46%; $p < 0.0001$) and 50COS + DON (68.57%; $p < 0.0001$) when compared with control group. In relation to goblet cell density in crypts, explants exposed to DON, 25COS + DON, and 50COS + DON showed a significant decrease of 38.97% ($p = 0.008$), 42.98% ($p = 0.003$), and 51.57% ($p = 0.001$), respectively, compared with the explants exposed to control treatment (Figure 2).

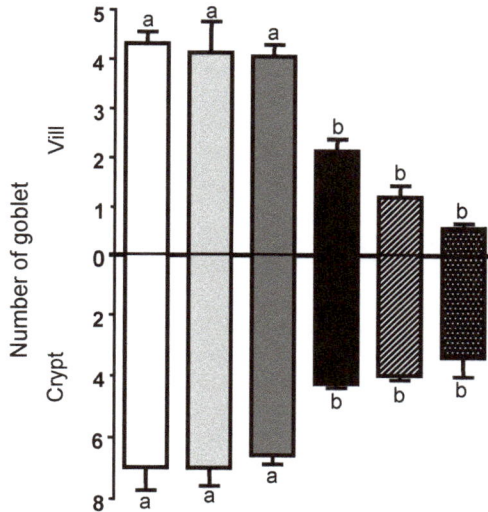

Figure 2. Mean goblet cell number on villi and crypts of swine jejunal tissue submitted to different treatments: control (□), 0.025 mg·mL^{-1} of COS (25COS) (▨), 0.05 mg·mL^{-1} of COS (50COS) (■), DON (10 μM) (■), 25COS plus DON (25COS + DON) (▨), and 50COS plus DON (50COS + DON) (▪). Values are mean ± SEM represented by vertical bars. Means with unlike letters ([a, b]) differ significantly by Tukey's test ($p < 0.05$).

3. Discussion

Functional oligosaccharides such as COS have been widely suggested as dietary supplements in post-weaning diets of piglets. While COS have been shown to improve growth performance, immunological status, gut microbiota, and intestinal morphology in weaned pigs [9], their effects on mycotoxins-induced intestinal toxicity have not been yet explored. Due to global distribution of DON, its permanence through feed and food processing, and its known intestinal toxicity, DON is considered a food security concern [3,5,24]. Studies on the potential protective effect of feed additives on the mycotoxins-induced intestinal toxicity have been conducted by our research group [25]. In the present study, we have assessed whether COS can prevent DON-induced intestinal toxicity using an ex vivo approach. Intestinal explants represent an adequate alternative model to toxicological studies [26]. This technique preserves the histological structure observed in vivo and allows for the reduction in the number of experimental animals [27]. To the best of our knowledge, it is the first work to analyze the action of COS facing a fusariotoxin challenge in piglets.

In previous studies, the effects of COS on intestinal health have been evaluated in piglets [9]. The range of COS effective doses is large (30 mg·kg^{-1}~5000 mg·kg^{-1}), and the results are variable [11,28]. In this study, the treatment with low levels of COS for 4 h induced no effects on the intestinal morphology (histological score, villi height, crypt depth, and villi height:crypt depth ratio). In accordance with those results, we demonstrated in a previous study that increasing doses of COS (0.025, 0.05, 0.10, and 0.15 mg·mL^{-1}) induced no change on the intestinal morphology of swine explants [29]. Accordingly, no effect on intestinal morphology was observed in weaned pigs fed diets containing increasing levels of COS (30 to 600 mg·kg^{-1}) for 14 days [18,28]. However, in piglets fed diets supplemented with 150 and 200 mg COS·kg^{-1} of feed for a 21-d and 26-d period, respectively, a significant increase on villi height and villi:crypt ratio was observed in jejunum of animals [17,19]. Although the mechanisms involved in COS action have not yet been fully elucidated, N-acetyl glucosamine, a basic component of this molecule can play an important role [13]. This radical can bind to determined strains of pathogens (bacteria), interfering with their adhesion capacity to the intestinal mucosa [11,30]. Moreover, in vivo studies indicate that COS is rapidly and efficiently utilized by beneficial intestinal microorganisms, increasing the proportions of *Lactobacillus* spp. and *Bifidobacterium* spp., especially in weaning pigs [17,30]. Thereby, changes in intestinal microbiota composition may provide a favorable environment for the proliferation of enterocytes as reported recently by Suthongsa et al. [19] and Thongson et al. [31]. Thus, short periods of treatment with COS would be insufficient to stimulate the intestinal cell proliferation and improve gut morphological parameters in weaned piglets.

Regarding animal feed and human food, the intestine is the first organ to be exposed to the toxic effect of mycotoxins [32]. In this study, DON induced a significant decrease in the histological parameters (histological score, villi height, crypt depth, and villi height:crypt depth ratio). The main histological changes were atrophy and fusion of the villi, loss of apical enterocytes, necrotic debris, and severe flattening of columnar epithelium. These results agree with previous in vivo and ex vivo studies that have evaluated intestinal exposure to DON [5,25,33]. DON at the cellular level causes inhibition of protein synthesis [34], inducing oxidative stress and cell apoptosis [35].

Co-treatment of COS and DON for 4 h did not prevent the lesions caused by DON as observed in the histological score (villi height, crypt depth, and villus:crypt ratio). It is important to highlight that studies about the effects of COS on the intestinal toxicity of DON are scarce, and in the available databases, no study concerning this aspect was found. Previous studies have evaluated the adsorption capacity of chitosan and chitosan polymers on mycotoxins in in vitro models. Recently, Solís-Cruz et al. [36], using an in vitro gastrointestinal model for poultry, identified that chitosan showed a lower binding activity against DON when compared to cellulosic polymers. Additionally, a poor adsorption efficiency of chitosan polymers for DON and T-2 toxin has been observed in a buffer system [37]. No results about the adsorption capacity of COS on DON was found. Thereby, we hypothesize that COS is not effective in reducing DON toxicity in swine jejunal explants due to its poor adsorbent capacity for mycotoxins. Moreover, it is important to note that short periods of exposure to COS can be insufficient to influence the intestinal population of *Lactobacillus*, which can counteract the adverse effects of DON in weaned piglets [38].

Considering that oligosaccharides from different natural sources show similar prebiotic activities in animals [39], it is important to note that the protective effect of milk-derived oligosaccharides (galacto-oligosaccharides (GOS)) has been identified on intestinal barrier function in a DON challenge. In that work, the pretreatment with GOS was responsible for preventing the decrease of DON-induced transepithelial electrical resistance in the Caco-2 cell monolayer, while the co-incubation of GOS and DON did not reduce the DON-induced intestinal barrier disruption. Similarly, when mice received GOS before DON, villi height of the proximal small intestine remained comparable to the control animals [40]. Thus, the treatment with functional oligosaccharides before exposure to mycotoxins is an important factor to consider in future studies.

Mucins secreted by goblet cells form the mucus layer present on the gastrointestinal mucosal surface and prevent adhesion of pathogens to enterocytes [41]. COS showed no effect on the goblet cell density of intestinal explants. Similarly, COS-supplemented diets (30 or 100 mg·kg^{-1}) induced no changes on goblet cell density in piglets fed for a period of 14 and 18 days, respectively [28,42]. In accordance, villi and crypts of swine intestinal explants exposed to increasing levels of COS (0.025, 0.05, 0.10, and 0.15 mg·mL^{-1}) showed no difference on goblet cell density among the treatments [29]. Conversely, 300 mg/kg of chitosan for 21 days resulted in a significant increase on the goblet cell density in the jejunal villi of weaned piglets fed a supplemented diet and challenged with enterotoxigenic *Escherichia coli* during a preliminary trial period [22]. Probably, higher doses of COS are necessary to induce changes on goblet cells density. On the contrary, DON induced a significant decrease on the number of goblet cells in intestinal explants. Reduction in the goblet cell density after a challenge with DON has already been reported in pigs and cultures of swine jejunal tissue [5,33,43]. While the effect of toxic doses of DON (10 µM) on goblet cells have been related to cell death in intestinal crypts [25], subtoxic doses of DON (1 μM) induced a reduction in the mucin production by down-regulation of the gene expression of these glycoproteins [44].

In this study, COS did not prevent the reduction in the goblet cell density induced by DON. Interestingly, a more pronounced decrease was observed on the goblet cell density in the villi of explants exposed both to COS and DON in relation to the other treatments. Previous studies have shown that chitosan induces a disruption of tight junctions (TJs) (CLDN4, zonula occludens 1 and occludin) affecting the epithelial permeability in the Caco-2 cell monolayer. These changes were transient and reversible after chitosan removal [45,46]. Similarly, Xiong et al., [28] showed that the expression of occludin in ileum and zonula occludens 1 in jejunum and ileum were decreased in piglets fed a diet supplemented with 30 mg·kg^{-1} of COS for a 14d-period. Similarly, in in vivo and ex vivo studies, DON induces a significant decrease in the expression of E-cadherin and occludin in the intestine of piglets [5,33]. Accordingly, considering our results and these previous studies, we hypothesize that COS acts similarly to DON on intestinal explants by regulating TJ expression, resulting in increased epithelial permeability, cell degeneration, and death.

In conclusion, we have shown that the exposure to low levels of COS induced no reduction in the toxic action of DON on the intestinal histological structure. The use of dietary supplements in animal feed with the objective of minimizing the toxic action of mycotoxins on intestinal tissue is of increasing interest. Due to the lack of results in the literature, additional studies to assess the effect of functional oligosaccharides on DON-induced intestinal toxicity are necessary. Experimental factors such as exposure time and host microbiota should be considered in future analyses.

4. Materials and Methods

4.1. Animals

After weaning, five crossbred (Landrace × Large White × Duroc) piglets were allocated in separate bays and received a standard diet from 21 to 24 days of age. Feed and water were provided *ad libitium*. A sample of feed was analyzed for mycotoxins by high performance liquid chromatography. Aflatoxins (B1, B2, G1, and G2), fumonisins B1 and B2, zearalenone, and deoxynivalenol were below the limit of detection (data not shown). After 3 days of feeding with solid feed, the animals were submitted to euthanasia using sodium pentobarbital (40 mg·kg^{-1} of body weight (BW)) intravenously. The techniques used in the procedures were previously approved by the Institutional Ethics Committee for Animal Experimentation (number 11361.2014.30).

4.2. Chito-Oligosaccharides

Mild chrysalis flour of the silkworm Bombyx mori L. (0.7 g·L^{-1}) was provided as the only carbon (chitosan) source and peptone (0.3 g·L^{-1}) as the nitrogen source to Bacillus subtilis DP4. The fermentation occurred at pH 9.6, at 28 °C, under agitation (110 rpm) for 96 h. The bacterial biomass was separated by centrifugation, and the supernatant was sterilized to be used in the assays as a crude extract containing 6.48 mg·mL^{-1} COS [29]. COS quantification was determined by the MBTH technique [47] using N-acetylglucosamine (0 to 100 μM) as standard.

4.3. Culture of Explants and Exposure to DON and COS

The procedures for obtaining jejunal explants followed the previously described technique [25]. Briefly, jejunum segments of 5 cm were washed with phosphate buffered saline (PBS), opened longitudinally, and explants sampled using a biopsy punch of 8 mm. Three explants per well were placed in six-well plates (EasyPath, São Paulo, Brazil) containing Dulbecco's modified Eagle's medium (DMEM-Gibco, Gaithersburg, MD, USA), antibiotics (penicillin/streptomycin—1.25 μL·mL^{-1}, Gibco and gentamicin—10 μL·mL^{-1}, Novafarma), fetal bovine serum (100 μL·mL^{-1}—Invitrogen, Carlsbad, CA, USA), and L-glutamine (0.4 μL·mL^{-1}—Sigma-Aldrich, São Paulo, Brazil). Explants were incubated at 37 °C under orbital shaking for 4 h in the following experimental groups: (1) Control: culture media;

(2) DON: culture media with 10 µM of DON (D0156, Sigma-Aldrich); (3) 25COS: culture media with 0.025 mg·mL^{-1} of COS; (4) 50COS: culture media with 0.05 mg·mL^{-1} of COS; (5) 25COS + DON: culture media with 25COS plus DON; (6) 50COS + DON: culture media with 50COS plus DON. The dose of DON used in this study was equivalent to an ingestion of feed contaminated with 3 mg DON·kg^{-1} of feed and was considered toxic in in vivo [5] and ex vivo [48] studies. The concentrations of COS used in this experiment corresponded to an ingestion of 25 mg COS·kg^{-1} and 50 mg COS·kg^{-1} of feed. Six explants (replicates) from each animal were collected for each treatment. After this period, explants were fixed in a 10% buffered formalin solution for morphological and morphometric evaluation.

4.4. Morphological and Morphometric Assessment

Samples for histological analysis were dehydrated in increasing concentrations of alcohol, diaphanyzed, and embedded in paraffin. Tissue slices (5 µm thickness) were stained with hematoxylin and eosin for morphological and morphometric evaluations. The periodic acid of Schiff (PAS) stain was used to assess the number of goblet cells in 10 villi and 10 crypts/explant at 400× magnification. The histological score previously described by Maidana et al. [49] and Gerez et al. [29] was used to compare histological changes between the different experimental groups. Briefly, the criteria used were enterocyte morphology, apical denudation of villi, changes in the lamina propia, villi fusion and atrophy, number of villi, and cell debris [43]. Samples with well-preserved histological structure showed a maximum score of 39 points, while the minimum score of 0 points was assigned to the explants with severe and diffuse lesions. For morphometric evaluation, villi height and crypt depth were measured using an image software system (Motic Image Plus 2.0, Motic Microscopy, Kowloon, Hong Kong) with 200× magnification as previously described [43]. The villi-height:crypt-depth ratio was also considered in the evaluation of intestinal integrity.

4.5. Statistical Analysis

A completely randomized design with five repetitions per treatment was employed. Six replicates from each animal were analyzed, resulting in one repetition. The data were represented as means ± SEM (standard error of the mean) and analyzed by free software Rstudio version 1.1.442—© 2009–2018 (Boston, MA, USA). Assumptions of residual normality (Shapiro-Wilk's test) and homoscedasticity (Bartlett's test) were checked and the data were submitted to analysis of variance (ANOVA) followed by Tukey's test. p-value $\leq$ 0.05 was regarded as statistically significant.

Author Contributions: J.G. analyzed the data and drafted the manuscript. L.B. conducted and assessed all experiments. V.H.M. contributed to the experiments. C.M.C. revised the manuscript critically. A.P.B. designed the experiments and contributed to the manuscript and has given final approval of the version to be published.

Funding: This research was funded by Fundação Araucária grant number [41.111]. A.P.R.L.B. was supported by fellowship from CNPq, Brazil. J.R.G. and L.Y.B. were supported by Capes/Fundação Araucária.

Acknowledgments: The authors are grateful to Raúl Jorge Hernan Castro-Gómez for having given the samples of COS. To Karina Basso and Thalita Evani Silva de Oliveira for helping in technical assistance for histological processing.

Conflicts of Interest: The authors have declared that no conflict of interest exists.

References

1. Shi, W.; Tan, Y.; Wang, S.; Gardiner, D.M.; De Saeger, S.; Liao, Y.; Wang, C.; Fan, Y.; Wang, Z.; Wu, A. Mycotoxigenic potentials of Fusarium species in various culture matrices revealed by mycotoxin profiling. *Toxins (Basel)* **2017**, *9*, 6. [CrossRef] [PubMed]
2. Kaushik, G. Effect of Processing on Mycotoxin Content in Grains. *Crit. Rev. Food Sci. Nutr.* **2015**, *55*, 1672–1683. [CrossRef] [PubMed]
3. Sugita-Konishi, Y.; Park, B.J.; Kobayashi-Hattori, K.; Tanaka, T.; Chonan, T.; Yoshikawa, K.; Kumagai, S. Effect of Cooking Process on the Deoxynivalenol Content and Its Subsequent Cytotoxicity in Wheat Products. *Biosci. Biotechnol. Biochem.* **2006**, *70*, 1764–1768. [CrossRef] [PubMed]

4. Streit, E.; Naehrer, K.; Rodrigues, I.; Schatzmayr, G. Mycotoxin occurrence in feed and feed raw materials worldwide: Long-term analysis with special focus on Europe and Asia. *J. Sci. Food Agric.* **2013**, *93*, 2892–2899. [CrossRef] [PubMed]

5. Bracarense, A.P.F.L.; Lucioli, J.; Grenier, B.; Drociunas Pacheco, G.; Moll, W.D.; Schatzmayr, G.; Oswald, I.P. Chronic ingestion of deoxynivalenol and fumonisin, alone or in interaction, induces morphological and immunological changes in the intestine of piglets. *Br. J. Nutr.* **2012**, *107*, 1776–1786. [CrossRef] [PubMed]

6. Pinton, P.; Tsybulskyy, D.; Lucioli, J.; Laffitte, J.; Callu, P.; Lyazhri, F.; Grosjean, F.; Bracarense, A.P.; Kolf-clauw, M.; Oswald, I.P. Toxicity of deoxynivalenol and its acetylated derivatives on the intestine: Differential effects on morphology, barrier function, tight junction proteins, and mitogen-activated protein kinases. *Toxicol. Sci.* **2012**, *130*, 180–190. [CrossRef] [PubMed]

7. Wu, L.; Liao, P.; He, L.; Ren, W.; Yin, J.; Duan, J.; Li, T. Growth performance, serum biochemical profile, jejunal morphology, and the expression of nutrients transporter genes in deoxynivalenol (DON)-challenged growing pigs. *BMC Vet. Res.* **2015**, *11*, 144. [CrossRef] [PubMed]

8. Yunus, A.W.; Ghareeb, K.; Twaruzek, M.; Grajewski, J.; Bohm, J. Deoxynivalenol as a contaminant of broiler feed: Effects on bird performance and response to common vaccines. *Poult. Sci.* **2012**, *91*, 844–851. [CrossRef] [PubMed]

9. Swiatkiewicz, S.; Swiatkiewicz, M.; Arczewska-Wlosek, A.; Jozefiak, D. Chitosan and its oligosaccharide derivatives (chito-oligosaccharides) as feed supplements in poultry and swine nutrition. *J. Anim. Physiol. Anim. Nutr.* **2015**, *99*, 1–12. [CrossRef] [PubMed]

10. Lodhi, G.; Kim, Y.; Hwang, J.; Kim, S.; Jeon, Y.; Je, J.; Ahn, C.; Moon, S.; Jeon, B.; Park, P. Chitooligosaccharide and Its Derivatives: Preparation and Biological Applications. *BioMed Res. Int.* **2014**, *2014*, 654913. [CrossRef] [PubMed]

11. Wang, J.P.; Yoo, J.S.; Kim, H.J.; Lee, J.H.; Kim, I.H. Nutrient digestibility, blood profiles and fecal microbiota are influenced by chitooligosaccharide supplementation of growing pigs. *Livest. Sci.* **2009**, *125*, 298–303. [CrossRef]

12. Maria de Souza, D.; Humberto Garcia-Cruz, C. Fermentative production of exocellular polysaccharides by bacteria. *Semin. Ciênc. Agrár.* **2004**, *25*, 331–340.

13. Kim, S.K.; Rajapakse, N. Enzymatic production and biological activities of chitosan oligosaccharides (COS): A review. *Carbohydr. Polym.* **2005**, *62*, 357–368. [CrossRef]

14. Sánchez, Á.; Mengíbar, M.; Rivera-Rodríguez, G.; Moerchbacher, B.; Acosta, N.; Heras, A. The effect of preparation processes on the physicochemical characteristics and antibacterial activity of chitooligosaccharides. *Carbohydr. Polym.* 2017; *157*, 251–257.

15. Fernandes, J.C.; Spindola, H.; De Sousa, V.; Santos-Silva, A.; Pintado, M.E.; Malcata, F.X.; Carvalho, J.E. Anti-inflammatory activity of chitooligosaccharides in vivo. *Mar. Drugs* **2010**, *8*, 1763–1768. [CrossRef] [PubMed]

16. Li, K.; Xing, R.; Liu, S.; Li, P. Advances in preparation, analysis and biological activities of single chitooligosaccharides. *Carbohydr. Polym.* **2016**, *139*, 178–190. [CrossRef] [PubMed]

17. Liu, P.; Piao, X.S.; Kim, S.W.; Wang, L.; Shen, Y.B.; Lee, H.S.; Li, S.Y. Effects of chito-oligosaccharide supplementation on the growth performance, nutrient digestibility, intestinal morphology, and fecal shedding of Escherichia coli and Lactobacillus in weaning pigs. *J. Anim. Sci.* **2008**, *86*, 2609–2618. [CrossRef] [PubMed]

18. Yang, C.M.; Ferket, P.R.; Hong, Q.H.; Zhou, J.; Cao, G.T.; Zhou, L.; Chen, A.G. Effect of chito-oligosaccharide on growth performance, intestinal barrier function, intestinal morphology and cecal microflora in weaned pigs. *J. Anim. Sci.* **2012**, *90*, 2671–2676. [CrossRef] [PubMed]

19. Suthongsa, S.; Pichyangkura, R.; Kalandakanond-Thongsong, S.; Thongsong, B. Effects of dietary levels of chito-oligosaccharide on ileal digestibility of nutrients, small intestinal morphology and crypt cell proliferation in weaned pigs. *Livest. Sci.* **2017**, *198*, 37–44. [CrossRef]

20. Huang, B.; Xiao, D.; Tan, B.; Xiao, H.; Wang, J.; Yin, J.; Duan, J.; Huang, R.; Yang, C.; Yin, Y. Chitosan Oligosaccharide Reduces Intestinal Inflammation That Involves Calcium-Sensing Receptor (CaSR) Activation in Lipopolysaccharide (LPS)-Challenged Piglets. *J. Agric. Food Chem.* **2016**, *64*, 245–252. [CrossRef] [PubMed]

21. Xiao, D.; Wang, Y.; Liu, G.; He, J.; Qiu, W.; Hu, X.; Feng, Z.; Ran, M.; Nyachoti, C.M.; Kim, S.W.; et al. Effects of chitosan on intestinal inflammation in weaned pigs challenged by enterotoxigenic *Escherichia coli*. *PLoS ONE* **2014**, *9*, e104192. [CrossRef] [PubMed]

22. Xiao, D.; Tang, Z.; Yin, Y.; Zhang, B.; Hu, X.; Feng, Z.; Wang, J. Effects of dietary administering chitosan on growth performance, jejunal morphology, jejunal mucosal sIgA, occluding, claudin-1 and TLR4 expression in weaned piglets challenged by enterotoxigenic *Escherichia coli*. *Int. Immunopharmacol.* **2013**, *17*, 670–676. [CrossRef] [PubMed]

23. Akbari, P.; Fink-Gremmels, J.; Willems, R.H.A.M.; Difilippo, E.; Schols, H.A.; Schoterman, M.H.C.; Garssen, J.; Braber, S. Characterizing microbiota-independent effects of oligosaccharides on intestinal epithelial cells: Insight into the role of structure and size: Structure–activity relationships of non-digestible oligosaccharides. *Eur. J. Nutr.* **2016**, *56*, 1919–1930. [CrossRef] [PubMed]

24. Zain, M.E. Impact of mycotoxins on humans and animals. *J. Saudi Chem. Soc.* **2011**, *15*, 129–144. [CrossRef]

25. Da Silva, E.O.; Gerez, J.R.; do Carmo Drape, T.; Bracarense, A.P.F.R.L. Phytic acid decreases deoxynivalenol and fumonisin B1-induced changes on swine jejunal explants. *Toxicol. Rep.* **2014**, *1*, 284–292. [CrossRef] [PubMed]

26. Kolf-Clauw, M.; Castellote, J.; Joly, B.; Bourges-Abella, N.; Raymond-Letron, I.; Pinton, P.; Oswald, I.P. Development of a pig jejunal explant culture for studying the gastrointestinal toxicity of the mycotoxin deoxynivalenol: Histopathological analysis. *Toxicol. In Vitro* **2009**, *23*, 1580–1584. [CrossRef] [PubMed]

27. Randall, K.J.; Turton, J.; Foster, J.R. Explant culture of gastrointestinal tissue: A review of methods and applications. *Cell Biol. Toxicol.* **2011**, *27*, 267–284. [CrossRef] [PubMed]

28. Xiong, X.; Yang, H.S.; Wang, X.C.; Hu, Q.; Liu, C.X.; Wu, X.; Deng, D.; Hou, Y.Q.; Nyachoti, C.M.; Xiao, D.F.; et al. Effect of low dosage of chito-oligosaccharide supplementation on intestinal morphology, immune response, antioxidant capacity, and barrier function in weaned piglets. *J. Anim. Sci.* **2015**, *93*, 1089–1097. [CrossRef] [PubMed]

29. Gerez, J.R.; Buck, L.Y.; Marutani, V.H.B.; Calliari, C.M.; Cunha, L.S.; Bracarense, A.P.F.R.L. Effects of chito-oligosaccharide on piglet jejunal explants: An histological approach. *Animal* **2018**, 1–6. [CrossRef] [PubMed]

30. Kong, X.F.; Zhou, X.L.; Lian, G.Q.; Blachier, F.; Liu, G.; Tan, B.E.; Nyachoti, C.M.; Yin, Y.L. Dietary supplementation with chitooligosaccharides alters gut microbiota and modifies intestinal luminal metabolites in weaned Huanjiang mini-piglets. *Livest. Sci.* **2014**, *160*, 97–101. [CrossRef]

31. Thongsong, B.; Suthongsa, S.; Pichyangkura, R.; Kalandakanond-Thongsong, S. Effects of chito-oligosaccharide supplementation with low or medium molecular weight and high degree of deacetylation on growth performance, nutrient digestibility and small intestinal morphology in weaned pigs. *Livest. Sci.* **2018**, *209*, 60–66. [CrossRef]

32. Grenier, B.; Applegate, T.J. Modulation of intestinal functions following mycotoxin ingestion: Meta-analysis of published experiments in animals. *Toxins (Basel)* **2013**, *5*, 396–430. [CrossRef] [PubMed]

33. Basso, K.; Gomes, F.; Bracarense, A.P.L. Deoxynivanelol and fumonisin, alone or in combination, induce changes on intestinal junction complexes and in E-cadherin expression. *Toxins (Basel)* **2013**, *5*, 2341–2352. [CrossRef] [PubMed]

34. De Walle, J.V.; Sergent, T.; Piront, N.; Toussaint, O.; Schneider, Y.J.; Larondelle, Y. Deoxynivalenol affects in vitro intestinal epithelial cell barrier integrity through inhibition of protein synthesis. *Toxicol. Appl. Pharmacol.* **2010**, *245*, 291–298. [CrossRef] [PubMed]

35. Mishra, S.; Dwivedi, P.D.; Pandey, H.P.; Das, M. Role of oxidative stress in Deoxynivalenol induced toxicity. *Food Chem. Toxicol.* **2014**, *72*, 20–29. [CrossRef] [PubMed]

36. Solís-Cruz, B.; Hernández-Patlán, D.; Beyssac, E.; Latorre, J.D.; Hernandez-Velasco, X.; Merino-Guzman, R.; Tellez, G.; López-Arellano, R. Evaluation of chitosan and cellulosic polymers as binding adsorbent materials to prevent Aflatoxin B1, Fumonisin B1, Ochratoxin, Trichothecene, Deoxynivalenol, and Zearalenone mycotoxicoses through an in vitro gastrointestinal model for poultry. *Polymers (Basel)* **2017**, *9*, 529. [CrossRef]

37. Zhao, Z.; Liu, N.; Yang, L.; Wang, J.; Song, S.; Nie, D.; Yang, X.; Hou, J.; Wu, A. Cross-linked chitosan polymers as generic adsorbents for simultaneous adsorption of multiple mycotoxins. *Food Control* **2015**, *57*, 362–369. [CrossRef]

38. Dalié, D.K.D.; Deschamps, A.M.; Richard-Forget, F. Lactic acid bacteria-Potential for control of mould growth and mycotoxins: A review. *Food Control* **2010**, *21*, 370–380. [CrossRef]

39. Singh, S.P.; Jadaun, J.S.; Narnoliya, L.K.; Pandey, A. Prebiotic Oligosaccharides: Special Focus on Fructooligosaccharides, Its Biosynthesis and Bioactivity. *Appl. Biochem. Biotechnol.* **2014**, *4*, 13–27. [CrossRef] [PubMed]

40. Akbari, P.; Braber, S.; Alizadeh, A.; Verheijden, K.A.; Schoterman, M.H.; Kraneveld, A.D.; Garssen, J.; Fink-Gremmels, J. Galacto-oligosaccharides Protect the Intestinal Barrier by Maintaining the Tight Junction Network and Modulating the Inflammatory Responses after a Challenge with the Mycotoxin Deoxynivalenol in Human Caco-2 Cell Monolayers and B6C3F1 Mice. *J. Nutr.* **2015**, *145*, 1604–1613. [CrossRef] [PubMed]

41. Kim, Y.S.; Ho, S.B. Intestinal goblet cells and mucins in health and disease: Recent insights and progress. *Curr. Gastroenterol. Rep.* **2010**, *12*, 319–330. [CrossRef] [PubMed]

42. Oliveira, E.R.; Da Silva, C.A.; Castro-Gómez, R.J.H.; Lozano, A.P.; Gavioli, D.F.; Frietzen, J.; Da Silva, E.O.; Novais, A.K.; Frederico, G.; Pereira, M. Chito-oligosaccharide as growth promoter replacement for weaned piglets: Performance, morphometry, and immune system. *Semin. Agrar.* **2017**, *38*, 3253–3269. [CrossRef]

43. Gerez, J.R.; Pinton, P.; Callu, P.; Grosjean, F.; Oswald, I.P.; Bracarense, A.P.F.L. Deoxynivalenol alone or in combination with nivalenol and zearalenone induce systemic histological changes in pigs. *Exp. Toxicol. Pathol.* **2015**, *67*, 89–98. [CrossRef] [PubMed]

44. Pinton, P.; Graziani, F.; Pujol, A.; Nicoletti, C.; Paris, O.; Ernouf, P.; Di Pasquale, E.; Perrier, J.; Oswald, I.P.; Maresca, M. Deoxynivalenol inhibits the expression by goblet cells of intestinal mucins through a PKR and MAP kinase dependent repression of the resistin-like molecule β. *Mol. Nutr. Food Res.* **2015**, *59*, 1076–1087. [CrossRef] [PubMed]

45. Smith, J.; Wood, E.; Dornish, M. Effect of Chitosan on Epithelial Cell Tight Junctions. *Pharm. Res.* **2004**, *21*, 43–49. [CrossRef] [PubMed]

46. Hsu, L.W.; Ho, Y.C.; Chuang, E.Y.; Chen, C.T.; Juang, J.H.; Su, F.Y.; Hwang, S.M.; Sung, H.W. Effects of pH on molecular mechanisms of chitosan-integrin interactions and resulting tight-junction disruptions. *Biomaterials* **2013**, *34*, 784–793. [CrossRef] [PubMed]

47. Horn, S.J.; Eijsink, V.G.H. A reliable reducing end assay for chito-oligosaccharides. *Carbohydr. Polym.* **2004**, *56*, 35–39. [CrossRef]

48. Lucioli, J.; Pinton, P.; Callu, P.; Laffitte, J.; Grosjean, F.; Kolf-Clauw, M.; Oswald, I.P.; Bracarense, A.P.F.R.L. The food contaminant deoxynivalenol activates the mitogen activated protein kinases in the intestine: Interest of *ex vivo* models as an alternative to in vivo experiments. *Toxicon* **2013**, *66*, 31–36. [CrossRef] [PubMed]

49. Maidana, L.; Gerez, J.R.; El Khoury, R.; Pinho, F.; Puel, O.; Oswald, I.P.; Bracarense, A.P.F.R.L. Effects of patulin and ascladiol on porcine intestinal mucosa: An ex vivo approach. *Food Chem. Toxicol.* **2016**, *98*, 189–194. [CrossRef] [PubMed]

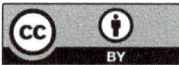

MDPI

St. Alban-Anlage 66

4052 Basel

Switzerland

Tel. +41 61 683 77 34

Fax +41 61 302 89 18

www.mdpi.com

Toxins Editorial Office

E-mail: toxins@mdpi.com

www.mdpi.com/journal/toxins

www.ingramcontent.com/pod-product-compliance
Lightning Source LLC
Chambersburg PA
CBHW051725210326
41597CB00032B/5606